Current Practice in Hand Surgery

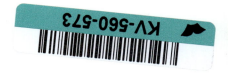

Current Practice in Hand Surgery

Edited by

Philippe Saffar
Institut Français de Chirurgie de la Main
Paris, France

Peter C Amadio
Mayo Clinic
Rochester, Minnesota, USA

Guy Foucher
SOS Main
Strasbourg, France

MARTIN ■ DUNITZ

© Martin Dunitz Ltd 1997

The copyright for Chapters 32 and 39 has been retained by their respective authors.

First published in the United Kingdom in 1997
by Martin Dunitz Ltd
The Livery House
7–9 Pratt Street
London NW1 0AE

A CIP record for this book is available from the British Library.

ISBN 1 85317 349 5

Composition by Scribe Design, Gillingham, Kent, UK
Printed and bound in Spain by Grafos, S.A. Arte sobre papel

CONTENTS

LIST OF CONTRIBUTORS

Sinna Alemzadeh
Service d'Orthopédie et Traumatologie
Cliniques Universitaires de Bruxelles
Hôpital Erasme
808 route de Lennik
B-1070 Brussels, Belgium

Jean-Yves Alnot
Centre Urgences Mains
Hôpital Bichat
46, rue Henri-Huchard
F-75877 Paris Cedex 18, France

Peter C Amadio
Mayo Clinic
200 First Street SW
Rochester, Minnesota 55905, USA

Stanley E Asnis
Department of Orthopaedic Surgery
Long Island Jewish Medical Center
Albert Einstein College of Medicine, and
Department of Surgery (Orthopaedics)
Cornell University Medical College
Orthopaedic Associates
800 Community Drive
Manhasset, New York 11030, USA

Arthur Atchabahian
Service d'Orthopédie
Hôpital Bichat
46 rue Henri Huchard
F-75877 Paris Cedex 18, France

Jacques Bardot
Department of Plastic Surgery
Centre Hospitalier Régional et Universitaire de
Marseille
CHU Timone
Boulevard Jean Moulin
13385 Marseille Cedex 5
France

Richard A Berger
Departments of Orthopedic Surgery and
Anatomy
Mayo Clinic
200 First Street SW
Rochester, Minnesota 55905, USA

Anil Bhatia
Sancheti Institute
16 Shivajinagar
Pune 411005
India

Allen T Bishop
Mayo Clinic
200 First Street SW
Rochester, Minnesota 55905, USA

William F Blair
Division of Hand and Microsurgery
Department of Orthopaedic Surgery
University of Iowa Hospitals and Clinics
Iowa City, Iowa 52242, USA

Remy Bleton
Centre Urgences Mains
Hôpital Bichat
46 rue Henri-Huchard
F-75877 Paris Cedex 18, France

Dieter Buck-Gramcko
Associate Professor of Hand Surgery
University of Hamburg, Germany, and
Wilhelmstift Children's Hospital
Liliencronstrasse 130
D-22149 Hamburg, Germany

Patricia E Burrows
830 Boylston Street, Suite 212
Chestnut Hill
Massachusetts 02167, USA

Dominique Casanova
Department of Plastic Surgery
Centre Hospitalier Régional et Universitaire de
Marseille
CHU Timone
Boulevard Jean Moulin
13385 Marseille Cedex 5
France

Erick Chevaleraud
Institut Français de Chirurgie de la Main
5 rue du Dôme
Paris XVIéme 75116, France

Andrew M Clarke
Hand Units of St Luke's and Sydney Hospitals
Sydney, Australia

Melissa Cohen
Department of Orthopaedic Surgery
University of Minnesota
420 Delaware Street SE
Minneapolis, Minnesota 55455, USA

W Bruce Conolly
University of New South Wales and University
of Sydney
Hand Units of St Luke's and Sydney Hospitals
Macquarie Street
Sydney 2000, Australia

John S Crombie
359 Veterans Boulevard
Rutherford, New Jersey 07070, USA

Landino Cugola
Via fontano del ferro 26/A
37129 Verona, Italy

Endre Cziffer
Department of Traumatology
Central Army Hospital
Robert K Krt 44
Budapest H-1553, Hungary

Fabienne Dhaene
Service d'Orthopédie et Traumatologie
Cliniques Universitaires de Bruxelles
Hôpital Erasme
808 route de Lennik
B-1070 Brussels, Belgium

Andrew Ellowitz
Department of Orthopaedic Surgery
University of Minnesota
420 Delaware Street SE
Minneapolis, Minnesota 55455, USA

David M Evans
The Hand Clinic
Oakley Green
Windsor SL4 4LH, and
Consultant Hand Surgeon
The Royal National Orthopaedic Hospital,
Stanmore
St Thomas' Hospital, London
Queen Mary's University Hospital, London, UK

Roslyn B Evans
Indian River Hand Rehabilitation
Suite D-101
777 37th Street
Vero Beach, Florida 32960, USA

Joseph M Failla
Department of Orthopaedic Surgery
Henry Ford Hospital
2799 West Grand Boulevard
Detroit, Michigan 48202, USA

Angel Farreres
Hospital Clinic i Provincial
Barcelona, Spain

Véronique Feipel
Laboratoire d'Anatomie Functionelle
Université Libre de Bruxelles CP 619
808 route de Lennik
B-1070 Brussels, Belgium

Diego L Fernandez
Department of Orthopaedic Surgery
Lindenhof Hospital
Bremgartenstrasse 117
CH-3012 Bern, Switzerland

Didier Fontes
Clinique du Sport
36 boulevard Saint-Marcel
F-75005 Paris, France

Guy Foucher
SOS Main
4 boulevard du Président-Edwards
F-67000 Strasbourg, France

Jan Fridén
Department of Hand Surgery
Sahlgrenska University Hospital
University of Göteborg
S-413 45 Göteborg, Sweden

Marc Garcia-Elias
Institut Kaplan
Paseo Bonanova, 9, 2º, 2ª
08022 Barcelona, Spain

Richard K Green
Department of Orthopaedics
University of Utah
4500 Primary Children's Medical Center
100 North Medical Drive
Salt Lake City, Utah 84113, USA

Sean M Griggs
Department of Orthopaedics
Brown University School of Medicine
Rhode Island Hospital
2 Dudley Street, 2nd Floor
Providence, Rhode Island 02905, USA

Joseph L Grzeskiewicz
Division of Plastic Surgery
University of Missouri
One Hospital Drive
Columbia, Missouri 65212, USA

Timothy J Herbert
Sydney Hospital and Sydney Eye Hospital
187 Macquarie Street
Sydney, NSW 2000, Australia

William H Holmes
Department of Orthopaedics
University of Utah
4500 Primary Children's Medical Center
100 North Medical Drive
Salt Lake City, Utah 84113, USA

James H House
Department of Orthopaedic Surgery
University of Minnesota
420 SE Delaware Street
Minneapolis, Minnesota 55455, USA

Richard S Idler
The Indiana Hand Center
8501 Harcourt Road
PO Box 80434
Indianapolis, Indiana 46280, USA

Peter J L Jebson
Orthopaedic Surgery Section
Department of Surgery
University of Michigan Medical Center
Ann Arbor, Michigan 48109, USA

Jesse B Jupiter
Harvard Medical School and
Orthopaedic Hand Service
Massachusetts General Hospital
WAC 527, 15 Parkman Street
Boston, Massachusetts 02114, USA

L Andrew Koman
Department of Orthopaedic Surgery
Bowman Gray School of Medicine
Wake Forest University
Medical Center Boulevard
Winston-Salem, North Carolina 27157, USA

Gary R Kuzma
2718 Henry Street
Greenboro
North Carolina 27405, USA

David M Lamey
CV Starr Hand Surgery Center
St Luke's/Roosevelt Hospital
New York 10019, USA

Lewis B Lane
Department of Orthopaedic Surgery
Long Island Jewish Medical Center
Albert Einstein College of Medicine, and
Department of Surgery (Orthopaedics)
Cornell University Medical College
Orthopaedic Associates
800 Community Drive
Manhasset, New York 11030, USA

Dominique Le Viet
Institut de la Main
Clinique Jouvenet
6 square Jouvenet
F-75016 Paris, France

Richard L Lieber
Department of Orthopaedics and Bioengineering
University of California and VA Medical Center
San Diego, California 92161, USA

Gau-Tyan Lin
Orthopedic Surgery
Kaohsiung Medical College
100 Shih-Chuan First Road
Kaohsiung, Taiwan, ROC

Ronald L Linscheid
Orthopedic Surgery
Mayo Clinic
200 First Street SW
Rochester, Minnesota 55905, USA

Graham D Lister
2800 Ocean Drive
Vero Beach
Florida 32963, USA

Alberto L Lluch
Institut Kaplan
Paseo Bonanova, 9, 2º, 2ª
Barcelona, Spain

Göran Lundborg
Department of Hand Surgery
Malmö University Hospital
S-205 02 Malmö, Sweden

Nancy M Lynch
Orthopaedic Healthcare Northwest
1200 Hilyard #600
Eugene
Oregon 97401, USA

Guy Magalon
Service de Chirurgie Plastique et Reparatrice
Centre Hospitalier Régional et Universitaire de Marseille
Hôpital de la Conception
147 boulevard Baille
F-13385 Marseille Cedex 05, France

Marteinn Magnusson
212 Hollandsresan
75755 Uppsala
Sweden

Paul R Manske
Department of Orthopaedic Surgery
Washington University Medical Center
One Barnes Hospital Plaza, Suite 11300
St Louis, Missouri 63110, USA

Daniel Marcireau
Service Orthopédie
Hôpital Laudoisière
2 rue Amboise Paré
75010 Paris, France

Takashi Masatomi
Department of Orthopaedic Surgery
Osaka University Medical School
2-2 Yamadaoka
Osaka 565, Japan

Ulrich Mennen
Professor and Head, Department of Hand and Microsurgery
Medical University of Southern Africa
PO Box 186
Medunsa 0204, Republic of South Africa

Jayasanker Menon
Department of Orthopaedic Surgery
Kaiser Permanente Medical Center
9985 Sierra Avenue
Fontana, California 92335, and
Department of Orthopaedic Surgery
Loma Linda University Medical Center
Loma Linda, California 92359, USA

Antonino Messina
Head, Hand Surgery Centre
Clinica Fornaca
Torino, Italy

Jane C Messina
I Clinica Ortopedica Università
Milano, Italy

Hans-Christoph Meuli
Department of Orthopaedic Surgery
Lindenhof Hospital
Bremgartenstrasse 117
CH-3012 Bern, Switzerland

Masakuzu Murai
South Wakayama National Hospital
Tanabe, Japan

Christophe Oberlin
Service d'Orthopédie
Hôpital Bichat
46 rue Henri Huchard
F-75877 Paris Cedex 18, France

Toshihiko Ogino
Department of Orthopaedic Surgery
Yamagata University School of Medicine
Iida-Nishi 2-2-2
Yamagata 990-23, Japan

Rick F Papandrea
Department of Orthopaedic Surgery
Mount Sinai Medical Center
Cleveland, Ohio, USA

Clayton A Peimer
Hand Center of Western New York
University of Buffalo
Millard Fillmore Health System
3 Gates Circle
Buffalo, New York 14209, USA

Isabelle Pigeau
Institut Français de Chirurgie de la Main and
Clinique des Lilas and Boucicaut Hospital
5 rue du Dôme
Paris XVIéme 75116, France

Gary G Poehling
Department of Orthopaedic Surgery
Bowman Gray School of Medicine
Wake Forest University
Medical Center Boulevard
Winston-Salem, North Carolina 27157, USA

George Psaras
Wits Medical School
7 York Road
Parktown 2193, Republic of South Africa

Charles L Puckett
Division of Plastic Surgery
University of Missouri
One Hospital Drive
Columbia, Missouri 65212, USA

Matthew D Putnam
Department of Orthopaedic Surgery
University of Minnesota
420 Delaware Street SE
Minneapolis, Minnesota 55455, USA

Morris Ritz
19 Webb Street
Caulfield
3162 Victoria, Australia

Leonard K Ruby
Department of Orthopaedics
Tufts University School of Medicine
New England Medical Center
750 Washington Street
Boston, Massachusetts 02111, USA

David S Ruch
Department of Orthopaedic Surgery
Bowman Gray School of Medicine
Wake Forest University
Medical Center Boulevard
Winston-Salem, North Carolina 27157, USA

Jaiyoung Ryu
West Virginia University Department of
Orthopedics
Robert C Byrd Health Sciences Center South
PO Box 9196, Morgantown
West Virginia 26506, USA

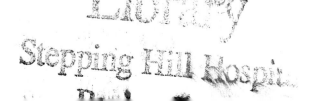

Philippe Saffar
Institut Français de Chirurgie de la Main
5 rue du Dôme
Paris XVléme 75116, France

Shelly M Sailer
Department of Orthopaedics
University of Washington
1959 NE Pacific Street
Seattle, Washington 98195, USA

Philippe Samson
Institut de la Main
Clinique Jouvenet
6 square Jouvenet
F-75016 Paris, France

Frédéric A Schuind
Service d'Orthopédie et Traumatologie
Cliniques Universitaires de Bruxelles
Hôpital Erasme
808 route de Lennik
B-1070 Brussels, Belgium

William H Seitz, Jr
Hand and Upper Extremity Surgery Clinics
Mount Sinai Medical Center and
Department of Orthopaedic Surgery
Case Western Reserve University School of
Medicine
Cleveland, Ohio 44106, USA

Donald C Sheridan
Orthopedic Surgery
Mayo Clinic
200 First Street SW
Rochester, Minnesota 55905, USA

Kozo Shimada
Osaka Kosei-Nenkin Hospital
Osaka, Japan

Beth P Smith
Department of Orthopaedic Surgery
Bowman Gray School of Medicine
Wake Forest University
Medical Center Boulevard
Winston-Salem, North Carolina 27157, USA

Thomas L Smith
Department of Orthopaedic Surgery
Bowman Gray School of Medicine
Wake Forest University
Medical Center Boulevard
Winston-Salem, North Carolina 27157, USA

Constantin Sokolow
Institut Français de Chirurgie de la Main
5 rue du Dôme
Paris XVléme 75116, France

T Greg Sommerkamp
Department of Orthopaedics
University of Cincinnati College of Medicine and
Hand Surgery Specialists Inc
20 Medical Village, Suite 177
Edgewood, Kentucky 41017, USA

Colin Song
Division of Plastic and Reconstructive Surgery
University of the Witwatersrand
PO Box 1264
Houghton 2041, Republic of South Africa

Tibor Szalontay
Department of Traumatology
Central Army Hospital
Robert K Krt 44
Budapest, Hungary H-1553

Ruggero Testoni
via Delle Menegone 10
37134 Verona, Italy

R Timothy Thurman
Department of Plastic Surgery
Wilford Hall Medical Center
Lackland Air Force Base
Texas 78236, USA

Huey-Yuan Tien
Kleinert Institute
1 Medical Center Plaza
225 Abraham Flexner Way, Suite 850
Louisville, Kentucky 40202, USA

Frédéric Tomei
Department of Plastic Surgery
Centre Hospitalier Régional et Universitaire de
Marseille
CHU Timone
Boulevard Jean Moulin
13385 Marseille Cedex 5
France

Michael A Tonkin
Department of Hand Surgery
Royal North Shore Hospital
St Leonards, Australia 2065

Steven M Topper
Hand Surgery and Reconstructive Microsurgery
4102 Pinon Drive Suite 100
United States Air Force Academy
Colorado 80840, USA

Thomas E Trumble
Department of Orthopaedics
University of Washington
1959 NE Pacific
Seattle, Washington 98195, USA

Tsu-Min Tsai
Kleinert Institute
1 Medical Center Plaza
225 Abraham Flexner Way, Suite 850
Louisville, Kentucky 40202, USA

Joseph Upton
830 Boylston Street, Suite 212
Chestnut Hill
Massachusetts 02167, USA

Philippe Valenti
Clinique La Francilienne
Pontault Combault, France

Ann E Van Heest
Department of Orthopaedic Surgery
University of Minnesota
420 SE Delaware Street
Minneapolis, Minnesota 55455, USA

David W Vickers
Division of Orthopaedics
University of Queensland
Watkins Medical Centre
225 Wickham Terrace
Brisbane, Australia 4000

Edward R Wang
Orthopaedic Hand Service
Massachusetts General Hospital
Boston, Massachusetts 02114, USA

Arnold-Peter C Weiss
Department of Orthopaedics
Brown University School of Medicine
Rhode Island Hospital
2 Dudley Street, 2nd Floor
Providence, Rhode Island 02905, USA

Terry L Whipple
Tuckahoe Orthopaedic Associates Ltd
1800 Glenside Drive
Suite 101
Richmond, Virginia 23226, USA

Michael B Wood
Orthopedic Surgery and Reconstructive
Microsurgery
Mayo Clinic
200 First Street SW
Rochester, Minnesota 55905, USA

Geoffrey J Yule
Division of Plastic Surgery
University of Missouri
One Hospital Drive
Columbia, Missouri 65212, USA

Carlos Zaidenberg
British Hospital
Buenos Aires Medical School
Perdriel 74
Buenos Aires, Argentina

PREFACE

Many hand surgeons tend to stick with the techniques they have first learned and find it hard to move to using new techniques. Microsurgery and arthroscopy, for example, were rejected at first by a number of surgeons, who have since been left behind by their more adaptable colleagues. However, the field of hand surgery is always moving on, and we all have to try – through meetings, and reading journals and books – to keep in touch with state of the art developments.

In *Current Practice in Hand Surgery* we have chosen the most interesting of the stream of new developments for examination; each chapter has an editorial commentary reflecting our personal experience and immediate reaction to the description of these new techniques. Obviously, for some new techniques the follow-up is fairly short and the results may have to be re-evaluated after some years. Many procedures have only been tried by the chapter authors themselves, and their use by other surgeons will be the keystone for evaluation of the technique. Reproducibility is the problem and, although some procedures are best performed by a small number of hyperspecialists, each surgeon should be able, after a learning period, to obtain the same results and to adopt the new technique or concept where appropriate. Major changes – such as robotization of surgery – are still to come and it is important that even the most reluctant surgeons are adaptable.

We would like to extend our thanks to all the international experts who have contributed to this book, and hope that readers will find it enjoyable and stimulating.

PS
PCA
GF
March 1997

1
Flexor sheath anaesthesia

Erick Chevaleraud

Introduction

Local digital anaesthesia, ring block or commissural block are useful techniques for finger surgery, often performed in emergency. Distal ischaemia,[1] although rare, has been described after local anaesthesia. Ring blocks provide inconstant results. A brachial plexus block or general anaesthesia seems excessive for short surgery performed on a finger. A description by David Chiu,[2] led us, in May 1991, to perform a digital anaesthesia by injecting the flexor sheath tendon. More than 1000 patients have now been treated, facilitating an assessment of this technique.

Anatomical review

David Chiu observed by chance a finger anaesthesia after the infiltration of a trigger finger with lidocaine and steroid. He performed cadaveric dissection of 10 fingers after an injection of blue dye in the flexor tendon sheath. He reported successful anaesthesia of the four digital nerves with one injection by this technique and described his own experience with 420 patients between 1985 and 1990.

We have used this technique since May 1991. Our results were not similar.[3] Only the palmar digital area was affected by this anaesthesia. Are French people different? We went back to anatomical books and performed cadaveric dissections. The flexor sheath distribution varies between the five fingers. The sheaths wrap the flexor tendons of the second, third and fourth digits from the distal interphalangeal joint to 1 cm proximal to the metacarpophalangeal joint. For the fifth finger, the sheath extends 4–5 cm proximal to the flexor retinaculum and enlarges

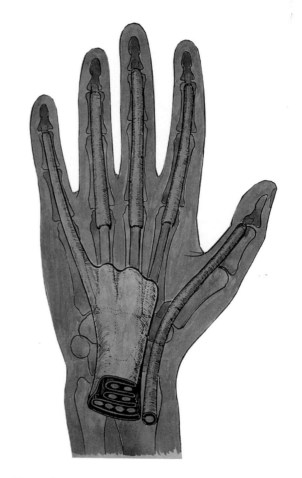

Figure 1

Flexor sheath distribution. (From Rouviere, *Anatomie Humaine*, (Masson: Paris, 1994).)

in the palm and carpal tunnel with anterior, posterior and intertendinous extensions. For the thumb, the sheath extends the length of the flexor pollicis longus (Figure 1).

An injection of 0.5 ml fluid is needed to fill the sheath. We did not observe finger anaesthesia with this volume. With 1 ml, hypoaesthesia is observed. Reliable anaesthesia is achieved with 2 ml of an anaesthetic solution. For the thumb and the fifth finger, the sheath extends to the wrist and we used a 4 ml injection which is always enough to obtain anaesthesia of the palmar digital nerves of these two digits.

Technique

After preparation of the skin with iodine alcohol or povidone iodine, the tendon flexor sheath is

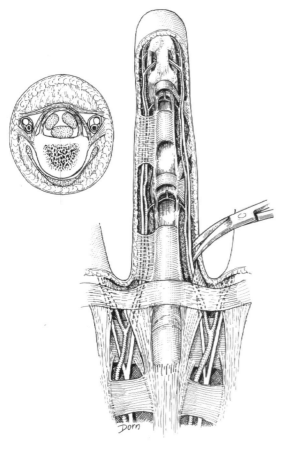

Figure 2

Vasculonervous pedicles alongside the flexor tendon. (From Tubiana R, McCullough CJ, Masquelet AC, *An Atlas of Surgical Exposures of the Upper Extremity* (Martin Dunitz and Lippincott, London and Philadelphia, 1990) with permission.)

Neurovascular bundles run along the flexor tendon sheath (Figure 2). The digital innervation is based on a double structure, palmar and dorsal. The palmar digital nerves supply sensory fibres to the volar aspect of the fingers and the dorsal aspect of the second and third phalanx of the second, third and fourth fingers. Dorsal digital nerves provide innervation to the dorsal aspect of the thumb and fifth finger and the first phalanx of the second, third and fourth fingers.

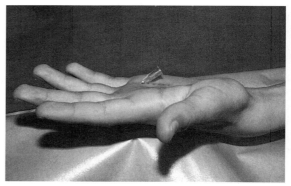

a

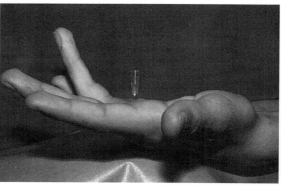

b

Figure 3

Technique of flexor sheath anaesthesia. (a) The needle is in a good position when it is moved upright by active movement of the finger (b).

punctured at the level of the metacarpopha-langeal joint. Active movement of the finger puts the needle upright (Figure 3), which indicates that the needle is in a good position. We use a 25 (0.5 × 16 mm) or 27 (0.40 × 13 mm) gauge needle and a 2.5 or 5 ml syringe with 2% lidocaine or, better, 0.5% bupivacaine without adrenaline, 1 ml for a child and 3–4 ml for an adult. This puncture and injection is painful and we use a cold spray or EMLA cream to reduce the discomfort. The onset of anaesthesia takes a few minutes, and skin incision is possible in five minutes.

Results

Our first discovery was that only the area of the lateral nerves is anaesthetised. The second discovery was the long duration of anaesthesia obtained with plain bupivacaine 0.5%: more than 10–12 hours and sometimes (20% of cases) around 24 hours of analgesia. This simple anaes-thesia is reliable with a 100% success rate,[3,4] providing there is a good understanding of finger innervation. Surgery of the palmar lateral nerve area is possible: nail pathology, wounds, tumours, removal of material or foreign body, tenolysis, neurolysis, and tenodermodesis, for example. Surgical extension on the dorsal digital nerve area requires a dorsal block for the first phalanx of the long finger and a truncular block, radial or ulnar, on the wrist for the thumb and fifth finger.

In addition to the restricted operating area, a second constraint of this technique is the time limitation of hand tourniquet. After 20–30 minutes the tourniquet tolerance is difficult. Intravenous sedation is possible but illogical in a one-day surgery centre. If a ring tourniquet cannot be used, time is a limiting factor of this technique, which should be reserved for proce-dures lasting less than 20 minutes.

Finally, the risk of infection should be discussed. The flexor sheath phlegmon is an arguable risk. Chiu did not mention any infec-tious complication for 420 patients treated between 1982 and 1987. In our first series of 350 patients between May 1991 and December 1992 we did not observe any problem. We did not use this technique for the infected finger (whitlow). The lack of infectious complications in our series of locoregional anaesthesia for hand surgery with a total of 46 822 patients in 10 years, and the antibacterial activity of local anaesthetics which has been reported,[5–7] reinforce our choice.

We have now performed more than 1000 injections of the flexor sheath, with complete success and no incident or accident.[3,4] We have extended the indication of this technique to localized finger sepsis (perionyxis). We use this technique primarily when the area and operat-ing time are compatible and, secondarily, to obtain a long period (18–24 hours) of postoper-ative analgesia.

Discussion

It is the diffusion around the puncture point to the palmar lateral nerves which is primarily responsible for the anaesthesia. Injection in front of the sheath provides the same anaesthesia, but of shorter (4–6 hours) duration. The long duration of anaesthesia (18–24 hours) observed in some cases is possibly due to diffusion along the sheath to the nerves.

The opening of the sheath by a distal wound does not disturb the block and it is not necessary to increase the anaesthetic volume.[8] For an infected finger, injection in front of the sheath is also possible.

The neurovascular bundles are not at risk since they are on both sides of the flexor tendon sheath.

Conclusion

Flexor sheath anaesthesia, besides its simplicity and reliability (full success), offers a good toler-ance with 3–4 ml bupivacaine, and an excellent and prolonged anaesthesia, without any particu-lar risk. Usable in the emergency room, it allows the management of many finger injuries. Well suited to one-day surgery, this technique is adaptable to infants.

We recommend this technique to surgeons and anaesthetists, aware of its anatomical limitations.

References

1 Vilain R, Michon J, *Infection de la Main chez l'Adulte et l'Enfant* (Masson: Paris, 1972) 82–5.
2 Chiu DTW, Transthecal digital block flexor tendon sheath used for anesthetic infusion, *J Hand Surg* (1990) **15A**:471–3.
3 Chevaleraud E, Ragot JM, Brunelle E, et al, Anesthésie locale digitale par la gaine des fléchisseurs, *Ann Fr Anesth Réanim* (1993) **12**:237–40.
4 Chevaleraud E, Anesthésie locale digitale par la gaine des fléchisseurs, *Cahiers Anesthésiol* (1993) **41**:647–8.
5 Schmidt RM, Rosenkranz HS, Antimicrobial activity of local anesthetics lidocaine and procaine, *J Infect Dis* (1970) **121**:597–607.
6 Noda H, Saionji K, Miyazaki T, Antibacterial activity of local anesthetics, *Jpn J Anesth* (1990) **39**:994–1000.
7 Kirk GA, Koontz FP, Chavez AT, Lidocaine inhibits growth of *Staphylococcus aureus* in propofol, *Anesthesiology* (1992) **77A**:407.
8 Boulay G, Dupont X, Anesthésie digitale transthécale en cas de section de la gaine du fléchisseur, *Ann Fr Anesth Réanim* (1995) **14**:310.

2
Local anaesthesia for thumb ulnar collateral ligament repair

Erick Chevaleraud

Introduction

Severe sprains of the ulnar collateral ligament of the metacarpophalangeal joint of the thumb are frequent, particularly with skiing accidents. The surgical treatment is based on precise indications[1]: Stener injury or displacement of a bone chip at the base of the first phalanx on radiography, associated volar plate lesion and palmar subluxation. For other indications, spontaneous healing with a conservative treatment may be used. Anaesthesia is useful in several ways. First, as a help for diagnosis, for clinical examination or stress radiographs. Second, in the operating theatre and third, for postoperative analgesia.

Anatomical review

Sensitive innervation of the thumb is provided on the dorsal aspect by the superficial branch of the radial nerve, and on the palmar aspect by the digital nerve, a branch of the median nerve. Truncular infiltration provides a reliable thumb anaesthesia. The superficial branch of the radial nerve arises from the radial nerve at the level of the lateral humeral epicondyle. It courses distally deep to the brachioradialis muscle, until it emerges between the tendon of brachioradialis and the extensor carpi radialis longus, and goes through the forearm fascia. It becomes subcutaneous at a mean of 9 cm proximal to the radial styloid.[2] It progresses distally and usually divides into two branches. The major branch continues distally to become the dorsoradial digital nerve of the thumb. It often divides into smaller

cutaneous branches that extend to the palmar distal part of the forearm, the wrist and the proximal radial thenar eminence. Anastomoses between these branches and branches from the lateral antebrachial cutaneous nerve are well known. The major dorsal branch continues distally, branching into the dorsoulnar digital nerve to the thumb and the dorsoradial digital nerves of the index and long fingers. The terminal branches of the median nerve arise distally to the carpal ligament. The digital nerves close to the long flexor tendon innervate the palmar skin of the thumb to the borders of the nail.

Technique

The superficial radial branch nerve block is reliable: at the forearm, between its emergence at the brachioradialis and its division at 5 cm from the radial styloid (Figure 1a); at the wrist, in the area of the radial styloid process and Lister's tubercle (Figure 1b). A subcutaneous infiltration of local anaesthetic, without paraesthesia, offers good anaesthesia of this branch.

For the palmar digital nerve, we use the flexor sheath anaesthesia, described by Chiu[3] (Figure 2).

We reported on the use of this technique and its limitations after we had performed more than 1000 local anaesthesias using this approach.[4] Anaesthesia occurs by diffusion from the puncture point to the digital nerves. The filling up of the sheath and secondary diffusion to the digital nerves may explain the long duration of the analgesia (18–24 hours) sometimes observed. An infiltration at the level of the sheath gives an

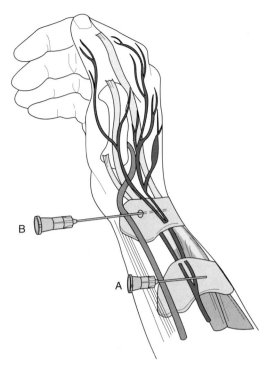

Figure 1

A, Radial block at the forearm. B, Radial block at the wrist.

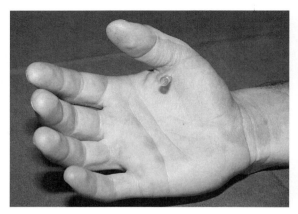

a

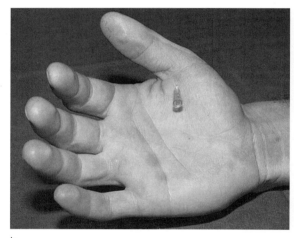

b

Figure 2

(a) Flexor sheath anaesthesia. (b) Good position of the needle in the sheath (made vertical by flexion of the finger).

equivalent anaesthesia but an analgesia of 6–8 hours with bupivacaine 0.5%. We use 25 (0.5 × 16 mm) or 27 (0.4 × 13 mm) gauge needles, a 5 ml syringe and bupivacaine 0.5% without adrenaline, 3–5 ml for each injection. If we do not want to perform a flexor sheath anaesthesia, because of a significant haematoma for example, it is possible to achieve a truncular block of the median nerve at the wrist.

Results

Anaesthesia and analgesia obtained with this technique are excellent.[5] The success rate is around 100%, but a significant palmar haematoma may impede the flexor sheath anaesthesia. This success rate is better than for plexus anaes-

thesia, where radial territory anaesthesia is insufficient in 15–20% of cases.[6] The duration of the procedure is a limiting factor—the tourniquet tolerance is poor after 20–30 minutes. Intravenous sedation is possible but illogical in a one-day surgery centre. A local infiltration under the tourniquet or a selective block of the brachial cutaneous nerve is possible but not always efficient. For specialized surgeons the interval of 20 minutes is sufficient for ulnar lateral ligament repair. The tourniquet is inflated before the incision is made, and adapted to patient morphology and blood pressure.

Postoperative analgesia is better than that observed after brachial plexus block with 1.25% lidocaine and 0.25 mg adrenaline, which we use for hand and upper limb surgery for outpatients. Paracetamol with codeine per os is prescribed if necessary at home.

We have not observed any incident or accident with this technique in a series of 450 patients who underwent thumb surgery.

Conclusion

This simple and easy technique provides an excellent thumb anaesthesia. Used as a first choice, it offers a good success rate and excellent postoperative analgesia. It adapts well for surgery of short duration, outpatient surgery and often in emergency situations. As no motor block is employed, the mobilization is immediate. The iatrogenicity is weak, 8–10 ml of subcutaneous bupivacaine 0.5% are tolerated well. The technique may also be used when a plexus block provides insufficient anaesthesia in the radial nerve sensitive area.

This technique may be used outside the operating theatre, in emergency or radiography rooms, and is suitable for children.

References

1   Lenoble E, Ebelin M, Lemerle JP, et al, Les entorses graves récentes de l'articulation métacarpophalangienne du pouce. Un accident fréquent en pratique sportive, *J Traumat Sport* (1989) **6**:55–62.
2   Abrams R, Brown R, Botte M, The superficial branch of the radial nerve, an anatomic study with surgical implications, *J Hand Surg* (1992) **17**:1037–41.
3   Chiu D, Transthecal digital block flexor tendon sheath used for anesthetic infusion, *J Hand Surg* (1990) **15**:471–3.
4   Chevaleraud E, Ragot JM, Brunelle E, et al, Anesthésie locale digitale par la gaine des fléchisseurs, *Ann Fr Anesth Réanim* (1993) **12**:237–40.
5   Chevaleraud E, Lenoble E, Anesthésie simplifiée pour le traitement chirurgical des entorses graves de l'articulation métacarpophalangienne du pouce, *Ann Chir Main* (1994) **13**:60–3.
6   Lanz E, Theiss D, Jankovic D, The extent of blockade following various techniques of brachial plexus block, *Anesth Analg* (1983) **62**:55–8.

Commentary

Chapter 1

In a one-day surgery center, the anaesthetist should adapt his or her technique to the patient's and surgeon's needs. This versatility may be adapted to the area where the surgery will be performed, the duration assigned for the procedure and the patient's temperament. Truncular, local and locoregional anesthesia may be combined. This sheath anesthesia represents an important tool for this type of surgery.

PS

Chapter 2

A very useful technique for this frequent winter injury.

PS

3

Flexor tendon repair: A historical perspective on early motion protocols and rationale for the early active motion rehabilitation program

R Timothy Thurman*, Thomas E Trumble and Shelly M Sailer

Introduction

A number of clinical studies which report early active motion after zone II flexor tendon repair have been published. Becker described early active flexion following a beveled multistrand peripheral suture technique in 1978.[1] With the use of Lister's criteria,[2] outcome assessment of 110 zone II flexor tendon repairs revealed 70% good-to-excellent results with a 10% incidence of tendon rupture.[3] Injuries were mixed and involved both superficialis and profundus tendons. Postoperative splinting maintained a neutral wrist position. Gentle unrestricted active flexion and extension inside a pain free range began with 24 hours of repair. The delayed return of extension noted is not surprising owing to the beveled repair which necessitated advancement of the tendon 1–1.5 cm. Conclusions regarding this method of repair and rehabilitation are hindered by relatively short patient follow-up and the lack of subsequent reports.

By means of a double loop locking suture technique, Lee allowed active flexion/extension after zone II repairs to the point of feeling 'tight'.[4] A dorsal block splint held wrist and metacarpophalangeal joint (MP) flexion at 30° and 60° respectively while it allowed unrestricted interphalangeal joint (IP) extension. Total active

motion (TAM) outcome assessment by the method of Strickland and Glogovac[5] of the 11 zone II repairs demonstrated one good and 10 excellent results.

Savage and Risitano found 100% excellent results for isolated flexor digitorum profundus and 70% good-to-excellent results for combined flexor digitorum superficialis/flexor digitorum profundus (FDS/FDP) repairs in an active motion protocol initiated within 24 hours of their particular six-strand flexor tendon repair technique.[6] Outcome assessment was in accordance with the scoring system of Buck-Gramcko et al.[7] Postoperative positioning maintained the wrist at neutral and MP flexion at 90°. Small force active and active-assisted MP and IP motion through an easy range continued for 6 weeks. The author does not comment on the role of early passive motion. More vigorous active, passive, resisted, and blocked exercises began 6 weeks after repair.

Strickland reported early favorable results for zone II flexor tendon repairs actively mobilized with a dorsal tenodesis splint.[8] This splint is based on reports from Cooney et al[9] and Savage[10] which show that if the wrist is placed in 30° of extension this actually decreases the force of flexion rather than increases it, and also increases differential tendon glide. These studies may revolutionize the thinking behind splinting for tendon injuries. These patients are first started on a 'flex and hold program'. The fingers are passively flexed with the contralateral hand. Gentle contraction of the flexors is maintained for approximately 5 seconds in this position with

*The opinions expressed in this chapter reflect those of the authors and do not represent those of the Department of Defense or the United States Air Force.

passive flexion maximized. During periods of inactivity, the extremity is placed in a standard dorsal blocking splint (DBS) with the wrist positioned in 20° of palmar flexion, the MPs in 50° of flexion and the IPs in neutral position for protection. Reports on functional outcome have not been published.

Silfverskiöld and May described their active motion protocol after zone II FDS/FDP repair with a two-strand modified Kessler plus a cross-stitch epitendinous technique.[11] The wrist was splinted in neutral position and the MP between 50° and 70° of flexion and motion was started 1–3 days after repair. This motion allowed active MP and IP extension within the restraints of the splint. Dynamic passive flexion was produced by rubber band flexion which incorporated all four fingers through a palmar bar. Similar to Strickland's protocol, active flexion is initiated with the IPs passively flexed as much as possible with the other hand. This program continued for 6 weeks with the force of flexion being modulated biweekly. By TAM outcome assessment criteria,[5] the authors noted 71% excellent and 25% good results. Two tendons ruptured for an incidence of 4.5%. Again, these investigators used intra-tendinous metal markers to evaluate tendon excursion radiographically. Retrospectively compared to a group previously managed with passive motion alone,[12] the actively mobilized group demonstrated a 9% improvement in mean active joint range of motion at 6-month follow-up (157° versus 144°). Particularly notable was 33% and 100% greater excursion per 10° motion at the PIP and DIP joints respectively.

How strong do flexor tendon repairs have to be?

In vivo measurements of human flexor tendon forces of contraction are illustrated in Table 1. Both studies were performed on patients who underwent open carpal tunnel release with local anesthesia. They differ somewhat in the device used to obtain measurements and the presence of tourniquet pressure in Urbaniak's group.[13] Forces reported by Schuind et al were obtained approximately 15 minutes after tourniquet deflation.[14] The higher values may indicate post-ischemic recovery of muscle power. These

Table 1 In vivo measurements of human flexor tendon forces (kilogram-force).

	Urbaniak et al[13]	Schuind et al[14]
PROM wrist	—	0.1–0.6
PROM digits	0.2–0.3	≤ 0.9
Active flexion (mild resistance)	≤ 0.9	Index DIP (FDP): 0.1–2.9 (1.9)* Index PIP (FDS/FDP): 0.3–1.3 (0.9)* Thumb IP (FPL): 0.4–3.5 (1.8)*
Active flexion (moderate resistance)	1.5	—

*Mean value; PROM, passive range of motion; DIP, distal interphalangeal; PIP, proximal interphalangeal; FDP, flexor digitorum profundus; FDS, flexor digitorum superficialis; FPL, flexor pollicis longus; IP, interphalangeal joint.

studies suggest that to be safe, a tendon repair should be able to resist 1.0 kilogram-force (kgf) for passive motion and 2.5 kgf for active motion, especially since associated edema and stiffness would be likely in a digit several days after tendon repair, thereby increasing the work of flexion. Both studies put into perspective the potential range of tensile forces imposed upon a tendon repair during passive and active motion of an uninjured digit.

How strong are the different tendon repairs?

There are many studies which compare gap and tensile strength but unfortunately they emphasize a particular repair technique. The different techniques tested, materials and models used, and methods of outcome assessment make extrapolation of the data into a specific clinical situation difficult.

A survey conducted by Strickland found 70% of responders favored a 'core' suture repair technique and 96% incorporated an epitendinous suture.[15] In terms of single core suture strength, Table 2 illustrates gap and tensile load to failure values measured by several investigators.[11,14–17] Some of these values fall short of that proposed for active,

Table 2 'Core' suture repair strength, human cadaver model (kilogram-force).

Reference	Core alone	Core + periphery
Urbaniak et al[13]	3.97 (fail)	—
Wade et al[16]	—	3.15 (fail)
		2.54 (gap)
Wade et al[17]	2.26 ± 0.63 (fail)	4.27 ± 1.38 (fail)
	0.86 ± 0.52 (gap)	3.73 ± 0.92 (gap)
Pruitt et al[18]	2.28 ± 0.25 (fail)	2.71 ± 0.42 (fail)
	0.89 ± 0.18 (gap)	2.28 ± 0.47 (gap)
Lee[19]	2.25 (fail)	—
	1.0 (gap)	

unresisted motion previously noted in Table 1 and do not account for potential loss of repair strength secondary to tendon softening over time.

To summarize these biomechanical studies:

(1) Increasing the number of suture strands in the repair increases the initial strength of the tendon repair.
(2) Gap formation is the initial means of failure of the tendon repair.
(3) Epitenon sutures provide added repair strength and decrease gap formation.
(4) Cyclic loading best models in vivo forces.
(5) The repair strength during the first 3 weeks after tendon repair is the most critical.

Early active motion protocol for zone II flexor tendon repair

The active motion zone II flexor tendon rehabilitation program in use at The University of Washington/Harborview Medical Center follows closely the splinting and motion guidelines described by Strickland.[8] A dorsal block splint is used during periods of rest and passive motion. Active and active-assisted motion is performed with a dorsal tenodesis splint which is hinged and which thereby permits the wrist position to be varied between flexion and extension. Wrist extension in the dorsal tenodesis splint optimizes differential flexor tendon glide and resistance to digital flexion which results from intrinsic extensor tendon 'tone'. Investigations by Savage[10] and Cooney et al[9] have provided the measurements of tendon excursion and forces resisting digital flexion on which this wrist position is based.

Active motion protocol

Initial 24–48 hours postoperatively

• The patient's postoperative dressing is removed.
• A custom dorsal protective splint is fabricated in the standard position (wrist in 20–30°

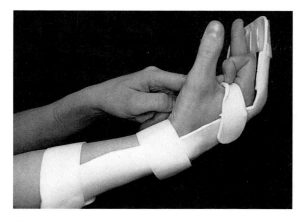

Figure 1

Use of the contralateral hand to perform passive range of motion exercises within the dorsal block splint.

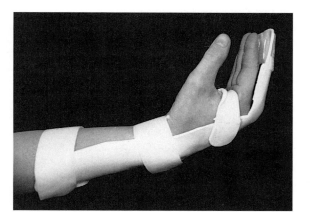

Figure 2

Active extension of the MP, PIP, and DIP joints within the restraints of the dorsal block splint.

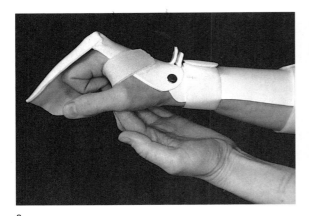

a

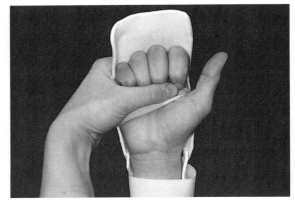

b

Figure 3

(a,b) Lateral and anterior views demonstrating passive wrist extension and digital flexion in a hinged dorsal tenodesis splint. Active small force flexion follows maximal passive digital flexion.

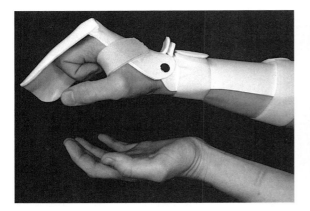

Figure 4

Active digital flexion in the dorsal tenodesis splint is maintained for approximately 5 seconds per cycle.

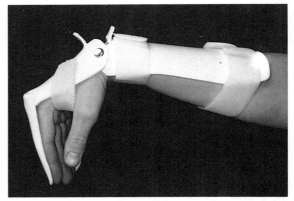

Figure 5

Relaxation phase following active flexion. The wrist passively volar flexes and the fingers assume an extended posture within the restraints of the dorsal tenodesis splint.

flexion, MPs in 60–70° flexion, and IPs neutral).
- The patient is instructed in passive range of motion exercises with the uninvolved hand, within the dorsal block splint (Figure 1).
- Twenty-five repetitions of passive PIP, DIP, and composite joint flexion and extension are performed each waking hour.

- Active extension of the PIP and DIP joints to the limits of the dorsal blocking splint is allowed (Figure 2).
- Coban® wrap (3M, St Paul, MN) is used to help decrease edema. Patients are instructed to wrap fingers at night and as able during the day.

From 24–72 hours to 4 weeks postoperatively

- When the patient has achieved adequate passive range of motion, and in the absence of severe edema, the tenodesis splint is fabricated (with the MPs in 60–70° flexion and the IPs neutral).
- The patient begins each hourly exercise session with passive range of motion exercises in the dorsal block splint, as previously described.
- Instruction in the active 'place and hold' exercises in the tenodesis splint is as follows. With the tenodesis splint securely in place, the wrist is passively brought into 30° extension (the two extension blocking tabs come together), while the fingers are pushed into full composite flexion (Figure 3a and b). The patient then gently contracts the finger flexors and attempts to hold the flexed position for 5 seconds (Figure 4). After 5 seconds the patient relaxes the muscle contraction and allows the wrist to drop into flexion and the fingers extend to the limit of the dorsal finger block of the splint (Figure 5). Twenty-five repetitions of this exercise are performed each hour.
- After each hourly session the patient returns to the dorsal block splint.
- Digital level edema control is continued between exercise sessions with the wrap or tubular elastic sleeves. It can be worn at all times except during active range of motion exercises as it can add increased resistance to finger flexion.
- These exercises are continued until the fourth week postoperatively.

Four weeks postoperatively

- The tenodesis splint is discontinued. The patient returns to a dorsal block splint after each exercise session.
- The hourly exercise sessions continue with initial passive range of motion exercises to the fingers to improve flexibility.

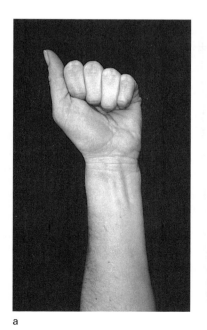 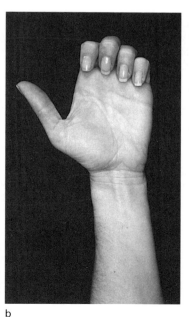 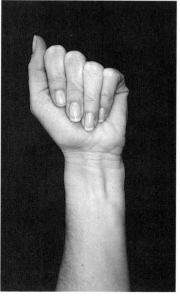

a   b   c

Figure 6

Maximum tendon gliding is facilitated as the patient actively moves between (a) a 'full', (b) a 'hook', and (c) a 'straight' fist.

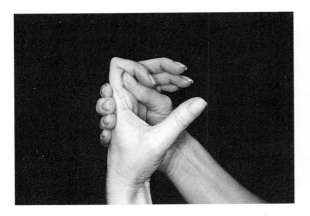

Figure 7

PIP joint blocking exercise.

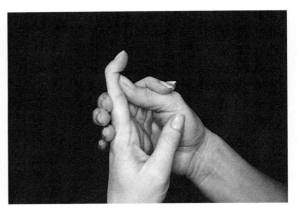

Figure 8

DIP joint blocking exercise.

- The same 'place and hold' exercises that were previously performed in the tenodesis splint are now performed without the guidance of the splint. The fingers are passively brought into flexion with the wrist brought into extension. Active muscle contraction is used to hold this position, then the muscles are relaxed and the hand falls into wrist flexion and finger extension, in a tenodesis pattern.

Fourth week

- Active movement from a full fist (Figure 6a), to a 'hook fist' (Figure 6b), to a 'straight fist' (Figure 6c) to full finger extension is used to facilitate maximum tendon gliding.
- The previous exercises are continued.
- The dorsal protective splint continues to be used between exercise sessions.

Five weeks

- The previous exercises continue and in addition, active wrist and finger flexion followed by wrist and finger extension is allowed.

Six weeks

- The dorsal blocking splint is discontinued.
- Active finger flexion exercises with joint

blocking at both the PIP (Figure 7) and DIP (Figure 8) joints are added to facilitate tendon gliding in patients with limited range of motion (ROM) (those not flexing to at least 3 cm from the distal palmar flexion crease). Note: blocking exercises to the small finger are not recommended.
- Buddy taping may be used to facilitate full flexion.

Seven weeks

- Passive extension exercises and extension splints may be used when indicated.

Eight weeks

- Light strengthening exercises (for example squeezing a soft foam ball) are initiated.

Nine weeks

- Soft putty can be used for strengthening.

From 10–14 weeks

- A progressive resistive strengthening program is used to return the patient to preoperative strength.
- Work simulation and reconditioning may be necessary in cases in which severe decondi-

tioning precludes a return to work in some occupations. A return to full unrestricted activity is allowed at 14 weeks.

The decision as to when to fabricate the tenodesis splint and proceed with the active exercises depends on the patient's level of pain and the level of edema in the involved fingers. It has been our experience that pain and edema can limit full passive range of motion significantly on the first day postoperatively, which would add increased resistance to active range of motion. It has worked well to delay the active range of motion and fabrication of the tenodesis splint until the second or third day postoperatively.

Once the patient is able to hold the fingers flexed to within 3 cm from the distal palmar crease, therapy visits can typically be reduced to once a week. It is also important that one can obtain full PIP extension. It has been our experience that patients can perform the exercises satisfactorily within 5–7 days postoperatively; PIP flexion contractures have not been a problem.

Contraindications

Contraindications to the use of this early motion program in our facility have been any conditions which severely impaired cognition or compliance, such as psychiatric conditions or substance abuse. Patients that appear unable to safely protect their hands while changing between the two different splints in the first 4 weeks have been treated with the modified passive flexion/active extension protocol, and remained in the dorsal block splint for the entire 6 weeks.

References

1   Becker H, Primary repair of flexor tendons in the hand without immobilization—preliminary report, *The Hand* (1978) **10**:37–47.
2   Lister GD, Kleinert HE, Kutz JE, et al, Primary flexor tendon repair followed by immediate controlled mobilization, *J Hand Surg* (1977) **2**:441–51.
3   Becker H, Orak F, Duponselle E, Early active motion following a beveled technique of flexor tendon repair: report on fifty cases, *J Hand Surg* (1979) **4**:454–60.

4   Lee H, Double loop locking suture: a technique of tendon repair for early active mobilization. Part II: Clinical experience, *J Hand Surg* (1990) **15A**:953–8.
5   Strickland JW, Glogovac SV, Digital function following flexor tendon repair in Zone II: a comparison of immobilization and controlled passive motion techniques, *J Hand Surg* (1980) **5**:537–43.
6   Savage R, Risitano G, Flexor tendon repair using a 'six strand' method of repair and early active mobilization, *J Hand Surg* (1989) **14B**:396–9.
7   Buck-Gramcko D, Dietrich FE, Gogge S, Bewertungskriterein bei Nachunterschungen von Beugesehnen-wiederherstellungen, *Handchirurgie* (1976) **8**:65–9.
8   Strickland JW, Flexor tendon repair—Indiana method, *Ind Hand Cen News* (1993) **1**:1–19.
9   Savage R, The influence of wrist position on the minimum force required for active movement of the interphalangeal joints, *J Hand Surg* (1988) **13B**:262–8.
10 Cooney WP, Lin GT, An K-N, Improved tendon excursion following flexor tendon repair, *J Hand Ther* (1989) **2**:102–6.
11 Silfverskiöld KL, May EJ, Flexor tendon repair in zone II with a new suture technique and an early mobilization program combining passive and active flexion, *J Hand Surg* (1994) **19A**:53–60.
12 Silfverskiöld KL, May EJ, Tornvall AH, Tendon excursion after flexor tendon repair in zone II: results with a new controlled-motion program, *J Hand Surg* (1993) **18A**:403–10.
13 Urbaniak JR, Cahill JD, Mortenson RA, Tendon suturing methods: analysis of tensile strengths. In: *AAOS: Symposium on Tendon Surgery in the Hand* (CV Mosby: St Louis, 1978) 70–80.
14 Schuind F, Garcia-Elias M, Cooney WP, et al, Flexor tendon forces: in vivo measurements, *J Hand Surg* (1992) **17A**:291–8.
15 Strickland JW, Opinions and preferences in flexor tendon surgery, *Hand Clin* (1985) **1**:187–91.
16 Wade PJF, Muir IFK, Hutcheon LL, Primary flexor tendon repair: the mechanical limitations of the modified Kessler technique, *J Hand Surg* (1986) **11B**:71–6.
17 Wade PJF, Wetherell RG, Amis AA, Flexor tendon repair: significant gain in strength from the Halsted peripheral suture technique, *J Hand Surg* (1989) **14B**:232–5.
18 Pruitt DL, Manske PR, Fink B, Cyclic stress analysis of flexor tendon repair, *J Hand Surg* (1991) **16A**:701–7.
19 Lee H, Double loop locking suture: a technique of tendon repair for early active mobilization. Part I: Evolution of technique and experimental study, *J Hand Surg* (1990) **15A**:945–52.

4

New suture techniques for flexor tendon repair

Gau-Tyan Lin

Introduction

Repair of the flexor tendon is a challenging problem for the hand surgeon. Because of the parallel tendon fibers, the required tendon suture technique is different from that in other soft tissue; the suture may quite easily be cut out from the tendon end. Since early mobilization has proved to be the most important principle to prevent adhesions of the repaired tendon,[1,2] a strong suture technique is essential for a successful tendon repair. Gap formation at the repaired tendon is another concern. Poor contact of the ruptured tendon ends may delay the healing process and increase the possibility of adhesions to surrounding tissue. This chapter reviews a personal method to improve the strength of tendon repair and facilitate tendon gliding postoperatively.

tendon, and then goes in again at the lateral side of the tendon, keeping the transverse thread volar to the longitudinal thread. The same maneuver is repeated four times, as the first and third suture loops grasp a short segment of the tendon, while the second and fourth suture loops grasp long segments of the tendon. The continual suture ends up with only one tying knot. This has several advantages: it reduces the chance of loosening of the knot; when the tendon sustains tensile load the thread will tighten automatically; and the tensile strength is evenly distributed to all four suture loops, avoiding failure due to stress concentration.

The transverse thread should be superficial to the longitudinal thread, to ensure the grasping power of the suture loop (Figure 2a).

New suture techniques

Core suture

The dynamic compression suture technique uses the 'near to far, far to near' principle, which brings the tendon ends closer when the tendon experiences tensile loads. Nylon 3-0 monofilament suture with a cutting needle is used. The suture technique is based on the modified Kessler[3] and Pennington (locking loop)[4] technique (Figure 1). The needle starts from one tendon end, going out the volar side of the

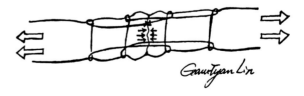

Figure 1

Dynamic compression suture technique, based on the 'near to far, far to near' principle; it uses a continual suture and only one suture knot, which is buried between the tendon ends.

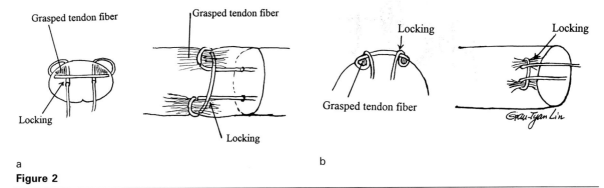

a

Figure 2

(a) Core suture. (b) Epitenon running suture.

Running locking suture

A 6-0 nylon or absorbable suture material is used for the running suture. The suture technique is described briefly. The first stitch goes through the end of the tendon and then comes out on the tendon surface. The following maneuver is the reverse to that of the core suture, keeping the transverse thread under the longitudinal thread to ensure locking of the suture loop[5] (Figure 2b). The running suture technique may be used when the repaired tendon surface is not smooth, especially on the volar side, which faces the pulley.

Synergistic wrist motion

This rehabilitation program was developed to increase tendon excursion without increased tension of the repaired tendon.[6,7] The basic principle was synergistic motion of the fingers and wrist: the fingers extend when the wrist flexes, and vice versa. The patient must fully understand this point, otherwise rupture of the repaired tendon may occur.

Several designs of dynamic splint have been introduced, but the fabrication of the splint is time consuming, the technique demanding and splints are not always effective. Currently we teach patients individually to perform synergistic

exercise without a splint. We start with the intact hand, until we make sure the patient understands the synergistic motion of wrist and fingers, and then shift to the operated hand (Figure 3).

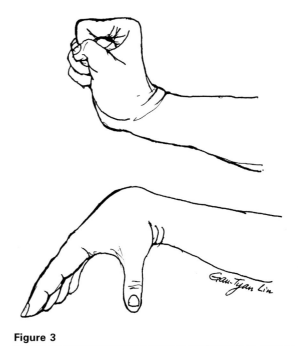

Figure 3

Synergistic wrist motion.

Discussion

Early motion is the most important factor in the prevention of adhesions. There are many suture techniques but none have the same tensile strength as intact tendon. Uncontrolled finger motion may jeopardize the repaired tendon. The actual tendon excursion is greater in active motion than passive motion of the finger joint. That is the effect of friction of the tendon and pulley. Running sutures were used only in some cases in which the repaired flexor tendon ends were not smooth.

Dynamic compression suture technique has two main advantages: it reduces the formation of a gap between the tendon ends, and it provides more tensile strength, partly due to four strands which grasp the tendon fibers.

According to our own results,[8] and those of other reports,[9] no matter what suture technique is used, an increase in suture strands will increase tensile strength.

Conclusion

A new suture technique was introduced to increase tensile strength and reduce the gap between the tendon ends. Early active motion based on synergistic wrist motion may increase tendon excursion and avoid adhesion.

References

1   Hitchcock TF, Light TR, Bunch WH, et al, The effect of immediate controlled digital motion on the strength of flexor tendon repairs, *Orthop Trans* (1986) **9**:270–1.
2   Gelberman RH, Woo SL-Y, Lothringer K, et al, Effects of early intermittent passive mobilization on healing canine flexor tendons, *J Hand Surg* (1982) **7**:170–5.
3   Kleinert HE, Kutz JE, Atasoy E, et al, Primary repair of flexor tendons, *Orthop Clin North Am* (1973) **4**:865.
4   Pennington DG, The locking loop tendon suture, *Plast Reconstr Surg* (1979) **63**:648–52.
5   Lin GT, An KN, Amadio PC, et al, Biomechanical studies of running suture for flexor tendon repair in dogs, *J Hand Surg* (1988) **13A**:553–8.
6   Cooney WP, Lin GT, An KN, Improved tendon excursion following flexor tendon repair, *J Hand Therapy* (1989).
7   Horii E, Lin GT, Cooney WP, et al, Comparative flexor tendon excursion after passive mobilization: An in vitro study, *J Hand Surg* (1992) **17A**:559–66.
8   Lin GT, Wu HC, Chian SH, et al, A biomechanical study of suture technique for flexor tendon repair, *J Appl Biomech* (1995) **10**:138–43.
9   Kubota H, Aoki M, Pruitt DL, et al, The tensile strength of various peripheral circumferential repair techniques in canine flexor tendons, *J Orthop Sci* (1996) **1**:136–9.

5
Repair of finger flexor pulleys – 1

Gary R Kuzma

Introduction

The importance of an intact and competent flexor tendon sheath for efficient and normal digital function has gradually become more appreciated from both laboratory research and clinical observation.

The pulley system is composed of annular (A) pulleys with fibers oriented transversely to the longitudinal axis of the bone and cruciate (C) pulleys with fibers oriented obliquely to the longitudinal axis of the bone. Anatomically they may be grouped in a proximal (P) followed by a distal (D) grouping, resulting in a proximal complex (i.e. AP_1 CP AP_2 AP_3) acting on the proximal interphalangeal joint, and a distal complex (i.e. AD_1 CD AD_2 AD_3) combination acting on the distal interphalangeal joint.[1] An alternative theory of grouping is represented by a system of orderly repeats of annular and cruciate pulleys (A1, C0 (variable), A2, C1, A3, C2, A4, C3, A5).[2] A more functional system modifies this latter convention and highlights the functional importance of the second annular pulley attached to the proximal one-half of the proximal phalanx and the fourth annular pulley attached to the proximal one-half bone of the middle phalanx for providing near normal joint function.[2]

In the normal digit, tendon balance and normal joint motion are dependent on the stout annular pulleys. Experimental studies have shown near normal digital motion will occur if the second (A2) and fourth (A4) annular pulleys are intact.[2] The contribution to normal digital function provided by the third annular pulley is debated. The remaining annular and cruciate pulleys play only a supportive role. These biomechanical data support either the theory of a proximal pulley/distal pulley system, i.e. a proximal subset for the proximal interphalangeal joint and a distal subset for the distal interphalangeal joint, or a theoretical balanced pair system on either side of the joint preventing bowstringing.

Until recent reports of closed rupture of the flexor tendon sheath,[3] the most usual reason for repair or reconstruction of the pulley system was following acute or late repair of flexor tendon lacerations. In reviews of pulley reconstruction techniques, no technique has been found to be equal in breaking strength to the normal annular pulley. Comparisons have been performed in the laboratory to assess the experimental comparative strengths of the various described repairs. Widstrom et al have compared single loop, volar plate, tendon weave, extensor retinaculum, palmar plate tunnel and loop and one-half repairs.[4] The palmar plate reconstruction was mechanically most effective while the extensor retinacular graft was mechanically least effective. Breaking strength varied from a mean strength of 2.8 kgf for the weave repair to 22.5 kgf for the loop and one-half repair. The weave most closely recreates the normal length of an annular pulley. A variation of the loop reconstruction using multiple loops around the phalanx is able to simulate the anatomy and biomechanics of the normal pulley but also falls short of normal annular pulley breaking strength.[2]

Technical aspects

In our series of closed pulley ruptures, all patients showed normal function initially, but slowly developed bowstringing and proximal interphalangeal (PIP) flexion deformity over time. The flexion contracture was the common complaint rather than bowstringing or altered strength. The diagnosis of flexor tendon

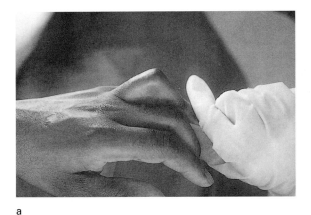

a

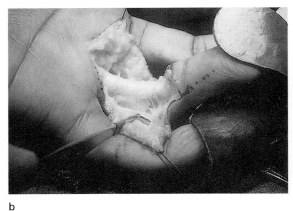

b

Figure 1

(a) Physical examination of patient with rupture of the flexor pulley resulting in bowstringing of flexor tendon and flexion deformity of the proximal interphalangeal joint. (b) Same patient at surgery showing incompetent flexor sheath.

bowstringing is made on physical examination visually and even more readily by palpation of the flexor sheath (Figure 1), especially under load. The flexion contracture of the proximal interphalangeal joint is readily appreciated. Routine radiographs of the involved digit are normal. Magnetic resonance imaging can confirm the diagnosis (Figure 2). In our cases of closed rupture of the sheath, pulleys A2–A3 and (in two-thirds of the cases) A4 were involved. This correlates with the relative breaking strengths of the annular pulleys found in laboratory studies. The frequency of digital involvement in our series was ring > little > middle which also correlates with the laboratory predictions of relative finger digital sheath strength for various fingers.

Reconstruction

The technique employed for reconstruction in our series was the tendon weave through the remaining thickened lateral margin of the stretched and scarred flexor sheath. In some cases, this reconstruction was combined with the reconstruction using a band of extensor retinaculum passed around the proximal and/or middle phalanx as a reinforcement. The weave technique is applicable only when sufficient stout lateral margins of the flexor sheath are present. One benefit of this repair is that it can be fashioned to produce a longer sheath reconstruction than any other method. Multiple loop reconstructions may also provide a broader reconstruction more similar to the natural A2 pulley. Extensor retinacular graft reconstruction has the capacity to provide a synovial lining.

Regardless of repair, the positioning of the reconstruction should be at the location of maximal curvature of the proximal or middle phalanx.[2] This positions the reconstruction at the normal location of the original A2 and A4 pulleys and should allow for the maximal potential for recovery of flexor tendon function. The most common cause of failure for the extensor retinaculum reconstruction is caused by the inability to adjust tension on the graft, resulting in a loose repair. This can be improved by modifying this

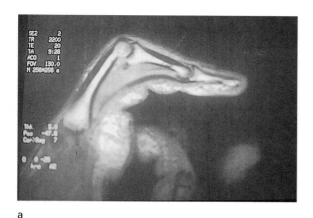
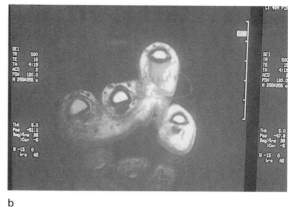

a   b

Figure 2

(a) Sagittal and (b) coronal magnetic resonance images of patient with incompetent pulley system.

technique to the belt-loop technique. This is done by passing one end of the extensor retinacular graft through itself. This allows the tension to be more easily applied and adjusted. The tension of any reconstruction should be as tight as possible.

Stretching of any of these repairs is anticipated with the potential for recurrence of tendon bowstringing. Following repair of the sheath, the PIP joint should be pinned in full extension for 3 weeks. Upon removal of the pin, active range of motion exercises are begun in a supervised therapy program. The reconstruction is protected with flexor tendon pulley ring supports externally. Recovery of motion may be slow and may take up to 1 year to regain optimal motion, especially flexion.

To date, results have been very encouraging. The active range of motion to the PIP joint in our series of closed rupture reconstruction has averaged 100° of motion. Distal interphalangeal joint motion has averaged 50° of motion.[3] No patient has had recurrence of the PIP joint flexion contracture or flexor tendon bowstringing. In the case of closed rupture, early recog-

nition may allow conservative treatment with external tendon pulley rings. I have treated one case successfully using this technique. An early diagnosis in acute cases is made by history and examination. All patients complain of a tearing sensation in the palmar aspect of the finger when an extension force is placed on an acutely flexed and fully loaded flexor mechanism. No case of flexor tendon rupture or avulsion was encountered. A high index of suspicion is necessary to make an accurate and correct diagnosis.

In the situation where the sheath is available for repair, i.e. following tendon repair or reconstruction, a simple running suture with nonabsorbable material has been effective. The repair frequently will require protection with external pulley rings if a major portion of A2 or A4 is involved.

In situations where there has been partial loss of an annular pulley, I have used the redundant portion of tenosynovium proximal to the A1 pulley as a graft. Use of a simple running nonabsorbable suture technique to the remaining annular pulley in this situation has been successful in a small number of cases.

Conclusion

With the increased awareness of the importance of the flexor sheath for flexor tendon nutrition and gliding, and the pulley system for maintenance of tendon range of motion, power and prevention of altered joint mechanics, stronger and more effective methods of repair and reconstruction of the annular pulleys and possibly a method to reconstruct cruciate pulleys may be forthcoming.

References

1   Strauch B, de Moura W, Digital flexor tendon sheath: an anatomic study, *J Hand Surg* (1985) **10A**:785–9.

2   Amadio PC, Lin GT, An KN, Anatomy and pathomechanics of the flexor pulley system, *J Hand Ther* (1989) **2**:138–41.

3   Bowers WH, Kuzma GR, Bynum DK, Closed traumatic rupture of finger flexor pulleys, *J Hand Surg* (1994) **19A**:782–7.

4   Widstrom CJ, Johnson G, Doyle JR, et al, A mechanical study of six digital pulley reconstruction techniques: Part I Mechanical effectiveness and Part II Strength of individual reconstruction, *J Hand Surg* (1989) **14A**:821–9.

6
Repair of finger flexor pulleys – 2

Dominique Le Viet and Philippe Samson

Introduction

Repair of digital pulleys is one of the major problems in flexor tendon surgery. Absence of one or more pulleys, secondary to trauma or surgical excision, should lead to bowstringing of flexor tendons. This results in serious functional trouble by limitation of flexion as well as a secondary loss of finger extension.

As early mobilization is one of the keys to success in flexor tendon repair, we think that the initial strength of a reconstructed pulley must allow early protected active motion. The situation is different when a staged reconstruction is selected, because no early stress is applied on the pulleys.

Technical aspects

It must be stressed that the exposure of the digital tunnel for the tenolysis or the tendon grafting preceding the pulley repair has to be atraumatic. The intact pulleys must be located and preserved, using a meticulous technique.

Material for pulley reconstruction

We prefer to use tendon grafts. When possible, an excised flexor tendon is used to repair the pulleys. The A4 pulley can be reconstructed with a 6 cm strip of flexor superficialis tendon remaining inserted on the middle phalanx and looped two times subcutaneously around the tendons and the phalanx.

When no tendinous remnant is available, we use the palmaris longus which must be harvested including its peritenon. When the palmaris longus is absent we use the extensor digitorum longus tendon to the third toe.

Reconstruction of digital flexor pulleys (thumb excepted)

The importance of reconstructing A2 and A4 pulleys has been emphasized by all authors. We use a multiple-loop technique (Figure 1), as advocated by Okutsu et al.[1] For the A2 pulley a three-loop graft is passed around the phalanx and the flexor tendon. Dorsally we pass the graft between the phalanx and the extensor hood, in contrast to Okutsu et al who pass it subcutaneously. For the A4 pulley we use a double-loop graft that is dorsally passed subcutaneously around the extensor tendon. A2 and A4 reconstructed pulleys are placed at the union of the proximal and middle thirds of the corresponding phalanx. The degree of tension of the loops is evaluated by pulling the flexor tendon in the palm. The pulleys must not strangle the tendon while permitting a complete flexion of the finger, without bowstringing.

The main advantages of this method are its ease in adjustment of the pulley location and tension, and its initial strength allowing early protected active motion.[2] We have discarded methods in which the graft is passed through a drill hole in the phalanx. These procedures are tricky, moreover the hole must be small enough not to weaken the phalanx, allowing only one loop of the graft.

In Karev's 'belt loop' procedure the flexor tendon is passed through slits in the volar plate of metaphalangeal and proximal interphalangeal joints.[3] Although efficient, the location of these

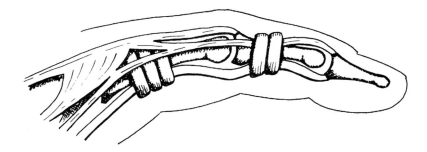

Figure 1

Reconstruction of finger A2 and A4 pulleys. The three loops are passed between the extensor and the phalanx at A2 level, while two loops are passed subcutaneously at A4 level.

reconstructed pulleys is not ideal and we believe the finger function is not as good as in an A2/A4 reconstruction in an anatomical place. Furthermore, it seems that the initial strength of this reconstruction does not allow early active mobilization. The use of extensor retinaculum seems to provide a stiff reconstructed pulley whose initial strength is poor.[4] Finally, we prefer the modification of the method of Okutsu et al because of its technical simplicity and its quite constant effectiveness.

Reconstruction of thumb flexor pulleys

The most important flexor pulleys of the thumb are the metacarpophalangeal or A1 pulley, and the oblique pulley which is an expansion from adductor pollicis. Presence of at least one of these two pulleys is necessary to obtain a complete active flexion of the thumb.

If both A1 and oblique pulleys are absent, and if a radial stump of A1 pulley exists, we reconstruct the A1 pulley using a tendinous plasty from adductor pollicis tendon (Figure 2).[5] The ulnar neurovascular bundle is retracted, allowing a good view of the distal insertions of adductor pollicis on the ulnar sesamoid and on the ulnar side of the proximal phalanx. Using a #11 scalpel blade, a proximally based anterior flap is raised from the tendon inserting on the phalanx. To obtain a flap long enough, dissection must be carried on proximally, including anterior muscular fibers in the flap. Two parallel incisions are made in the tendon inserting on the ulnar sesamoid, creating a small tunnel. The flap is

then passed through this tunnel, over the flexor tendon, and secured to the radial stump of the A1 pulley using three 2/0 polyamide sutures. Sutures must not be in contact with the flexor tendon. The metacarpophalangeal joint is immobilized in a splint for 4 weeks.

This technique of reconstruction has proven to be satisfactory and is strong enough to allow early active controlled motion of the interphalangeal joint. The adductor pollicis tendon flap used is vascularized, reducing the risks of adhesion. Its length can be easily adjusted, and no sequel has been observed at the donor site.

If no radial stump of A1 pulley is present, the adductor flap is too short to reconstruct the whole pulley. In this case we choose the double-loop method, the tendon graft being passed dorsally between the proximal phalanx and the extensor tendon.

Conclusion

Digital pulley reconstruction is usually performed at the time of tenolysis or grafting of a flexor tendon. It can also be necessary if bowstringing of the flexor tendon results in loss of complete active flexion. This secondarily leads to a limitation of finger extension because of fibrosis between the volar plate and the dislocated tendon. During surgery this fibrous callus must be resected to allow full finger extension and to permit direct appliance of the tendon on the phalanx and the volar plate.

An isolated rupture of the A2 or A4 pulley, as sometimes seen in rock climbers, does not generally lead to functional limitation. Surgery is

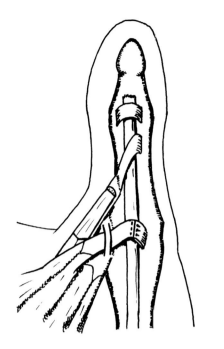

Figure 2

Thumb A1 pulley reconstruction.

usually necessary only when all the pulleys from A2 to A4 are torn.

Repair of the A1 pulley of the thumb is usually indicated for bowstringing of the flexor pollicis longus tendon resulting in a loss of complete flexion of the thumb interphalangeal joint. The diagnosis can be made when the loss of flexion is corrected after pressure is applied on the volar aspect of the thumb proximal phalanx.

References

1   Okutsu I, Ninomiya S, Hiraki S, et al, Three-loop technique for A2 pulley reconstruction, *J Hand Surg* (1987) **12A**:790–4.

2   Lin GT, Amadio PC, An KN, et al, Biomechanical analysis of finger flexor pulley reconstruction, *J Hand Surg* (1989) **14B**:278–82.

3   Karev A, The 'belt loop' technique for the reconstruction of the pulleys in the first stage of tendon grafting, *J Hand Surg* (1984) **9A**:923–4.

4   Lister GD, Reconstruction of pulleys employing extensor retinaculum, *J Hand Surg* (1979) **4**:461–4.

5   Le Viet D, Ebelin M, Un procédé de reconstruction de la poulie métacarpo-phalangienne du pouce, *Rev Chir Orthop* (1982) **68**:347–50.

7

Flexor tendon grafting and tenolysis in the pediatric patient

Nancy M Lynch and Richard S Idler

Introduction

Flexor tendon injuries in children can be difficult to diagnose due to the child's inability to cooperate with a thorough examination. As a result, some of these injuries may go undiagnosed for a period of time. Even when recognized in a timely fashion, the treatment of flexor tendon injuries may be appropriately delayed, such as in the face of mutilating trauma or infection. Under such circumstances, tendon grafting may be required. In the pediatric population, compliance with postoperative therapy is often difficult to enforce and requires modification of adult protocols. Likewise, indications for flexor tenolysis must be tempered given a child's difficulty with participating in operative and therapy protocols. Little has been written on the indications, techniques and results of flexor tendon grafting and tenolysis in children. Most series on the subjects fail to isolate the pediatric patient as a subset with special considerations. As such, the preoperative selection of patients for these procedures and counselling of their parents remains difficult.

Indications and requirements

Tendon grafting

Flexor tendon grafting was once advocated for all zone II lacerations regardless of the age of injury. However, as in adults, it has been shown that the results of primary repair of flexor tendon injuries in children using current repair techniques are superior to grafting in any zone.[1] Present recommendations reserve grafting for delayed recognition of a flexor tendon injury in which primary flexor tendon repair is not possible, rupture of a primary repair, injuries or infection resulting in segmental loss of tendon substance, or with staged flexor tendon reconstruction. Application of the Boyes classification,[2] which grades the severity of tissue damage of the digit, may help determine which patients will benefit from a one- versus a two-stage procedure. A one-stage procedure is most appropriately performed in a digit with minimal flexor sheath scarring which will not require joint releases, nerve reconstruction, or reconstruction of a deficient pulley system. An absolute prerequisite for a one-stage procedure is full passive range of motion in the affected digit preoperatively. Compromise of surrounding soft tissue, neurovascular and/or bony integrity requires a two-stage procedure. Prior to the second stage of a two-stage procedure, soft tissue equilibrium and full passive motion must be obtained.

Indications for grafting in zone I injuries are not well established. Although good results have been reported, tendon grafting in zone I with an intact flexor digitorum superficialis is controversial.[3] Collapse of the A4 pulley may require a pulley reconstruction. To achieve maximum flexion at the DIP joint may require a secondary flexor tenolysis. In the absence of a functional deficit, a 'superficialis' finger may be preferable to flexor tendon grafting which requires intensive therapy, possible additional surgery, or an outcome inferior to the initial preoperative status.

Tenolysis

Patients with limited active flexion but with a passive potential for full digital motion following primary repair or grafting may benefit from tenolysis. General guidelines suggest that a plateau in motion 3–6 months postoperatively which renders the digit unable to touch the palm is an indication for this procedure. Additionally, soft tissues must be in a state of equilibrium, fracture healing must be complete, and the neurovascular function of the digit must be adequate. In children, consideration must also be given to their ability to participate in their care.

Maturity in handling the intraoperative environment and postoperative therapy in spite of the anticipated discomfort is one of the keys to success. Active intraoperative participation by the patient in tenolysis helps limit the necessary amount of surgical intervention. Immediate participation in postoperative therapy is a requirement for a successful outcome. Preoperative evaluation by a hand therapist may assist the hand surgeon in eliminating poor operative candidates. If a general anesthetic is required to perform the tenolysis, consideration should be given to whether the procedure should be delayed until the patient has reached a more mature age.

It has not been conclusively demonstrated that a delay in this procedure diminishes the chance of a successful outcome with surgery at a later date. Improvement in range of motion has been seen over time in some younger patients treated nonoperatively. In one series, younger patients undergoing flexor tenolysis demonstrated a gradual long term loss of motion despite initial promising results. Although open to influence based on the maturity of the individual patient, we have found children under the age of 11 are poor candidates for tenolysis.

Technical aspects

Tendon grafting

If available, a local source for the tendon graft is preferred. The tendon graft may be obtained from the flexor digitorum superficialis of the involved finger if both tendons are lacerated. An alternative local source is the tendon of the palmaris longus which is usually of sufficient length to reach from the finger to the wrist. The plantaris tendon may be harvested, but its presence cannot be detected preoperatively. A fourth potential source, the long toe extensor,

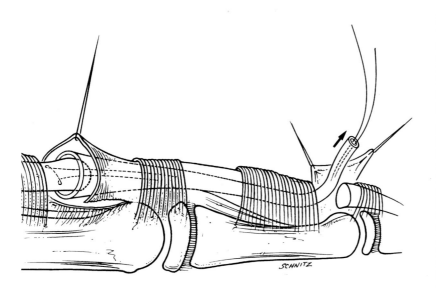

SCHNITZ

Figure 1

A #5 pediatric feeding tube may be cut down to size and used to facilitate passage of the flexor tendon through the tendon sheath to the repair site. Core sutures are first placed in the end of the tendon. The small end of the feeding tube is fed through the flexor sheath to the repair site. The core sutures of the flexor tendon are then passed through the tube emerging out at the repair site. By traction on the core sutures the flexor tendon can be drawn up to the funnel end of the feeding tube and sometimes within the tube. Simultaneous traction on the distal end of the feeding tube and core sutures allows the tendon to be passed through this sheath to the repair site.

may be of limited length. Other alternative sources of tendon graft include the extensor indicis proprius, accessory slip of the extensor digiti minimi quinti, or partial harvest of the flexor carpi radialis tendon. Experimental studies by Abrahamsson and Gelberman suggest better results may be obtained by the use of tendon grafts with a tenosynovial lining.[4] An alternative to tendon grafting in the thumb with an adequate flexor sheath is a superficialis tendon transfer.

The pediatric patient creates special surgical challenges for tendon grafting. The placement of core sutures in small tendon grafts may be technically difficult and requires appropriately-sized suture material. All pulleys must be patent and the graft not oversized. The graft must be atraumatically threaded through the flexor sheath. Passage may be facilitated with the use of a pediatric feeding tube (Figure 1).

Part of the art of tendon grafting lies in securing the graft and setting proper tension on the flexor system. This is most easily accomplished by first securing the tendon graft at the distal phalanx. A 3.0 polypropylene or slow absorbing monofilament suture is placed through the distal end of the graft with a Bunnell weave, then passed through oblique drill holes in the terminal phalanx to exit dorsally where it may be tied directly onto the nail or over a bolster (Figure 2). Care should be taken to avoid placing drill holes through the physis when the transosseous technique is used.

Alternatively, an extraosseous technique may be used for the small terminal phalanx. The suture from the distal end of the tendon graft is passed through the stump of the profundus tendon and along the side of the phalanx, to exit at the tip of the digit (Figure 3). The ends are then tied over a bolster.

Proximally a Pulvertaft weave is performed in the palm or wrist joining the graft to the profundus tendon of the involved digit when present and possesses adequate excursion of 2–2.5 cm. If the original profundus muscle is not available, then a transfer into the profundus of an adjacent digit may be performed. Tension is set on the system through the Pulvertaft weave such that the affected digit rests in a slightly greater posture of flexion than the adjacent digits. With passive wrist extension the grafted digit should flex as much or slightly greater than the other digits by a tenodesis effect.

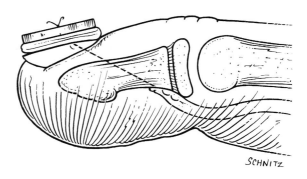

Figure 2

When the terminal phalanx is of sufficient size it is possible to use a transosseous passage of the core sutures to the button on the dorsum on the nail plate. It is important to avoid injury to the physis during this procedure.

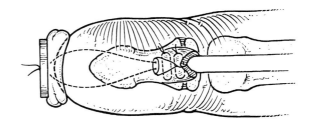

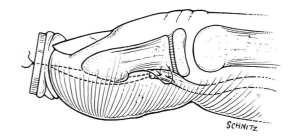

Figure 3

In the small terminal phalanx an extraosseous passage of the core sutures around the terminal phalanx can be performed. As with the transosseous technique the core sutures are secured over a button at the tip of the digit.

Several factors in young children preclude a rehabilitation program for tendon grafting which emphasizes early motion. Effective composite and isolated passive range of motion is not reliably performed on the smaller digits of children. Fabrication of a protective splint which can be secured in place in the absence of supervision is difficult for the pediatric extremity. A long arm cast with the wrist flexed 20–30°, the MP joints in 60–80° of flexion and the IP joints in extension is applied for 3 weeks. After this interval, a protective dorsal blocking splint may be utilized for protection. An attempt is made to encourage functional use of the hand. Supervised play therapy which emphasizes activities which involve grasping or individual digit motion may be beneficial. By 6–8 weeks unrestricted use is usually tolerated.

The technique of staged reconstruction involves an initial excision of all damaged tendons and scar tissue within the remaining sheath. Any existing joint contractures must be released. The hand must be of sufficient size to at least accommodate the smallest silicone rod, which is 2 mm. Pulley reconstruction is performed with remnant flexor tendon, from other sources of tendon graft, or extensor retinaculum from the wrist, and should recreate at least the A2 and A4 pulleys. Additional pulley reconstruction is indicated to correct tendon bowstringing with flexion across any of the digital joints. The tissues used for pulley reconstruction may be anchored to any remaining rim of the pulley or may be placed around the phalanx. Placement of grafts through drill holes in the bone should be avoided in the pediatric patient due to the small size of the phalanx. Soft tissue equilibrium and full passive motion must be present before the second stage of flexor tendon reconstruction is started and usually requires at least 3 months to achieve.

Rehabilitation after the first stage of a two-stage reconstruction emphasizes passive motion. This will require regular participation by the parent in performing these exercises with the child. If the hand is of sufficient size, buddy strapping may be beneficial. Night extension splinting is important to maintain full digital extension. During the second stage, for the first 3 weeks postoperatively, protection of the tendon graft in a long arm cast (as previously described) is recommended. Subsequent therapy is identical to that for children following primary tendon grafting. Because of the potential for late contracture of the tendon pseudosheath, long term digital extension splinting is advisable.

Tenolysis

Patients old enough to undergo surgery with a local anesthetic supplemented by intravenous sedation are good candidates for flexor tenolysis. This is true for both adult and pediatric patients. Tourniquet discomfort can be minimized by the use of sequential upper arm and forearm tourniquets or a supplemental bier block during the initial phase of the procedure. A method of flexor tenolysis described by Strickland is effective.[5] For the surgical approach, a midlateral incision is favored whenever possible, but previous incisions may dictate the approach.

Preservation of the annular pulleys, particularly A2 and A4, is important. To accomplish a thorough tenolysis, annular pulleys may be incised but only cruciate pulleys should be excised. If the integrity of the pulley system cannot be maintained, pulley reconstruction should be undertaken to eliminate bowstringing. To commence the tenolysis, the borders of the flexor tendons are defined outside the zone of original injury and lysis progresses towards the site of maximum pathology. Use of small joint arthroscopy or ophthalmic knives may be helpful to release adhesions beneath the pulleys. The technique should be as atraumatic as possible. Use of excessive force when traction lysis of adhesions is performed may lead to pulley rupture in the pediatric patient. If the patient is awake this allows periodic active flexion checks to minimize the surgery necessary to restore active range of motion. The operative goal is to achieve active motion equal to the passive potential for digital motion. Should intraoperative findings identify an unsuspected tendon rupture or excessively scarred tendon bed with incompetent pulleys, the surgeon should be prepared to proceed with a staged flexor tendon reconstruction.

The postoperative regimen following tenolysis emphasizes early active, active assisted, and passive range of motion, beginning within 24 hours of surgery. Ideally therapy should be performed on an hourly basis under the supervision of a therapist or educated adult. Program modifications for tendons of poor quality or in situations where pulley reconstructions have been performed will be difficult to enforce. Measures for edema control and interval extension splinting are used between exercise sessions. Once sutures have been removed, early use of the hand can be a supplement to therapy. Functional electrical stimulation and continuous passive motion devices are helpful if the child can understand their use. Unrestricted use of the hand is possible by 6 weeks. Long term night extension splinting for 3–6 months is advisable to prevent late digital contracture.

Results

Tendon grafting

In the largest series reported to date of children who have undergone primary flexor tendon grafting, 80% had a good or fair result.[1] Two-stage reconstruction has a higher complication rate and higher failure rate in children when compared to adults.[6] While some concern exists that the growth of a finger may be affected by the loss of its flexor system, clinically this has not been reported as a significant problem and it is appropriate to defer treatment until the patient is older and able to participate in adult treatment protocols.

Tenolysis

Only one series which specifically addresses flexor tenolysis in children exists in the literature.[7] In this series, children under the age of 11 showed no substantial improvement in motion compared to their preoperative measurements. On the other hand, 13 out of 21 patients aged 11 or older demonstrated good or excellent results following flexor tenolysis. Two patients showed

a diminished long-term result and the author has recommended periodic long-term follow-up for pediatric patients who have undergone tenolysis. Tenolysis following grafting had a less favorable result than following primary tendon repair.

Conclusion

The absolute surgical indications for flexor tendon grafting and tenolysis in the pediatric population are the same as those in adults. The presence of open growth plates and smaller structures to be handled surgically necessitates some modification in surgical technique. With a cooperative child and supportive family primary flexor tendon grafting and even staged flexor tendon reconstruction can be successfully accomplished in the young patient. Flexor tenolysis, however, requires a maturity level on a par with an adult. Delaying treatment until such time will enhance outcome in complicated flexor reconstructions or tenolysis in the pediatric population.

References

1   Vahvanen V, Gripenberg L, Nuutinen P, Flexor tendon injury in the hand in children: a long-term followup study of 84 patients, *Scand J Plast Reconstr Surg* (1951) **15**:43–8.
2   Boyes JH, Flexor-tendon grafts in the fingers and thumb, *J Bone Joint Surg* (1950) **32A**:489–99.
3   Bora FW, Profundus tendon grafting with unimpaired sublimus function in children, *Clin Orthop* (1970) **71**:118–23.
4   Abrahamsson SO, Gelberman R, Maintenance of the gliding surface of tendon autografts in dogs, *Acta Orthop Scand* (1994) **65**:548–52.
5   Strickland JW, Flexor tenolysis: a personal experience. In: Hunter JM, Schneider LH, Mackin EJ, eds, *Tendon Surgery in the Hand* (CV Mosby: St Louis, 1987) 216–33.
6   Amadio PC, Staged flexor tendon reconstruction in children, *Ann Hand Surg* (1992) **11**:194–9.
7   Birnie RH, Idler RS, Flexor tenolysis in children, *J Hand Surg* (1995) **20A**:254–7.

Commentary

Chapter 3

This paper accurately captures the current state of affairs in flexor tendon rehabilitation. The authors have carefully married techniques from a variety of sources to provide up-to-date listings of what's "in": synergistic motion and early active 'place and hold' exercises.

PCA

Chapter 4

Gau-Tyan Lin came to the Mayo Clinic as a visiting scientist about 10 years ago and brought with him two fascinating concepts, both of which have since been widely adopted. The first is the use of multiple strand techniques to improve the quality of tendon repair sufficient to the point where early active motion may be used. His thoughts on that subject are reproduced here.

Doctor Lin also brought to Mayo the concept of synergistic motion as an adjunct to tendon rehabilitation. In this technique, wrist flexion is combined with finger extension and wrist extension combined with finger flexion in order to improve tendon gliding after tendon repair.

Both techniques have proved to be valuable in improving the quality of results after tendon surgery.

PCA

Chapters 5 and 6

Finger flexor pulley reconstruction is not necessarily new but is something old that is definitely quite useful. Here Doctors Leviet, Samson and Kuzma outline the current state of affairs for this classic hand surgery topic. There is some more scientific evidence coming to help us with our pulley reconstructions. Work done by Gelberman, Seiler and at my own institution, the Mayo Clinic, has shown that pulley reconstructions that take advantage of tissues which have a synovial surface create less friction than pulley reconstructions by tissues which do not have a synovial surface. For example, an extensor retinaculum (assuming the synovial face is towards the tendon) would have less friction between it and the underlying tendon than would a pulley reconstruction created from a palmaris longus tendon graft. Tensioning of the pulley reconstruction can also be an issue and in our own work we have found that a tension of approximately 150 g provides sufficient snugness so that the reconstructive pulley is closed opposed to the underlying tendon, but not so tight as to increase the friction when the tendon tries to glide. Although not so scientific as the elegant work presented by Lieber elsewhere in this volume, such laboratory work, coupled with the clinical observations such as those presented here, should help make our pulley reconstructions more predictable in the future.

PCA

Chapter 7

Although the surgical techniques of tendon grafting and tenolysis do not change, it is critical to take into account the age of the patient when deciding whether, and when, to perform the procedure. As these authors emphasize, the critical factor is the ability of the child to cooperate with the postoperative rehabilitation program. In my own practice I have found two important considerations. One, of course, is the emotional maturity of the child. Occasionally, one will encounter a child as young as 4 or 5 years old who is mature enough and well behaved enough to cooperate with a complicated tendon rehabilitation program. This is rare. Most commonly, children do not possess the requisite maturity until age 10, and this is the age at which one would generally recommend reconstruction to parents of a very young child who has sustained a severe hand injury. It is true that hands without normal tendon function will not grow normally, but the development of a hand with a failed, complicated tendon reconstruction is usually even worse.

The second circumstance that is often noted in these children relates to the fact that the injuries are uncommon, and become progressively more uncommon as better primary care of tendon injuries is provided in smaller and smaller communities. Often the most severe injuries occur in patients who live a long distance away from major hand surgery treatment centers and this can pose an additional problem with rehabilitation. It has been my experience that rehabilitation that cannot be carefully supervised by the treating surgeon will often produce poorer results than rehabilitation which the surgeon has the opportunity to supervise. Again this may pose a serious difficulty for patients of any age who must travel a great distance for medical care. This is another area which must be comprehensively discussed with the patient and the patient's family before a complex reconstructive effort is embarked upon.

PCA

8

Advances in management of the open and repaired zone III extensor tendon injury

Roslyn B Evans

Introduction

The acutely repaired central slip (extensor zone III) injury treated traditionally with 4–6 weeks of immobilization is often compromised by loss of extensor tendon excursion, extensor lag at the proximal interphalangeal (PIP) joint level, and loss of flexion at the interphalangeal (IP) joints. These problems are expensive and time consuming in terms of the extensive rehabilitation often required, additional surgery, and loss of work. Clinical experience and literature review indicate that the following factors influence the complications and final outcome of the acutely repaired and immobilized central slip injury:

(1) the broad tendon–bone interface in zone IV,
(2) splinting the PIP joint at less than absolute full extension during the immobilization phase,
(3) the effects of stress deprivation on connective tissue about the PIP joint (i.e. tendon, ligament, cartilage), and the high incidence of complex injuries in zones III and IV.

Poor final results have moved a few clinicians to recommend early passive motion for the zone III and IV extensor injury with a variety of passive protocols and dynamic splints which are either hand-based or forearm-based. Early motion in these zones has not been widely accepted because the majority assume that early motion will lead to attenuation, if not rupture, of the central slip. The sceptical are indeed correct if the postoperative protocol is not closely monitored with attention to proper splinting so that the PIP joint rests at absolute 0°, and motion

is precisely controlled to allow only 3–4 mm of excursion of the repaired tendon.

Based on theoretical work, a carefully defined early active short arc motion (SAM) protocol was defined and tested clinically.[1,2] Standard rehabilitation methods were compared to the SAM protocol and evaluated in terms of:

(1) PIP joint and distal interphalangeal (DIP) joint flexion,
(2) PIP joint extension lag,
(3) total active range of motion (TAM) as calculated by the Strickland–Glogovac formula, and
(4) treatment time.

Materials and methods

The results of open and repaired zone III extensor tendon injuries (64 digits in 55 patients) treated by myself in a private hand rehabilitation practice over a 7 year period were analyzed.[2] The patients were referred by 23 different orthopedic or plastic surgeons with no controls on surgical management.

The patients were divided into two groups depending on postoperative management technique. The patients in group I (30 patients) were treated with 3–6 weeks (mean 33 days) of continuous immobilization before any PIP joint motion was initiated. The patients in group II (25 patients) were treated with immediate active short arc motion (SAM) initiated between 2 and 11 days postoperatively (mean 5 days). Group I patients treated during the first 2 of the 7 years reviewed

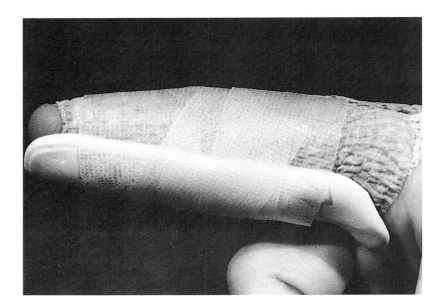

Figure 1

The involved digit is splinted in a volar thermoplastic splint immobilizing the proximal interphalangeal and distal interphalangeal joints at 0°. Dorsal pressure is applied over both joints with one inch Transpore™ tape. (Reprinted with permission from Evans RB.[2])

were evaluated retrospectively. All patients treated during the last 5 years reviewed were evaluated prospectively (some group I, all group II). Patients were excluded only for insufficient follow-up or associated flexor tendon injury.

A number of variables were considered for each patient. Age, gender, digit, treating surgeon, postoperative day that motion was initiated, day of discharge from therapy, PIP extension lag, PIP and DIP joint flexion at various time intervals, and complexity of injury were recorded. Simple injury was defined as extensor tendon laceration with or without lateral band injury and repair. Complex injury was defined as tendon laceration with associated injury to cartilage, ligament, bone, or distal joint.

Group I consisted of 38 digits in 30 patients with injury to 10 index, 16 long, 6 ring, and 6 small digits. Twenty-six patients were male (87%) and 4 female (13%), with an average age of 40 (range 14–70) years. Complex injuries occurred in 76% of this group, with 15 of the 38 digits (39%) being saw injuries.

Group II consisted of 26 digits in 25 patients with injury to 13 index, 11 long, 0 ring, and 2 small digits. Twenty patients were male (80%) and 5 female (20%), with an average age of 42

(range 12–68) years. Complex injuries occurred in 80% of this group, with 11 of 26 digits (42%) being saw injuries.

Postoperative management with immobilization: Twenty-three cases were referred to hand therapy after the immobilization phase with a variety of physician-applied splints. Seven patients were referred to hand therapy early and were immobilized in digital casts which included only the PIP and DIP joints. Controlled motion was initiated between 3 and 6 weeks (mean 33 days), dependent on the date of referral to therapy, with standard rehabilitation protocol.[3]

Postoperative management with immediate active short arc motion: In group II the PIP and DIP joints of the involved digit were immobilized in complete extension in a volar static thermoplastic splint. One inch Transpore™ tape (3M Medical Surgical Division, St Paul, Minnesota 55144) was applied directly over the PIP and DIP joints to insure that both rested at 0° of extension (Figure 1). A home exercise program was prescribed for the patient in which two template splints were used to control excursion and stress application for the zone III and IV extensor tendon. Template splint 1 (Figure 2) is a volar static splint with a 30° PIP joint flexion angle and a 20–25° DIP flexion

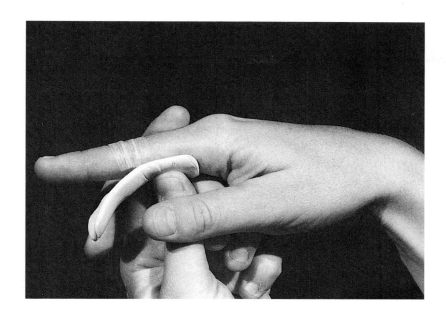

Figure 2

Template splint 1 allows 30° flexion at the proximal interphalangeal joint and 20–25° flexion at the distal interphalangeal joint, preventing the patient from overstretching the repair site by allowing only precalculated excursion of the central slip. The proximal interphalangeal joint is actively flexed and extended in this controlled range while the wrist is positioned in 30° of flexion, the metacarpophalangeal joint at 0° of extension, and the affected digit is supported at the proximal phalanx level by the contralateral hand. (Reprinted with permission from Evans RB.[2])

angle. Template splint 2 is a volar static extension splint which positions the PIP joint in full extension and is cut away at the DIP joint.

The patients were instructed to exercise within the template splints at least eight times per day with 20 repetitions of active flexion and extension for the PIP and DIP joints. The exercise position for the short arc motion protocol was 30° of wrist flexion and 0° to slight flexion for the MP joint. The patients were instructed to manually support the proximal phalanx of the involved digit in template splint 1 with the unaffected hand. The digit was then actively flexed and extended through the allowed range for the PIP and DIP joints (Figure 2). The patients were instructed that each exercise should be performed slowly and that the digit should be sustained briefly in the fully extended position. Template splint 2 was then applied with manual pressure over the PIP joint stabilizing this joint at 0° of extension. If the lateral bands were not repaired, the DIP joint was flexed fully and extended to 0°; if the lateral band(s) were repaired, the DIP joint was flexed only to 30–35° with active extension emphasized.

Between exercise sessions the PIP and DIP joints of the injured digit were held at 0° of extension in the digital protective splint (Figure 1). Patients were instructed to reapply the Transpore™ tape if it stretched to prevent the joints from resting in a posture of slight flexion. If no lag developed after 2 weeks of controlled motion at 30°, then template splint 1 was altered to allow 40° at the PIP joint during the third postoperative week and 50° during the fourth postoperative week.

The wrist, MP joint of the affected digit, and other digital joints were free to move through a normal range of motion (ROM) during the healing phase; only the IP joints of the injured digit were immobilized. Controlled mobilization and splinting at 4 weeks provided protection for the healing tendon as PIP joint flexion was gradually increased. Digital edema was controlled with a single layer of Coban™ (3M, St Paul MN) wrap for the first 4 weeks and the usual anti-edema measures (elevation, ice, retrograde massage) were utilized.

Results

Group I digits were compared with Group II digits with each category considered separately for statistical significance.* These results have been reported in detail elsewhere[2] and are summarized in Tables 1 and 2. The results for each digit were calculated using the Strickland–Glogovac formula which excludes the MP joint:

$$\frac{(\text{sum of active PIP joint and DIP joint flexion}) \text{ minus extensor lag}}{175} \times 100$$

= % normal combined PIP joint/DIP joint flexion

These results should be considered in light of the high percentage of complex injuries in both groups (76% of group I, 77% of group II). Group I averaged 63% of normal, group II 75% of normal. The mean day for initiation of motion, day of discharge, PIP flexion, DIP flexion, total active motion (TAM), and extensor lag were all highly significant ($P < 0.01$) in favor of the patients treated with the SAM protocol over those treated with immobilization. No patient in group II developed a boutonnière deformity, and no tendon ruptured. The patients in group II had an average of 3° of PIP extensor lag, with a maximum of 10° extensor lag. The early motion group experienced less extensor lag, better flexion at both digital joints, shorter treatment time, and no skin or wound problems.

The results of this preliminary study continue to be supported in my clinical experience. As of the time of writing I have treated another 16 cases of open and repaired central slip injuries with excellent results in regard to time of treatment necessary to establish a good result (average 6 weeks), PIP extension lag (3°), and TAM (146°).

Discussion

The rationale for early motion

The rationale for early motion following tendon repair is based on numerous research studies that demonstrate that some stress at a tendon repair site is beneficial both biochemically and biomechanically to the repaired tendon and that some degree of controlled motion will reduce complications associated with immobilization by maintaining homeostasis in the adjacent connective tissues. Biochemically, the immobilized tendon experiences a loss of glycosaminoglycan concentration, loss of water, decreased fibronectin (FN) concentration, and decreased endotenon healing. Biomechanically, the immobilized tendon loses tensile strength in the first 2 weeks postrepair and gliding function by the tenth day postrepair. Controlled motion during the healing phase has been demonstrated to increase FN concentration, fibroblast chemotaxis, repair site DNA, tensile strength, gliding properties, synovial diffusion, and peri-tendinous vessel density and configuration for tendon. Numerous clinical studies support the practice of early motion for protocols for tendon at all levels with the exception of zone I extensor.

Experimental work has demonstrated significant decreases in tendon excursions and increases in work requirement for the complex tendon injury as compared to the simple tendon injury. Extensor injury at the zone III and IV levels is more often than not complex.[2]

Defining the problems

The zone III and IV injury often produces poor functional results especially in the more complex cases associated with crush or periosteal injury. Newport et al,[5] in a report of long-term results of extensor tendon repair, found that extensor tendon injuries within the digit treated with immobilization had high percentages of fair and poor results as compared to those of more proximal injuries, and that injuries in zones III and IV had higher percentages of resultant extensor lag (35%) and loss of flexion (71%). Other researchers have reported similar findings.

The unfavorable ratio of tendon to bone interface in zone IV, the complex gliding requirements of the extensor system on the dorsal aspect of the digit, and the often complex nature of this injury yields functional problems associated with adhesions.[6] The immobilized repair in zone III devoid of the benefits of greater intrinsic

*Statistical significance testing was performed by Isadore Enger, MA, MS, statistician, Department of Orthopaedics and Rehabilitation, University of Miami School of Medicine, Miami, Florida.

Table 1 Final results and statistical analysis comparing Groups I and II. (Reprinted with permission from Evans RB.[2])

Results	Group I (Immb)	Group II (SAM)	Statistical significance	
			(t Test)	(χ^2)
Number digits	38	26		
Mean age	39.9	42.2	>0.5 NS	
Male sex (%)	86.8	80.8		>0.5 NS
Complex injury (%)	76.3	76.9		>0.5 NS
Mean day motion initiated	32.9	4.59	<0.001 S	
Mean day injury to D/C	76.07	51.38	<0.001 S	
PIP ext. lag on 1st motion day	13°	3°	<0.01 S	
PIP ext. lag on D/C day	8.13°	2.96°	<0.01 S	
PIP motion at 6 weeks	44°	88°	<0.001 S	
PIP motion at D/C	72°	88°	<0.01 S	
TAM (PIP & DIP) at D/C	110.7°	131.5°	<0.01 S	
DIP motion at D/C	37.63°	45°	<0.01 S	

D/C, discharge; Immb, immobile for 3–6 weeks; S, significant; NS, non-significant.

healing and strengthening associated with early motion may attenuate or gap when motion is initiated at 4–6 weeks because its proximal segment is adherent and non-gliding. This increased resistance or drag in zone IV elevates the extensor tension in zone III and may exceed the tensile strength of the repair. We observe this in the immobilized central slip that begins to lag in extension with late mobilization programs as flexion parameters are increased.

Another contributing factor to extensor lag is the improperly applied splint. It is not uncommon for the immobilized central slip injury not followed in therapy until the late mobilization phase to have been splinted incorrectly in some flexion with resultant extensor lag. Aluma-foam splints with adhesive tape proximal and distal to the PIP joint encourage swelling and allow the PIP joint to rest in flexion; finger casts that are not checked frequently allow the PIP to rest in flexion as edema decreases. The edematous joint associated with complex injury will posture in 30–40° of flexion to more comfortably accommodate the increased volume of edema. In this position effusion or edema under the central slip will increase its moment arm, place tension on the repair, and may cause gapping or attenuation of the repair with resultant extensor lag.

The effects of stress deprivation on connective tissues have been well documented. Immobilization may result in functional limitation of

not only tendon, but of ligament and cartilage with loss of both PIP and DIP motion. The clinical portion of this study has demonstrated that a large percentage of injuries in zones III and IV are complex (77% of 64) and that many have associated injury to adjacent soft tissue, the PIP, or DIP joint. The complex injury can be expected to

Table 2 Classification of results comparing Groups I and II (Strickland–Glogovac formula). (Reprinted with permission from Evans RB.[2])

Classification	Group I (immobilization)	Group II (early active short arc motion)
Excellent (85–100%, ≥ 150°)	5 (13%)	5 (19%)
Good (70–84%, 125°–149°)	11 (29%)	12 (46%)
Fair (50–69%, 90°–124°)	12 (32%)	7 (27%)
Poor (0–49%, > 90°)	10 (26%)	2 (8%)

Note: Group I had 38 digits, Group II had 26 digits.

produce an increased fibroblastic response, thus some controlled motion is especially critical with these cases to maintain soft tissue gliding. Age, lengthy immobilization, or associated osteoarthritis may turn a simple injury into a complex one.

Will the repaired central slip tolerate some controlled motion during the healing phase?

The SAM protocol described in this study creates approximately 4 mm of extensor tendon excursion through zones III and IV at 0–30° active flexion and extension (as calculated by radians).[1] Distal joint motion addresses the problem of lateral band adherence.[1] Force application or applied resistance at the repair site has been calculated mathematically with 0–30° of active PIP motion (with the wrist flexed to reduce the resistance of the flexor system) at 291 g.[1] This internal tendon tension is 200 g less than the lowest tensile strength measured for extensor tendon repairs through the healing process that would create a 2 mm repair site gap.

A detailed study of the dynamic anatomy of the extensor mechanism at this level indicates that the exercise position of wrist flexion at 30°, MP joint position of 0° to mild flexion and active PIP motion from 0–30° of flexion followed by active extension creates a work requirement or internal tendon tension that will be tolerated by repairs at this level. The position of wrist flexion reduces the workload of the extensor digitorum communis (EDC) by reducing the resistance of the extrinsic finger flexors, and by facilitating the interossei which work in the position of wrist flexion to help extend the PIP joint. The position of MP extension transmits physiologic tension to the EDC in zones III and IV because the sagittal bands glide proximally with MP extension. When the MP is flexed the sagittal bands glide distally and the EDC is able to transmit virtually no force distal to the MP joint because of its insertion on the dorsal hood/sagittal band complex. Thus, the position of MP joint extension facilitates EDC function, yet minimizes its work requirement because in this position the lumbricals assist IP joint extension both directly through the action on the PIP joint and indirectly by neutralizing the viscoelastic resistance of the

flexor digitorum profundus (FDP). The position of MP extension further reduces the workload of the EDC through action of the interossei on the two distal joints.

Timing and duration of exercise are critical components of the SAM protocol. Basic science research suggests that wound activity and tensile strength are enhanced by very early motion. Some authors feel that immediate constrained digital motion following repair may allow progressive healing without the intervening phase of tendon softening described in early studies on tensile strength. Clinical results are improved with motion initiated by day 2 or 3, even over cases where motion is delayed until day 6 or 7.[2] Frequent exercise is suggested based on an experimental study on canine flexor tendon which concluded that tensile properties, as represented by linear slope, ultimate load, and energy absorption, were significantly improved in tendons treated with a higher frequency of passive motion, and on a multicenter clinical study of repaired zone II flexor tendons which demonstrated that greater durations of daily passive motion resulted in increased active IP motion.

It is not necessary to splint the wrist or MP joint with this injury, and indeed it may be contraindicated because controlled physiologic motion is necessary to maintain glide in zones III and IV.[1,2]

Conclusion

The SAM protocol for the open and repaired central slip injury addresses the problems as defined for extensor injury at this level:

(1) adhesion formation in zone IV,
(2) incorrect position of immobilization, and
(3) connective tissue stress deprivation.

The defined exercise parameters create an internal tendon tension at the repair site that will be tolerated by conventional extensor tendon repair. This technique has proven itself to be safe, simple, effective, comfortable, and inexpensive. Attenuation of the repaired central slip with this highly controlled rehabilitation program has not been a problem.

References

1 Evans RB, Thompson DE, An analysis of factors that support early active short arc motion of the repaired central slip, *J Hand Ther* (1992) **15**:187–201.

2 Evans RB, Early active short arc motion for the repaired central slip, *J Hand Surg* (1994) **19A**:991–7.

3 Evans RB, An update on extensor tendon management. In: Hunter JM, Mackin EJ, Callahan AD, eds, *Rehabilitation of the Hand: Surgery and Therapy*, 4th ed (CV Mosby: St Louis, 1995) 565–606.

4 Evans RB, Immediate active short arc motion following extensor tendon repair, *Hand Clin* (1995) **11**:483–512.

5 Newport ML, Blair WF, Steyers CM, Long term results of extensor tendon repair, *J Hand Surg* (1990) **15A**:961–6.

6 Brand PW, Thompson DE, Micks JE, The biomechanics of the interphalangeal joints. In: Bowers WH, ed, *The Interphalangeal Joints* (Churchill Livingstone: New York, 1987) 21–54.

9

Extensor pollicis longus rupture: A new method of surgical repair

Joseph M Failla

Introduction

A new method of surgical repair is here described for extensor pollicis longus (EPL) tendon rupture, combining direct repair of the tendon ends with step cut lengthening of the distal end. This technique eliminates the need for harvesting a tendon transfer or free graft. It is suitable for chronic EPL rupture, in which the proximal tendon stump has retracted to form a gap. It also facilitates reconstruction of proper tendon length. This technique is only possible when the tendon stumps can be directly repaired by mobilization of the stumps or passive extension and adduction of the thumb.

Materials and methods

A linear incision is made over the EPL tendon and then curved radially distal to Lister's tubercle to follow the tendon to MP joint level (Figure 1a). Branches of the radial sensory nerve are dissected and preserved. The proximal and distal EPL stumps are isolated and the gap between them measured, with the thumb passively flexed to the palm. The thumb is then hyperadducted and hyperextended maximally and Allis clamps are used to advance the distal stump proximally in order to oppose the tendon stumps (Figure 1b); if the stumps can be opposed they are repaired with a core or mattress 4-0 nonabsorbable suture (Figure 1c). The distal tendon stump was previously prepared for a step cut lengthening 1 cm distal to the suture line (Figure

1d). The length of the step cut is one-half the length of the measured gap plus 1 cm; with lengthening, each side of the step cut tendon will fill half the gap, with the extra centimeter being for overlap and suture.

The distal tendon is then lengthened by sliding open the step cut incision. A provisional simple suture is placed, and the tension tested by the tenodesis effect on the EPL tendon with wrist flexion and extension. The step cut tendon is then sutured side-to-side with 4-0 mattress nonabsorbable sutures (Figure 1e). The tendon end-to-end suture and distal step cut are depicted diagramatically in Figure 2.

The thumb is immobilized with a plaster thumb spica splint in adduction and extension, with the wrist extended for 4 weeks. An orthoplast thumb spica splint is used for an additional 2 weeks, with gentle active thumb motion without resistance monitored by a hand therapist.

Discussion

Surgical repair of EPL tendon rupture was first reported by Duplay (1876), who used transfer of the extensor carpi radialis longus (ECRL). Riddell (1963), Moore et al (1987), Saffar and Fakhoury (1987), Mannerfelt et al (1990), and Hove (1994) used the ECRL or the extensor indicis proprius (EIP) as a motor; Mannerfelt et al preferred to leave the EIP intact in rheumatoid patients who might need it for reconstruction of future tendon ruptures. Steindler (1946) and Harrison et al

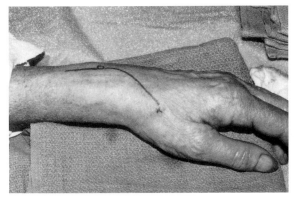

a

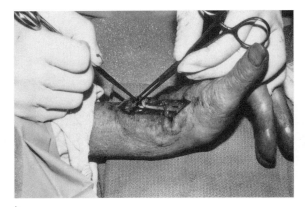

b

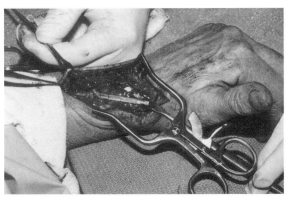

c

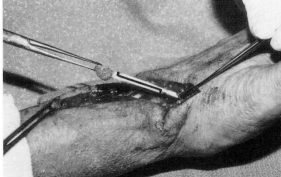

d

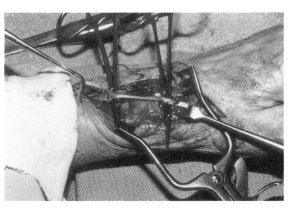

e

Figure 1

(a) Incision (X = palpable distal stump EPL). (b) The tendon ends are opposed with Allis clamps. (c) EPL repair with the thumb hyperextended and adducted, and the wrist extended. (d) Planned step cut in the distal stump. (e) Completed repair, with the proximal suture line above the left hemostat and the distal step cut suture line above the right hemostat.

(1972) recommended transfer of the extensor pollicis brevis. Moore (1936), Bunnell (1948), Backhouse (1981) and Chitnis and Evans (1993) used the abductor pollicis longus. Rare choices for tendon transfer include use of the palmaris longus by Moore et al (1987), an unexpectedly encountered anomalous extensor digitorum brevis manus by Varian and Pennington (1977), and the extensor digitorum communis of the little finger by Hove (1994).

Direct suture is rarely possible with chronic EPL tendon rupture, but suture with tolerance of a gap was reported by Trevor (1950). Filling the gap with a free tendon graft was suggested by Steindler (1946), Hamlin and Littler (1977), Saffar and Fakhoury (1987), Magnell et al (1988), and Mannerfelt et al (1990); the latter group showed results with tendon graft comparable to those after EIP transfer.

The technique described in this report is unique and has not been previously reported. Advantages of the technique are:

(1) Elimination of the need for harvesting a normal musculotendinous unit for transfer, or a free graft to fill in a gap between tendon ends. Repair is accomplished simply by rearranging the intact elements of the EPL tendon.
(2) Facilitation of adjustment of tension in the tendon transfer, by sliding open the step cut tendon to the appropriate length.

The disadvantage of the technique is that it would not be possible if the stumps could not be approximated.

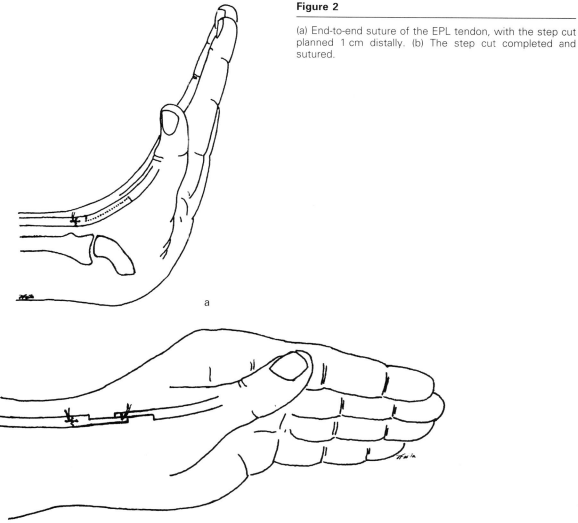

a

b

Figure 2

(a) End-to-end suture of the EPL tendon, with the step cut planned 1 cm distally. (b) The step cut completed and sutured.

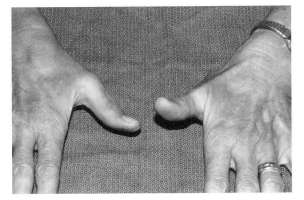

a

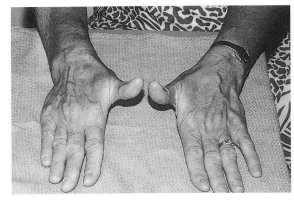

b

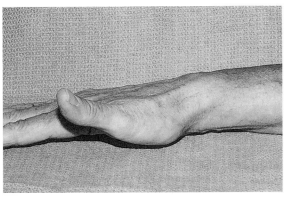

c

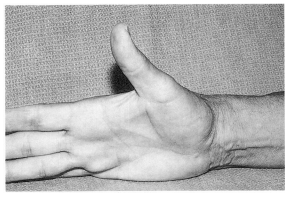

d

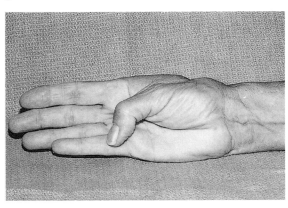

e

Figure 3

(a) Loss of right thumb extension after nondisplaced Colles' fracture. The EPL contour is absent and the patient cannot elevate the thumb metacarpal off the table; intrinsic interphalangeal joint extension is present. (b,c) Restored ability to elevate the thumb metacarpal 4 years after repair. (d) Active thumb extension and (e) flexion 4 years after repair.

The method is based on previously established principles that have been used successfully. Specifically, it is consistent with the good results obtained by tendon graft, for it can be seen in Figure 2 that the portion of the EPL tendon between the proximal suture line and the distal step cut suture line is essentially a free graft from the EPL tendon itself. The method is also conceptually similar to that used for repair of chronic flexor pollicis longus (FPL) tendon rupture by

Urbaniak and Goldner (1973), in which the FPL is advanced distally and step cut lengthened proximally. In contrast, the EPL is advanced proximally and step cut lengthened distally.

In conclusion, chronic EPL tendon rupture can be repaired in some cases by proximal advancement and distal step cut lengthening.

References

Backhouse KM (1981) Abductor pollicis longus musculo-tendinous split as a replacement motor for ruptured extensor pollicis longus, *The Hand* **13**:271–5.

Bunnell S (1948) *Surgery of the Hand*, 2nd edn (JB Lippincott: Philadelphia) 668–9.

Chitnis SL, Evans DM (1993) Tendon transfer to restore extension of the thumb using abductor pollicis longus, *J Hand Surg* **18B**:234–8.

Duplay S (1876) Rupture sous-cutanee du tendon du long extenseur du pouce de la main droite, au niveau de la tabatiere anatomique, *Bull Mem Soc Chir Paris* **2**:788.

Hamlin C, Littler JW (1977) Restoration of the extensor pollicis longus tendon by an intercalated graft, *J Bone Joint Surg* **59A**:412–14.

Harrison S, Swannell AJ, Ansell BM (1972) Repair of extensor pollicis longus using extensor pollicis brevis in rheumatoid arthritis, *Ann Rheum Dis* **31**:490–2.

Hove LM (1994) Delayed rupture of the thumb extensor tendon, *Acta Orthopaed Scand* **65**:199–203.

Magnell TD, Pochran MD, Condit DP (1988) The intercalated tendon graft for treatment of extensor pollicis longus tendon rupture, *J Hand Surg* **13A**:105–9.

Mannerfelt L, Oetker R, Ostlund B, et al (1990) Rupture of the extensor pollicis longus tendon after Colles' fracture and by rheumatoid arthritis, *J Hand Surg* **15B**:49–50.

Moore JR, Weiland AJ, Valdata L (1987) Tendon ruptures in the rheumatoid hand: analysis of treatment and functional results in 60 patients, *J Hand Surg* **12A**:9–14.

Moore T (1936) Spontaneous rupture of extensor pollicis longus tendon associated with Colles' fracture, *Br J Surg* **23**:721–6.

Riddell DM (1963) Spontaneous rupture of the extensor pollicis longus. The results of tendon transfer, *J Bone Joint Surg* **45B**:506–10.

Saffar P, Fakhoury B (1987) Secondary repair of extensor pollicis longus, *Ann Chir Main* **6**:225–9.

Steindler A (1946) *Orthopedic Operations*, 3rd edn (Charles C Thomas: Springfield) 112.

Trevor D (1950) Rupture of the extensor pollicis longus tendon after Colles' fracture, *J Bone Joint Surg* **32B**:370–5.

Urbaniak JR, Goldner JL (1973) Laceration of the flexor pollicis longus tendon: delayed repair by advancement, free graft, or direct suture, *J Bone Joint Surg* **55A**:1123–48.

Varian JPW, Pennington DG (1977) Extensor digitorum brevis manus used to restore function to a ruptured extensor pollicis longus, *Br J Plast Surg* **30**:313–15.

10

The by-pass extensor musculo-tendinous transfer: A salvage technique for substance loss of the extensor apparatus in the fingers*

Christophe Oberlin, Arthur Atchabahian and Anil Bhatia

Introduction

Loss of substance of the extensor apparatus on the proximal phalanx is a difficult problem to deal with, especially after repeated operations. Anatomical repair is no longer possible, and the variety of reconstructive techniques that have been described bears witness to the failings of all of them. We have developed a technique based on a different premise.

Technical aspects

The aim of this technique is to avoid adhesions and joint stiffness, and to allow the tendon to loosen slightly without losing extension. In large substance losses we have no choice but to use a tendon graft, and in standard procedures temporary pinning of the proximal interphalangeal (PIP) joint is routinely necessary. Our technique allows immediate mobilization in order to avoid the necessity of a secondary tenolysis (Figure 1).

Loosening of the extensor tendon by as little as 3 mm following existing techniques can cause a lag of 20° (Evans and Burkhalter 1986) without

any hope for self-restoration. We therefore use a muscle other than extensor digitorum communis to allow a certain amount of self-adaptation to this loosening. The best muscle seemed to be the extensor indicis, since the extensor digiti minimi is not always powerful enough and if it is used, the remaining band from the extensor digitorum communis to the little finger is too feeble to sustain extension of the digit.

The first step of the operation (Figure 2) is to cut the distal end of the tendon of the extensor indicis through a dorsal incision at the metacarpophalangeal (MP) level. It is freed and delivered through another incision more proximally. The palmaris longus tendon is then harvested by two volar incisions and is fixed to the end of the extensor indicis tendon by a Pulvertaft-type suture.

The dorsal aspect of the middle phalanx is then exposed by a longitudinal incision straight to bone, splitting the remains of the extensor apparatus, if any, in two. The tendon graft is passed subcutaneously from the dorsum of the hand toward the dorsum of the middle phalanx. Three strong threads are passed through three transosseous tunnels and tied around the tendon graft. The tension of the transferred tendon is adjusted to produce a mild overextension of the PIP joint with regard to the adjacent fingers. The extensor apparatus is resutured over the tendon. The tourniquet is released and haemostasis is achieved followed by skin closure. A below-elbow plaster slab is applied on the volar aspect extending from the proximal forearm to the PIP joint,

*This chapter is a revised version of an article originally published as Oberlin C, Atchabahian A, Salon A, Bhatia A and Ovieve JM (1995) The by-pass extensor tendon transfer, *J Hand Surg* **20B**:392–7.

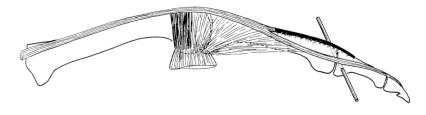

a

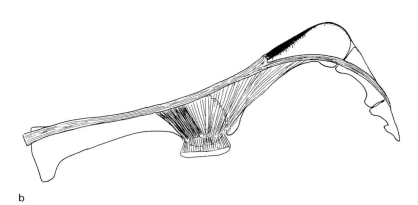

b

Figure 1

Causes of failure of standard procedures to restore a normal function. (a) PIP joint immobilization by a Kirschner wire. (b) Tendon stretching after rehabilitation begins because of adhesions, producing a dropping finger.

holding the wrist in 40° of extension and the MP joints in 0° of extension.

Postoperatively, immediate active mobilization of the interphalangeal joints of the finger is allowed. The orthosis is retained full-time for 3 weeks followed by night-time immobilization for a further 2 weeks.

Pros and cons compared to classical techniques

Many techniques have been advocated for the late treatment of lesions of the central slip of the extensor tendon of the finger. Some of them, such as tenotomies and so-called anatomical repairs, are relevant only for a boutonnière deformity, and could not be considered for our patients presenting with a loss of substance of the extensor apparatus. Four key papers have described the use of a tendon graft (Figure 3): Fowler (quoted by Littler 1964) used the lateral bands or, in the case of severe substance loss, the flexor digitorum superficialis as motor for a graft fixed on to the base of the middle phalanx.

Nichols (1951) attached the graft to the common extensor tendon itself. Tubiana and Valentin (1969) split the graft in three, thus grafting the central band and preventing the lateral bands from going apart. Flatt (1963) used a palmaris longus graft harvested in continuity with an aponeurosis flap, and wrapped the lateral bands in the aponeurosis flap in order to hinder development of a boutonnière deformity.

Many other authors use a tendon rearrangement (Figure 4). The central band can be split in two, either longitudinally (Snow 1976) or sagittally (Foucher quoted by Michon 1987), or both lateral bands (Hellmann 1964, Aiache et al 1970) or only one of them (Michon 1987) is split and used to restore the PIP joint extension. Some techniques link tenotomies to reconstructive procedures: Littler's technique (1964) involved cutting one of the lateral bands distally and fixing it on the base of the middle phalanx. In 1967 he improved his technique by simultaneously splitting the other lateral band and suturing one half of it to the contralateral band. Matev (1964, 1969) cut the lateral bands at different levels to use the proximal part of one of them to restore the extension of the PIP joint, and the

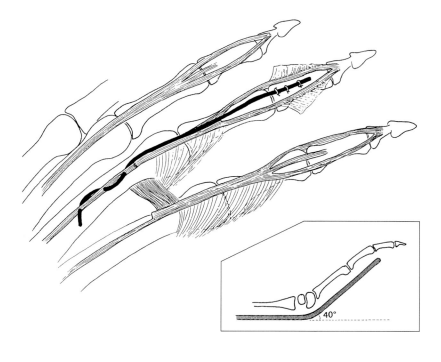

Figure 2

Technique of the by-pass musculotendinous transfer. The principles are as follows. First, the
motor is an independent muscle
which 'by-passes' the attachments of the normal extensor
apparatus such as sagittal bands;
it can thus adapt its strength and
excursion to produce full PIP
extension. Second, extension of
the wrist reduces the tension on
the transfer, allowing the PIP joint
to be left free; immediate active
and passive mobilization of this
articulation prevents stiffness.

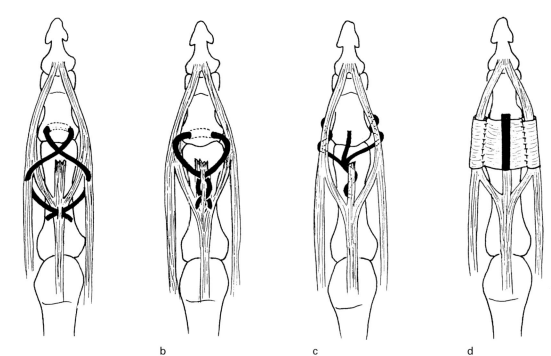

a   b   c   d

Figure 3

Graft procedures used for repair of a substance loss of the extensor apparatus according to (a) Fowler (in Littler 1964);
(b) Nichols (1951); (c) Tubiana and Valentin (1969); (d) Flatt (1963).

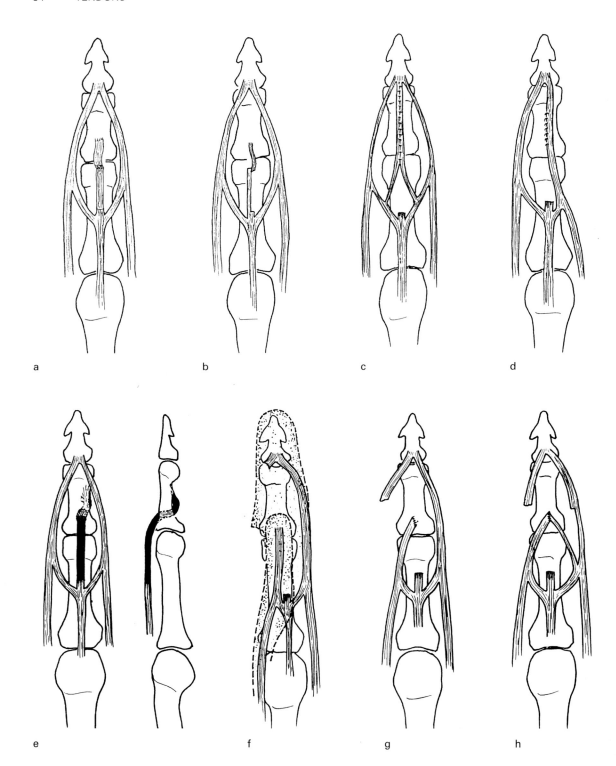

a

b

c

d

e

f

g

h

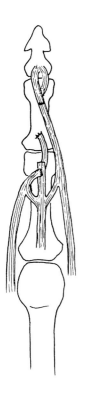

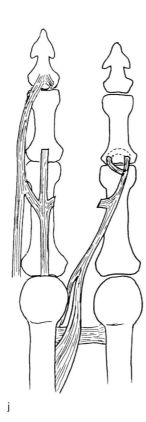

i

j

Figure 4

Plasty procedures used for repair of a substance loss of the extensor apparatus, according to (a) Snow (1976); (b) Foucher (in Michon 1987); (c) Aiache et al (1970); (d) Michon (1987); (e) Stack (1971); (f) Joshi (1981); (g) Littler (1964); (h) Littler and Eaton (1967); (i) Matev (1969); (j) Snow (1976).

distal part sutured to the proximal part of the other lateral band lengthens it as is required in chronic boutonnière deformity where there is a retraction of the lateral bands. Snow (1976) described an interesting technique, consisting of transfer of the lateral band of an adjacent finger. Other lesser known techniques include the use of the flexor digitorum superficialis tendon: retrograde (Stack 1971), or anterograde (Ardao quoted by Burton 1988) and the cutaneo-tendinous flap of Joshi (1981), filling in for both the tendon and the skin substance losses.

Those procedures often require very good soft tissue conditions, and are thus not useful in a multi-operated finger with a large tendon substance loss. None of these techniques provides the patient with a tendon solid enough to allow immediate mobilization, and in all cases the PIP joint is temporarily fixed in extension with a Kirschner wire for 3 weeks. This period of immobilization allows development of joint stiffness and strong adhesions of the tendon graft or transfer. When rehabilitation begins, the effort to flex the PIP joint progressively stretches the tendon and the final result is a dropping finger (Figure 1).

When reviewing the literature for this chapter, we discovered that our technique is not quite original. Joshi (1981) mentioned, at the end of his paper on tendinocutaneous flap, a procedure consisting of an extensor digiti minimi transfer elongated with a free tendon graft and transferred to the base of the middle phalanx. He used it for two patients in whom his procedure with a tendocutaneous flap was a failure, with an excellent final outcome.

Results

Six patients were operated upon by this technique. For each patient, we assessed the pre- and

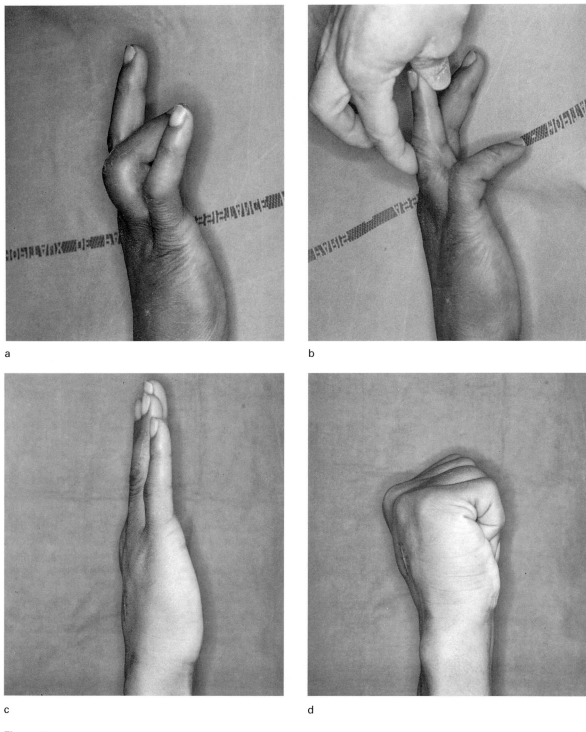

a

b

c

d

Figure 5

Clinical case (Patient 2): (a,b) preoperative status; (c,d) postoperative motion.

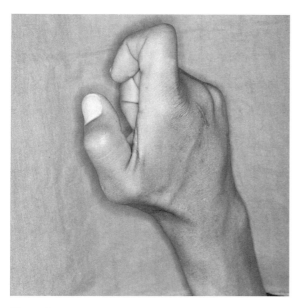

Figure 6

Independent postoperative index finger extension.

postoperative ranges of motion of the PIP joint (active and passive before the operation, and only active after it) and the active and passive motion of the distal interphalangeal (DIP) joint. The mobility of the MP joint was full in five patients. In one it had been fused because of a traumatic total destruction.

The results, together with age, sex, finger injured, injury type and number of previous operations, are reported in Table 1. The mean active PIP motion was 51/89° preoperatively and 11/86° postoperatively. Three results could be considered excellent (0/85°, 0/90°, 10/100°), two good (15/90°, 0/80°), the second of these after a dorsal tenoarthrolysis, and one fair (40/85°).

The additional tendon is routinely subluxed with the MP joint, producing a mild cosmetic blemish, but no functional impairment. An excellent result is shown in Figure 5. In each patient the extension of the index finger remained independent (Figure 6).

Table 1 Results of by-pass extensor musculotendinous transfer.

	Patient 1	Patient 2	Patient 3	Patient 4	Patient 5	Patient 6
Age	19	32	41	23	14	30
Sex	F	M	M	M	F	M
Occupation	Student	Locksmith	Mechanic (driver)	Joiner	Schoolchild	Musician
Finger	3 L	4 L	5 R	4 L	4 L	3 R
Injury	Traffic: skin tendon	Domestic: open PIP fracture	Work: open PIP fracture	Surfacing machine	Tumour	Domestic
Lateral bands	Absent	Fibrotic	Fibrotic	Absent	Fibrotic	Present
Previous operations	4 (skin flap)	3 (malunion tenolysis)	2 (arthrolysis)	1 (open PIP fracture, MP fusion)	2 (bone grafting)	1 (extensor repair)
Preop PIP joint mobility						
active:	50/80	55/90	70/100	40/80	40/85	45/100
passive	10/80	15/90	30/100	10/80	15/85	10/100
Preop DIP joint mobility:						
active	15/15	0/25	0/30	20/30	0/60	0/70
passive	Fusion	0/25	0/30	10/45	0/60	0/70
Postop PIP joint mobility: active	0/85	0/90	40/85	15/90	0/80 (secondary arthrolys.)	10/100
Postop DIP joint mobility: active	Fusion	0/30	0/10	10/30	0/40	0/60
Follow-up (months)	15 m:	14 m:	12 m:	13 m:	20 m:	12 m:
Result	Excellent	Excellent	Fair	Good	Good	Excellent

Indications

The by-pass musculotendinous transfer is helpful in the treatment of substance loss of the extensor apparatus in long fingers, after repeated operations. The results in terms of the PIP joint range of motion are satisfactory, with the slight inconvenience of limited DIP joint flexion. It is a salvage technique and simpler ways of restoring PIP joint extension are preferred if the soft tissue conditions permit.

References

Aiache A, Barsky AJ, Weiner DL (1970) Prevention of the boutonnière deformity, *Plast Reconstr Surg* **46**:164–7.

Burton RI (1988) Extensor tendons—late reconstruction. In: Green DP, ed, *Operative Hand Surgery*, 2nd edn (Churchill Livingstone: New York) 1465–1505.

Evans RB, Burkhalter WE (1986) A study of the dynamic anatomy of extensor tendons and implications for treatment, *J Hand Surg* **11A**:774–9.

Flatt AE (1963) *Care of the Rheumatoid Hand* (CV Mosby: St Louis) 38–46.

Hellmann K (1964) Die Wiederherstellung der Strecksehnen im Bereich der Fingermittelgelenke, *Langenbeck's Arch Klin Chir* **309**:36–8.

Joshi BB (1981) A salvage procedure in the treatment of the boutonnière deformity caused by a contact burn and friction injury, *The Hand* **14B**:33–7.

Littler JW (1964) Principles of reconstructive surgery of the hand. In: Converse JM ed, *Reconstructive Plastic Surgery*, 4th edn, Vol 4 (WB Saunders: Philadelphia) 1612–32.

Littler JW, Eaton RG (1967) Redistribution of forces in the correction of the boutonnière deformity, *J Bone Joint Surg* **49A**:1267–74.

Matev I (1964) Transposition of the lateral slips of the aponeurosis in treatment of long-standing 'boutonnière deformity' of the fingers, *Br J Plast Surg* **17**:281–6.

Matev I (1969) The boutonnière deformity, *Hand* **1B**:90–5.

Michon J (1987) La boutonnière, *Ann Chir Main* (French) **6**:307–14.

Nichols MH (1951) Repair of extensor-tendon insertions in the fingers, *J Bone Joint Surg* **33A**:836–41.

Snow JW (1976) A method for reconstruction of the central slip of the extensor tendon of a finger, *Plast Reconstr Surg* **57**:455–9.

Stack GH (1971) Buttonhole deformity, *Hand* **3**:152–4.

Tubiana R, Valentin P (1969) Les déformations en boutonnière des doigts, *Rev Chir Orthop* (French) **55**:111–24.

11

Clinical use of sarcomere length to gauge tension of tendon transfers

Richard L Lieber and Jan Fridén

Introduction

Surgical tendon transfers in the upper extremity are commonly used to restore lost function after trauma, head injury, stroke and neuromuscular disease. Traditional guidelines used to decide which specific donor muscle should be used for a particular tendon transfer include: morbidity caused by loss of the donor muscle, muscle availability, route of transfer, and functional synergy.[1] Less attention has been paid to the specific functional and structural characteristics of the donor muscles themselves or the specific length at which the muscle should be attached.[2,3] We have developed an intraoperative method for measuring sarcomere length in human skeletal muscle.[4] Measurement of sarcomere length is important because the sarcomere (Figure 1a) is the basic unit of force generation in skeletal muscle.[5] As a result, force generated by the sarcomere is highly dependent on its length. Since whole muscles are essentially large collections of sarcomeres, it follows that muscle force is highly dependent on sarcomere length (Figure 1b). It thus behooves the surgeon to transfer muscles at sarcomere lengths which result in maximal function. Unfortunately, it is not possible to gauge sarcomere length accurately by measuring or sensing muscle passive tension. Since the passive tension–sarcomere length relationship is not clearly defined for muscles of different architectures, passive tension alone does not provide the information needed to set muscle length.

Technical aspects

Intraoperative laser device

The device that we currently use consists of a 5 mW helium–neon laser beam aligned with a specially designed prism such that the beam projects normal to one prism face and reflects 90°, exiting the other prism face (Figure 2). The prism reflective surface is aluminum-coated to direct all available laser power through the muscle.

The device is calibrated using diffraction gratings of 2.50 μm and 3.33 μm grating spacings placed at the location of the muscle fiber bundle directly on the prism. Diffraction order spacings from the ±first order and the ±second order are measured to the nearest 0.1 mm using dial calipers which correspond to a spatial resolution of about 0.02 μm. In practice, repeated measurement of diffraction order spacing resulted in a sarcomere length variability of 0.10 μm ± 0.21.

Sarcomere length measurement protocol

After administration of anesthesia, the appropriate muscle is exposed and the overlying fascia removed. This is necessary since the fascia scatters laser light such that no diffraction pattern results. (To date, we have measured

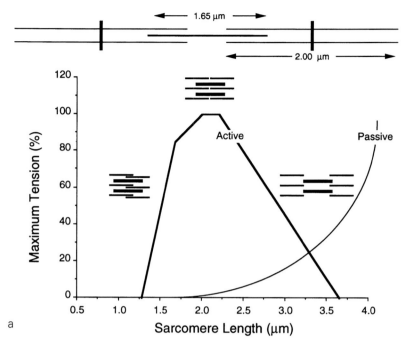

a

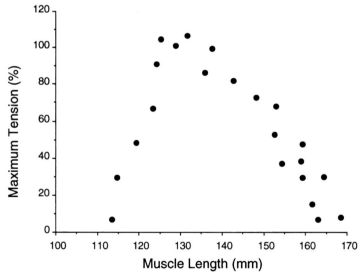

b

Figure 1

(a) Sarcomere length–tension relationship derived for frog skeletal muscle. Schematic at top of figure provides relative actin and myosin filament lengths. Note that maximum actual force exists when myofilament overlap is optimal. Cartoons above curve demonstrate relative myofilament overlap. Thin line represents the passive tension of an unstimulated frog semitendinosus muscle. (b) Typical muscle length–tension curve obtained to illustrate that muscle force is also highly dependent on length. Thus, the goal intraoperatively is to set muscle to the length at which force generation is optimal.

sarcomere length in exsanguinated tissue and we have evidence of laser light scattering by red blood cells. Thus, sarcomere lengths measured in the absence of a tourniquet show greater degrees of scattering.) After muscle exposure, a small muscle fiber bundle is isolated using delicate blunt dissection, with care not to over-stretch muscle fibers. In practice, the smaller the bundle, the more crisp the diffraction pattern.

The illuminating prism is inserted beneath the fiber bundle (Figure 2) and approximated into the normal plane of the muscle and the laser diffraction pattern imaged onto a glass slide. The diffraction angle (θ) relative to the undiffracted

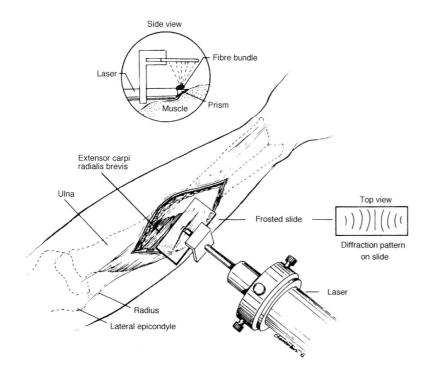

Figure 2

Device used for intraoperative sarcomere length measurement. The helium–neon laser is aligned normal to the transmitting face of the prism for optimal transmission of laser power into the muscle. Second order diffraction spacing was measured manually using calipers. Inset shows a transverse view of the illuminating prism placed beneath a muscle fiber bundle. (From Lieber et al[4] with permission.)

zero order beam is then calculated using the grating equation $n\lambda = d\sin\theta$, where λ is the laser wavelength (0.632 µm), d is sarcomere length, and n is diffraction order, assuming that the zero order bisected the orders on either side. For practical reasons (measurement resolution and diffraction pattern brightness) we typically use the second diffraction order (i.e. $n = 2$ in the grating equation).

Pros and cons compared to classic techniques

The classic technique used to gauge tension of tendon transfers relies on the experience of the surgeon to determine just how taut the transfer should be. Since the relationship between passive tension and optimal sarcomere length is not known for all muscles, this method has variable results. In practice, experienced surgeons become used to ensuring that certain transfers are not

stretched to too great an extent while other transfers must be placed quite taut. Of course, the use of direct sarcomere length measurement obviates the need for estimation of optimal length but still requires the surgeon to decide the length at which the muscle will be transferred. Currently, there are very few guidelines available in this regard but studies are underway in a number of laboratories to provide concrete guidelines for the various procedures.

Results

Sarcomere length change with joint rotation

We have measured sarcomere lengths in the extensor carpi radialis brevis and longus (ECRB and ECRL) muscles and the flexor carpi ulnaris (FCU) in a total of 69 patients. In the ECRB muscles of five patients,[4,6] with the wrist in full

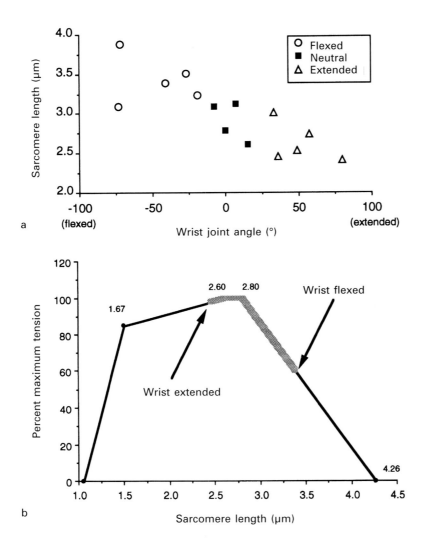

Figure 3

(a) Sarcomere length versus wrist joint angle relationship determined for the five experimental subjects. Negative angles represent wrist flexion relative to neutral while positive angles represent wrist extension. One-way ANOVA revealed a significant difference between wrist joint angles and sarcomere lengths in the three positions, (O) flexed angles, (■) neutral angles, (△) extended angles. (b) Hypothetical length–tension curve obtained using measured filament lengths and assuming the sliding filament mechanism proposed by Gordon et al (1966).[5] Shaded area represents sarcomere length change during wrist flexion (causing sarcomere length increase) and wrist extension (causing sarcomere length decrease). (Figure 3a from Lieber et al[4] with permission.)

extension, sarcomere length was about 2.6 μm (Figure 3a) which was significantly shorter (and thus would develop about 50% of the tension) than the 3.4 μm sarcomere length measured in the flexed position (*P* < 0.005). (Interestingly, sarcomere lengths measured by electron microscopy in the same fiber bundles of the same muscles were not identical to those obtained intraoperatively, suggesting that fixation and processing results in a situation quite different from that found in vivo.) The significance of these findings in the ECRB is that muscle force is not designed to be maximum in the neutral wrist position but would actually be maximal with the wrist fully extended. Thus, with the wrist fully flexed the ECRB would develop about 50% maximal tension while with the wrist fully extended the muscle generates maximal force (Figure 3b). The precise rationale for such a design is not clear but it emphasizes the fact that the intuitive proposed function of the musculoskeletal system may not actually be the correct one.

We have also made measurements in the FCU (Figure 4) muscle prior to and after transfer into the common extensor tendon in five radial nerve palsy patients.[7] This is an interesting transfer from an architectural point of view since the muscle fibers of the FCU are shorter than those of the extensor digitorum communis (EDC).[3,8] The most significant result was that the absolute sarcomere length and sarcomere length operating range of the FCU increased after transfer into the EDC complex ($P < 0.001$). Prior to transfer, with the wrist fully extended and fingers flexed, FCU sarcomere length was 4.22 ± 24 µm and decreased to 3.19 ± 0.05 µm as the wrist was fully flexed. This represented an overall sarcomere length range of 1.03 µm (Figure 5). After the tendon transfer, all sarcomere lengths were significantly longer ($P < 0.001$). Specifically, sarcomeres were 0.74 ± 0.14 µm longer with the muscle in its fully lengthened position (4.96 ± 0.43 µm) and 0.31 ± 0.16 µm longer with the FCU in the fully shortened position (3.50 ± 0.06 µm). At these sarcomere lengths, the FCU muscle was predicted to develop significant force only during movement involving synergistic wrist flexion and finger extension. These data indicate that overstretch of the FCU has profound consequences in tendon transfer since it is the shortest fibered muscle acting at the wrist. Of course, this accounts for much of the reason why use of the flexor carpi radialis or superficial digital flexor to the ring finger has been advocated for restoration of digital extension following radial nerve palsy.[9]

We also used biomechanical modeling to predict the sarcomere length that would result in maximum muscle forces with both the wrist and fingers extended (the desired purpose of the transfer). The model demonstrated that if the FCU were transferred at a longer sarcomere length (about 5 µm), dramatic increases in muscle force in the position of functional grasp could be obtained. This could result in a significant functional advantage to the patient. The disadvantage of inserting the FCU at the longer length is that less force is generated by the muscle when the wrist is in the more flexed position. Whether or not this would represent a functional loss to the patient remains to be determined. These results underscore the common notion that it is necessary to insert the FCU-to-EDC transfer under large tensions. Studies are underway investigating both normal muscle function and other patient populations to provide concrete guidelines for the tendon transfer procedures.

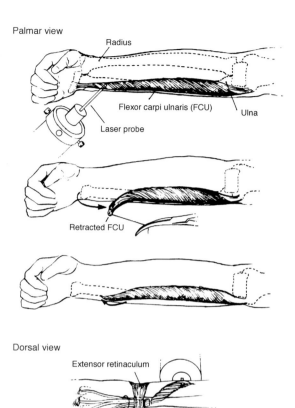

Figure 4

Artist's depiction of intraoperative laser diffraction of the flexor carpi ulnaris muscle during transfer into the common tendons of the extensor digitorum communis. (From Lieber et al[7] with permission.)

Indications

Indications for this procedure are the need to reattach or transfer muscles. This procedure is thus applicable to surgical tendon transfer of the upper extremity, digital flexor tendon repair, and tendon transplantation.

Acknowledgements

This work was supported by the Veterans Administration, NIH Grant AR31592, and the Swedish Medical Research Council.

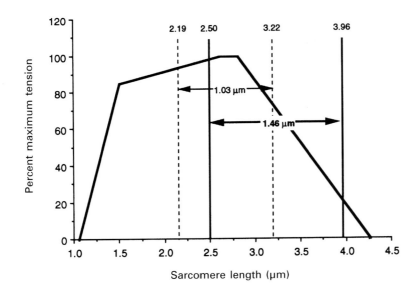

Figure 5

Schematic depiction of estimated sarcomere length operating ranges during wrist flexion and extension. Dashed vertical lines represent sarcomere length changes during normal flexor carpi ulnaris action as a wrist flexor. Solid vertical lines represent sarcomere length changes after the flexor carpi ulnaris is transferred into the extensor apparatus and the wrist joint is rotated. Increase in sarcomere length and sarcomere length operating range are predicted to decrease muscle force. (From Lieber et al[7] with permission.)

References

1   Brand PW, Hollister A, *Clinical Mechanics of the Hand*, 2nd edn (Mosby: St Louis, 1993).

2   Brand PW, Beach RB, Thompson DE, Relative tension and potential excursion of muscles in the forearm and hand, *J Hand Surg* (1981) **3**:209–19.

3   Lieber RL, Jacobson MD, Fazeli BM, et al, Architecture of selected muscles of the arm and forearm: anatomy and implications for tendon transfer, *J Hand Surg* (1992) **17**:787–98.

4   Lieber RL, Loren GJ, Fridén J, In vivo measurement of human wrist extensor muscle sarcomere length changes, *J Neurophys* (1994) **71**:874–81.

5   Gordon AM, Huxley AF, Julian FJ, The variation in isometric tension with sarcomere length in vertebrate muscle fibres, *J Physiol (Lond)* (1966) **184**:170–92.

6   Fridén J, Lieber RL, Physiological consequences of surgical lengthening of extensor carpi radialis brevis muscle-tendon junction for tennis elbow, *J Hand Surg* (1994) **19A**:269–74.

7   Lieber RL, Pontén E, Fridén J, Sarcomere length changes after flexor carpi ulnaris-to-extensor digitorum communis tendon transfer, *J Hand Surg* (1996) **21A**:612–18.

8   Lieber RL, Fazeli BM, Botte MJ, Architecture of selected wrist flexor and extensor muscles, *J Hand Surg* (1990) **15**:244–50.

9   Brand PW, *Tendon Transfers in the Forearm*, Vol 2 (Williams & Wilkins Co: Baltimore, 1975).

Commentary

Chapter 8

Zone 3 (boutonnière/central slip) injuries of the extensor mechanism have traditionally been treated with prolonged immobilization, even after surgical repair. Ms Evans, perhaps the most innovating and talented hand therapist now practising in the field of hand rehabilitation, outlines her technique for early mobilization, with improved functional results. This clearly seems an example of something which is new and very useful.

PCA

Chapter 9

This interesting technique has been used to advantage by Doctor Failla in two cases. It seems a worthwhile addition to the surgeon's 'bag of tricks'.

PCA

Chapter 10

This is an excellent addition to the hand surgeon's 'bag of tricks'. The only drawback I see is that, when there is loss of extensor substance over the proximal phalanx sufficient to justify this kind of procedure, skin quality is often also lacking. It has been my experience that tendon transfer in a poorly vascularized bed is likely to fail by adhesions even with a well-motored craft and despite early motion. Thus in some severe cases a two-stage approach might need to be considered: skin flap coverage as a first stage, followed by tendon grafting at some later point.

PCA

Another interesting technique to restore PIP joint extension; the possibility of immediate postoperative mobilization is certainly an advance. However, good results require complete passive preoperative extension of the PIP joint, which is not usually the case after several reconstructive procedures.

PS

Chapter 11

Tendon transfer surgery has historical roots which go back to the very beginning of orthopedic surgery and hand surgery. Thus far, there has been more art than science, particularly in the technical aspects of tendon transfer. Deciding on the proper tension at which to suture the transfer in particular has been an area where clinical experience has been the only guide to distinguish too tight from too loose. This may change in the future. Doctors Lieber and Fridén describe a technique by which sarcomere length can be measured in the operating room, forming a scientific foundation for gauging transfer length.

PCA

Recent trends and future prospects in mini external fixation

Endre Cziffer and Tibor Szalontay

Introduction

The world has changed considerably since 1976, when after much effort by the manufacturer (J Fréres, Switzerland) the first miniaturized sophisticated external bone fixator appeared on the medical market and Asche and colleagues introduced the Hoffmann-minifixator into clinical practice.[1] After a few published clinical series, in 1990 and 1994 two books attempted to summarize all the knowledge on mini external fixation of small bones and joints.[2,3] In the past 20 years the equipment and indication range of external fixation have radically changed. As static devices were replaced with dynamic fixators, the aim of the treatment was to achieve the more favourable biological, secondary callus formation instead of primary bone healing. The new devices offered this opportunity and the improved results encouraged biomechanical research into more effective devices. Besides the classical indications of open fracture treatment—osteomyelitis and segmental lengthening for congenital and acquired shortening—many new fields were reported where external fixators were beneficial. Despite this, many hand surgeons dislike external minifixation and do not even use it in the primary management of complex open injuries. The AO/ASIF method, after 20 years of success and domination among the treatment options in Europe, has spread to North America. The strong influence of osteosynthesis has limited the use of external fixation in hand surgery. However, although mini instruments, plates and screws are widely used and favoured nowadays, large series in the past 20 years have demonstrated that the infection rate for compound fractures treated with internal fixation can never be as it is low as with extrafocal fracture management.

Following the fast development of large scale fixators, and thanks to DeBastiani's school, the dynamic fracture treatment concept invaded the realm of mini external fixation as well, not only for dynamic fracture treatment, but also dynamic aftertreatment of small joints with single or double ball joints fixators.[4,5]

Extensive biomechanical studies have demonstrated that certain types of intraarticular fractures with severe comminution and small fragments, affecting mostly the proximal interphalangeal joint, preclude internal fixation and the possibility of early motion. The achievements of the famous Russian school of Ilizarov, Volkov and Oganesian have been developed further to maintain reduction, apply permanent traction to the joint using ligamentotaxis, and allow early postoperative motion under distraction.[6]

What follows is an overview of the current, theoretical and future possible application fields of external fixation in the hand with special emphasis on the polytraumatized hand and difficult reconstruction.

Indications for minifixation

General indications

Those orthopaedic trauma indications where external fixation provides an alternative solution to conservative management or internal fixation include the following:

1 Closed fracture fixation

Simple stable fractures can be treated conservatively. Simple unstable fractures can be managed with pins, screws or plates. Comminuted fractures of the phalanges and metacarpals are, by contrast, in our opinion best treated with extrafocal fixation and traction with minifixators. Many technical and septic complications can be avoided, including skin closure difficulties, postoperative fibrosis, tendon adhesions, and so on, if minifixation is chosen over multiple pins or obtrusive plates and screws. In the future we believe that increasing numbers of external fixators can be expected in this field.

2 Arthrodesis

According to Charnley's principle, joint fusion in small segments can also be achieved with external fixation. Temporary joint immobilization may be useful in juxta-articular fractures, while definitive arthrodesis is done in cases of major defects of the joint surface or inveterate joint destruction. In mild or moderate arthroses, distraction and mobilization of the joint can be tried. This indication is one of the latest developments in the field of external fixation. The so-called arthrodiastasis, or distraction arthroplasty, provides increasing range of motion after a few weeks of distraction and may postpone the definitive end stage treatments of arthrodesis or arthroplasty. This is one of the most promising fields of external fixation today. The method requires modern hinge fixators with a distraction capability.

3 Osteotomy fixation

Osteotomies are best treated with internal fixation and early postoperative motion. External fixation is an alternative possibility primarily for those surgeons who are highly skilled in techniques of external fixation.

4 Treatment of delayed bone union and pseudoarthrosis

These again are usually treated with osteosynthesis and bone grafts, but minifixators allow castless aftertreatment, early joint motion and simultaneous compression at the fracture site.

Primary indications

Those orthopaedic trauma indications, where external fixation is a method of choice.

1 Osteomyelitis

This is a classical indication for minifixation. Extrafocal fixation, sequestrectomy and local antibiotherapy are advised for treatment. There is no question in our minds that even in the future this indication will remain one of the most important for minifixation.

2 Repeated surgery after failed osteosynthesis

In comminuted fractures treated with internal stabilization, as mentioned above, if the synthesis becomes unstable or ineffective, or a fracture treated with many Kirschner wires becomes displaced again it is best in our opinion to remove all metal implants, realign the fracture and stabilize with external fixation. Repeated osteosynthesis carries the risk of a high infection rate.

Absolute indications

Those conditions in skeletal surgery, for which good results cannot be expected and there is no other practical alternative to external fixation.

1 Potentially infected fractures with soft tissue and bone loss

Comminuted, contaminated, displaced open fractures associated with significant soft tissue and bone loss are the major indications for using external fixation. The bony stability of the affected ray is lost, the segment is collapsed and shortened. To restore it to normal length, miniplates or improvizational solutions may be tried,

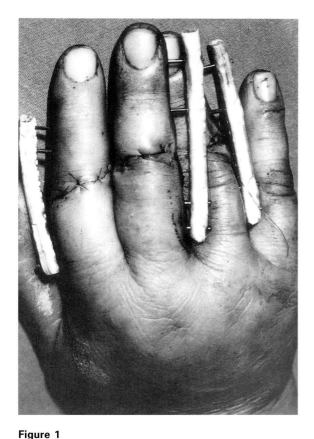

Figure 1

Multiple finger injuries treated with Manuflex single use fixators.

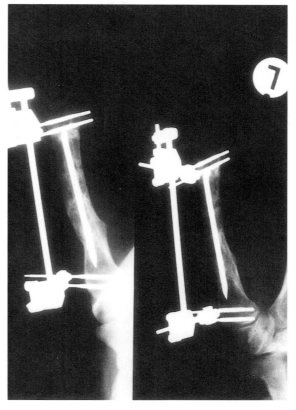

Figure 2

Distraction lengthening of the first metacarpal with a minifixator using the callotasis technique. The longitudinal intramedullary pin functions as a guide and prevents angular deformity during the elongation process.

but the plates are obtrusive and often there are no soft tissues to cover the wound; therefore internal fixation is not preferable in these cases. To align the fracture, restore the normal length of the finger, facilitate bone grafting, allow unlimited access to the wound, and permit maximum flexibility of skin replacement, minifixators are the only practical option. In cases of polytraumatized hand, where multiple digits are affected and the function of the hand as a whole is endangered, the treatment is also best done by choosing external fixation or combination with minimal internal fixation such as intraosseous wiring (Figure 1). Adjacent fingers can be treated and mobilized independently, although in such cases

the fixators may disturb simultaneous tendon reconstruction if that is necessary. After restoration of the normal length of the finger by traction, we sometimes face a significant bone defect. One must not be afraid of the bone defect, because it can be grafted safely at an early stage. In our practice we fill the bone gaps with gentamycin-loaded PMMA (polymethyl–methacrylate) beads (Septopal™, Merck Co., Darmstadt, Germany), and after 7–10 days primary delayed bone grafting is performed in a clean wound bed. If the conservative treatment is troublesome owing to wound conditions and the osteosynthesis is hazardous due to a high risk of infection, always choose external fixation!

2 Bone lengthening procedures

In cases of amputation, ineffective primary fracture management with unacceptable shortening, or in congenital malformations with short or missing digits, gradual, successive elongation can effectively be done only by the use of minifixators. The daily longitudinal adjustment of an 'artificial fracture' (subperiosteal corticotomy) by callotasis allows the surgeon to lengthen the segment gradually with external force and stretch the soft callus until the required length is achieved (Figure 2). To date no alternatives exist to the mini distraction devices using the Ilizarov–Matev–Kessler–Cowen–etc callotasis techniques. Internal stabilizers cannot fulfil these requirements. The gradual daily elongation is often done by the patients or parents at home. In longlasting elongation procedures pin site problems cannot be avoided, but with careful daily pin site care, superficial pin site drainage can be minimized and deep infections can be prevented.

3 Combined interventions

Simultaneous stabilization of a fracture or nonunion and mobilization of the neighbouring soft tissues like stiff joints, web spaces and skin contractures can only be performed with fixators. Major surgical intervention can be avoided by the use of pins and adjustable external frames.

4 Mass casualties, extreme circumstances

Under extreme circumstances, such as the management of man-made or natural catastrophes and in wartime, the best choice is often to use external stabilization for fracture treatment. In cases of closed fracture the external stabilizer can be a cast, but in compound fractures the minifixator is a method of choice. In such conditions the injuries must always be considered to be potentially infected. In mass casualties there is never enough time for individualized operations. Internal stabilization demands longer operation times and higher surgical dexterity than a simple preliminary external stabilization, which allows for rapid transport of the patients out of the catastrophe area. Furthermore, the surgical management in such conditions is mostly performed by surgeons less skilled in orthopaedic and hand surgery. Generally, the external fixators have great advantages in the management of extremity trauma in mass catastrophes. For these purposes standardized, uniform, well packed and arranged, presterilized single use fixators kits are preferable. The logistic aspects of the application of complicated devices increase the time and budget required for such applications and increase the organizational difficulties in the delivery of prompt and efficient care for large numbers of patients. In traditional armed conflicts the ratio of extremity injuries can be as high as 40–60%. In our peacetime practice 40–50% of all of our trauma patients are hand injuries. In catastrophe situations a significant number of hand injuries might be expected.

Difficult reconstructions

The management and reconstruction of complex hand injuries will often call upon one or more reconstruction methods. Digital ray shortening can be treated effectively with external fixators using the callotasis technique. Normal length can usually be restored in a few weeks or months. Finger joint and metacarpophalangeal joint defects can be replaced with different types of small prostheses. Different techniques of tendon reconstruction and transfer are also well known. The harvesting of nonvascularized and vascularized bones to fill bone cavities is a part of our everyday practice. To use these treatment options separately, in several steps, is always an option, but the reconstruction process and the rehabilitation period are then quite time-consuming. Scar formation after a series of operations may be extensive. Combined procedures reduce total recovery time but pose an additional set of problems. In combined one-stage reconstruction the different techniques may disturb each other, too many instruments or implants may clutter a small area like the hand, or extensive dissection may damage the blood supply. For these reasons combined reconstructions should be very well planned. In single-stage techniques, a combination of distraction lengthening, osteotomy, bone grafting, implant arthroplasty and tendon transfer cannot be performed without the assistance of permanent lengthening (Figure 3). This facilitates

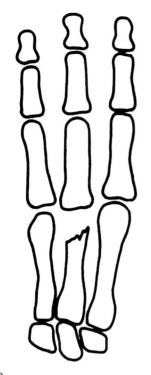

a

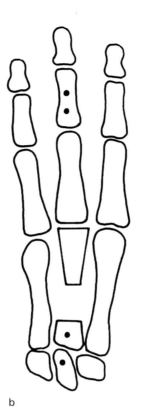

b

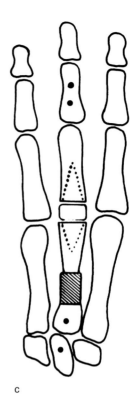

c

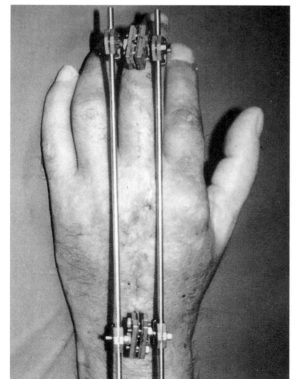

d

Figure 3

(a) Difficult combined one-stage reconstruction. Schematic representation of ray shortening due to a septic distal metacarpal defect. (b) Representation of the fixator pin sites. First the normal length of the injured ray was restored by traction. The base of the metacarpal was then rotated in the sagittal plane and moved distally after subperiosteal dissection. (c) Conventional Swanson-type finger joint implantation. Interposition of a corticocancellous bone graft from the iliac crest. The extensor indicis proprius tendon was transposed. (d) Early clinical picture and the double Hoffmann-minifixator frame.

the management of a complex injury with multiple tissue defects. Improvisation and a full 'bag of tricks' can often convert complicated, staged surgery into a single, less complex procedure and may shorten the rehabilitation period markedly.

Discussion

External fixators respect the blood supply and allow more biological, secondary bone healing with stronger callus formation. The modern, dynamic–ligamentotactic–hinged mini external fixators can provide advantages not only in the management of complex, compound injuries of the hand, but also by facilitation of the reconstructive procedures of congenital or acquired malformations. In cases of infection or potentially infected recent injuries, extrafocal fixation offers the best results. The indication range has widened in the last 10 years. Today mini external fixators are used not just in hand surgery, but for reconstructive operations of the feet and maxillo-facial surgery as well. They have great advantages and can be used with success for congenital malformations of the foot. The development of a new generation of small and mini external fixators can provide all the advantages that the sophisticated larger devices do. A concerted effort must be made to reduce the cost of the devices and surgical interventions and to develop professionally appropriate, cost-effective instruments to meet the needs of the enormous population of patients with hand injuries and their consequences.

References

1   Asche G, Haas HG, Klemm K, Erste Erfahrungen mit dem Minifixateur externe nach Jaquet, *Akt Traumatol* (1979) **9**:261.

2   Schuind F, Burny F, ed, *New Technique of Osteosynthesis of the Hand* (Karger: Basel, 1990).

3   Cziffer E, ed, *Minifixation. External Fixation of Small Bones* (Literatura Medica: Budapest, 1994).

4   Cziffer E, Dynamic minifixators. In: Cziffer E, ed, *Minifixation. External Fixation of Small Bones* (Literatura Medica: Budapest, 1994).

5   Pennig D, Gausepohl T, Lukosch R, The multidirectional minifixator. In: Cziffer E, ed, *Minifixation. External Fixation of Small Bones* (Literatura Medica: Budapest, 1994).

6   Hastings H II, Ernst JMJ, Dynamic external fixation for fractures of the proximal interphalangeal joint, *Hand Clin* (1993) **9**:659–74.

13

The use of suture anchors in the hand and wrist

Sean M Griggs and Arnold-Peter C Weiss

Introduction

Advances in metallurgy and machining techniques have increased the diversity of orthopedic implants. One recent development is the suture anchor.

Traditional methods of reattaching soft tissue to bone such as transosseous tunnels or drill holes can require awkward exposure to obtain the correct angle of approach, additional soft tissue stripping, and difficulty in passing the suture or biologic tissue. In the carpus, these issues become extremely important due to the substantial cartilage surfaces which are best preserved. Soft tissue anchors help to avoid these difficulties as they necessitate less soft tissue stripping and joint destruction and provide an excellent fixation post for soft tissue repair.

Suture anchors are themselves not without pitfalls and must be carefully applied to obtain optimal results. Loss of anchor fixation and migration is the single most troubling aspect of their use and this can be greatly diminished by attention to detail in anchor placement.

Review of anchor types

Many anchor systems are currently available for use in the hand and wrist and the number of available designs is sure to multiply over the next several years. This section will detail some of the most commonly used types of anchors.

Historically, the first anchor system was the Statak (Zimmer, Warsaw, Indiana) device introduced by Goble in 1988.[1] The original design was

large and not particularly useful in smaller bones. To remedy this situation, the mini-Statak anchor was developed.

The mini-Statak comprises a self-tapping threaded screw-type anchor with an eyelet for attachment of the suture. It has the following measurements: a 2.5 mm outer thread diameter, a 1.9 mm core diameter, and a length of 8.0 mm. It is available preloaded with #0, #2-0, or #3-0 nonabsorbable polyester suture but can also be obtained unloaded. When the mini-Statak is inserted into dense cortical bone, the insertion site must be predrilled to prevent anchor breakage during insertion. This extra step makes it only slightly less easy to use than originally intended. The strength of the mini-Statak in experimental studies (pull-out strength) is 32 lb (14 kg) in diaphyseal cortex (DC), 37 lb (17 kg) in metaphyseal cortex (MC), and 65 lb (30 kg) in cancellous trough. An even smaller version of the mini-Statak is also available. The Statak 1.5 has a 1.5 mm core diameter. It has a pull-out strength of only 13 lb (6 kg) in DC, 12 lb (5 kg) in MC and 21 lb (10 kg) in a metaphyseal trough.[2]

In 1989, the Mitek (Mitek Products, Westwood, Massachusetts) first generation (GI) suture anchor was introduced. The original Mitek was similar in function to a fishing hook. This original design evolved into a second generation anchor, the Mitek GII anchor.

The Mitek GII has two barbs at 180° to each other and functions similar to a harpoon. The GII is composed of a central titanium core with an arc made of nitenolol (an alloy of nickel and titanium) which has the biomechanical property of being able to deform during insertion and recoil to its original form once below the cortex.

This recoil causes the anchor to lock beneath the surface after insertion thus preventing pull-out. The insertion site for the Mitek suture anchor must be predrilled with a tapered drill and guide which is supplied by the manufacturer. Predrilling does not complicate its use and the system is easily used.

The GII measures 8.8 mm in length, 2.4 mm in diameter, and has an arc length of 7.8 mm (the arc length is the spread of the nitenolol barbs in their relaxed shape). The drill measures 2.4 mm by 14.2 mm. It has excellent pull-out strengths measuring 105 lb (48 kg) in DC, 66 lb (30 kg) in MC, and 82 lb (37 kg) in cancellous trough.[3] The GII is available preloaded with suture or can be loaded at the time of use. It can accommodate a #2 or smaller suture. The second generation Mitek is also available in a miniaturized version, the mini-GII. The mini-GII measures 1.8 mm in width by 5.4 mm in length with an arc length of 5.5 mm. The drill size is 2.0 mm by 9.7 mm. Experimentally, its pull-out strengths measure 47 lb (21 kg) in DC, 15 lb (7 kg) in MC, and 20 lb (9 kg) in cancellous trough.[3] It too can be purchased preloaded with suture or unloaded. It will accommodate a #0 or smaller suture. Its small size and excellent pull-out strengths make the mini-GII well suited for use in the surgery of the hand and wrist.

The Harpoon suture anchor (Arthrotek, Warsaw, Indiana) is a wedge design that is made of a titanium alloy with recoil properties similar to that described for the Mitek device. The Harpoon measures 3.2 mm by 10.0 mm and is introduced by direct impaction through the bone. No predrilling is required unless the cortex is very dense. Experimentally, it has pull-out strengths of 69 lb (31 kg) in DC, 47 lb (21 kg) in MC, and 40 lb (18 kg) in cancellous trough.[2] It is available preloaded with suture or it can be loaded at the time of its insertion. It will accommodate a #2 or smaller suture. A mini-Harpoon is also available which measures 2.0 mm by 6.0 mm. Its pull-out strengths are 57 lb (26 kg) in DC, 50 lb (23 kg) in MC, and 39 lb (18 kg) in cancellous trough.[2] It too is available preloaded or unloaded and will accommodate a size #1/0 or smaller suture.

The Anchorlock suture anchor (Wright Medical Technology, Arlington, Tennessee) is a screw-type anchor system which has the design feature of a suture eyelet recessed within the anchor itself. This eliminates the known risk of eyelet break-off due to the torque generated during anchor insertion. This anchor is available in a width of either 1.9 mm or 2.5 mm. No pull-out strength data are available for this device but it would be expected to perform comparably to a Statak of similar size.

The use of bioabsorbable implants in the repair of hand or wrist injuries is currently in the trial stages. They may not have as good a pull-out performance as metallic devices in cancellous troughs.[2-4] These implants may also cause unwanted local tissue inflammation with sterile abscess formation.[5]

Indications in hand and wrist surgery

With an adequate understanding of the technique of insertion and the biomechanical strengths and limitations of the chosen anchor, the surgeon should be able to use anchors effectively.

Tendon insertions

Avulsion injuries of the flexor digitorum profundus (FDP), and mallet or boutonnière injuries to the extensor digitorum communis can effectively be treated with soft tissue anchors if adequate bone stock is available for proper anchorage.[6,7]

Hallock was the first to report the use of a suture anchor to repair avulsion of the FDP tendon.[6] Rehak et al and later Skoff et al also reported use of a suture anchor to repair flexor tendon injuries at or near their insertions with good results.[7,8] Skoff et al also performed an in vitro study to compare the strength of anchor fixation of an avulsed FDP to that of the Bunnell technique. They found the two techniques to have comparable strengths with the limiting factor being the strength of the suture used.

A suture anchor can easily be used to gain purchase in an open mallet injury in which the soft tissue is compromised and its reinsertion is not amenable to traditional oversewing of the tendon into the area of insertion. The repair may be protected with either Kirschner wire distal interphalangeal joint fixation or a conventional splint, depending on the condition of the dorsal soft tissues.

Injuries of the scapholunate

Frequently, open repair of torn carpal ligaments is required to stabilize the carpus, and this surgery remains one of the most challenging technical tasks in hand surgery. Traditional techniques of ligament repair require a significant amount of surgical dissection and soft tissue stripping to allow the surgeon to safely and accurately drill interosseous tunnels for suture or tendon graft placement. In addition these techniques, by their nature, can lead to significant articular cartilage compromise.

In the limited confines of the wrist, suture anchors are ideal to accomplish the task of ligament reattachment to bone.[7,8] Reattachment of the ligament can be approached directly. The site of ligament avulsion can be exposed with minimal soft tissue stripping and the insertion site need only be secured in one plane for safe anchorage. Another of the advantages of the use of suture anchors in the carpus is the substantial time saving due to their relative ease of use.

Collateral ligament disruptions

Avulsions of the collateral ligaments of the thumb (skier's or gamekeeper's thumb) and those of the collateral ligaments at the proximal interphalangeal (PIP) or metacarpophalangeal (MP) joints are usually amenable to conservative treatment. However, some patients with instability and pain are best treated by operative repair of the ligament to bone. Suture anchors are an excellent choice for these ligament repairs.

General technical considerations

After adequate soft tissue exposure and identification of the disrupted soft tissues (Figure 1a), planning for accurate placement of the suture anchor device is essential. After determining appropriate device location, direct drilling or predrilling is undertaken under direct visualization protecting the neurovascular structures (Figure 1b). The anchor devices are always preloaded with the appropriate size suture and the anchor placed either through direct drilling or after a predrilling hole has been manufactured. The anchoring device should be tested by pulling on the sutures to ensure solid fixation (Figure 1c). The soft tissue structures are repaired directly with the suture from the anchor device and care is taken to try to get as much tension on the soft tissue repair as possible (Figure 1d). Postoperative anteroposterior and lateral radiographs should always be obtained to ensure appropriate positioning of the anchor device including depth prior to wound closure (Figure 1e and f).

Discussion

In general, suture anchors are of two design types: either a screw type or a harpoon type. The screw type is usually inserted without predrilling while the harpoon type usually requires predrilling. The suture anchors lock into position either by virtue of their screw threads or by their postinsertion configuration (barbs prevent pullout or migration). Both types have been shown to have adequate biomechanical pull-out strength in vivo and in vitro.[3,4,7] In biomechanical testing of various anchor types, Barber et al have shown that the most common mode of failure is suture breakage.[3,4] The anchor is therefore only as strong as the suture it is holding.

The insertion technique for the anchor is also very important. Burkhart compared the Deadman theory used in fence post anchorage and showed theoretically that the angle of insertion of the anchor should be less than or equal to 45° from the pull of the suture to maximize pull-out strength of the anchor while minimizing tension on the suture/tendon construct. This in theory would minimize the risk of failure at the weakest point, the suture.[9]

After insertion of any anchor, proper seating must be tested—the sutures are gently pulled to check for failure of the anchor's locking mechanism to engage. This step in the procedure will prevent early failures from poor insertion technique or the presence of inadequate bone stock.

Once suture anchor insertion is understood, the physician must understand the limitations of the device. Certain anchors perform poorly in cancellous trough bone which is precisely the type of bone stock left after tendon avulsion.

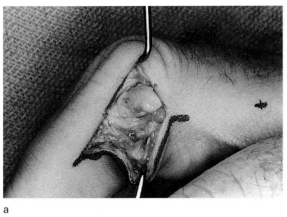

a

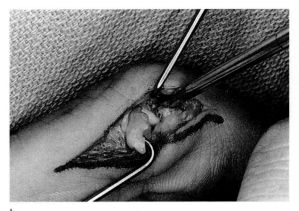

b

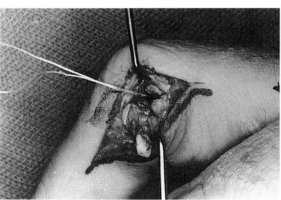

c

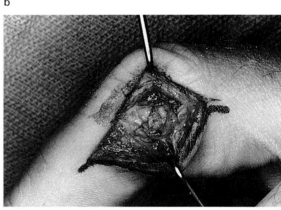

d

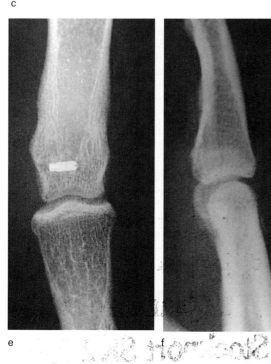

e   f

Figure 1

A 22-year-old college athlete with a chronic radial collateral ligament disruption of the proximal interphalangeal joint treated conservatively for 2 years with recurrent dislocations had operative exposure via the midlateral approach to expose the proximally disrupted radial collateral ligament (a). After the appropriate epicenter origin of the collateral ligament was determined, the anchor hole was predrilled under direct vision (b). After appropriate predrilling, a harpoon-type anchor was placed with its suture already attached. The pull-out of the suture anchor should be tested prior to soft tissue repair (c). Repair of the disrupted radial collateral ligament with as much tension on the soft tissues as possible was undertaken with the suture from the anchor device (d). Anteroposterior (e) and lateral (f) radiographs were taken to ensure appropriate localization and depth of the suture anchor device.

Also, the anchor should only act as a suture post and should not be expected to make up for loss of tissue or to give strength to attenuated tissue which, after healing, will be unable to withstand the forces placed upon it. The repaired soft tissue must be able to withstand the requirements of function once it has been given the chance to heal.

Before any anchor system is used, the surgeon must be well versed in the technique of insertion of the chosen implant as well as its limitations and advantages. It is prudent to know the technical aspects of insertion to prevent destruction of the bony insertion site, which would lead to anchor failure and possibly prevent use of a more traditional technique for salvage. The surgeon must know the size of the implant and the depth of its insertion drill to prevent over-penetration and extension of the implant through the cortex.[8] The understanding of the bony anatomy will help to prevent these complications. The surgeon must also remember that the placement of multiple anchors in close proximity to each other will actually weaken the insertion site and can lead to failure; fewer but well fixed anchors are preferable.

In summary, suture anchors provide the surgeon with an easy method for suture fixation to bone to allow soft tissue reconstruction. An appropriate size suture should always be chosen according to the requirements of the rehabilitation program to be instituted for the patient. With careful insertion of the anchors in terms of both appropriate alignment and depth, substantial operating time may be saved. With experience, the surgeon will find the use of suture anchors allows for less soft tissue stripping and decreased surgical time. This time saving should more than compensate for the cost of the devices themselves.

References

1 Goble EM, Somers MK, Clark R, et al, The development of suture anchors for use in soft tissue fixation to bone, *Am J Sports Med* (1994) **22**:236–9.

2 Barber FA, Herbert MA, Click JN, The ultimate strength of suture anchors, *Arthroscopy* (1995) **11**:21–8.

3 Barber FA, Herbert MA, Click JN, Suture anchor strength revisited, *Arthroscopy* (1996) **12**:32–8.

4 Barber FA, Deck MA, The in vivo histology of an absorbable suture anchor: a preliminary report, *Arthroscopy* (1995) **11**:77–81.

5 Bostman OM, Osteolytic changes accompanying degradation of absorbable fracture fixation implants, *J Bone Joint Surg* (1991) **73A**:679–82.

6 Hallock GG, The Mitek mini GII anchor introduced for tendon re-insertion in the hand, *Ann Plast Surg* (1994) **33**:211–13.

7 Skoff HD, Hecker AT, Hayes WC, et al, Bone suture anchors in hand surgery, *J Hand Surg* (1995) **10B**:245–8.

8 Rehak DC, Sotereanos DG, Bowman MW, et al, The Mitek bone anchor: application to the hand, wrist, and elbow, *J Hand Surg* (1994) **19A**:853–60.

9 Burkhart SS, The deadman theory of suture anchors: observations along a South Texas fence line. *Arthroscopy* (1995) **11**:119–23.

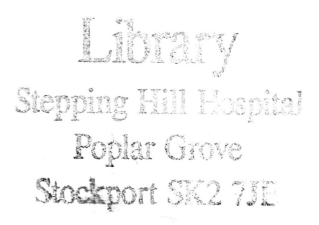

14

Use of a new dynamic compression screw in the hand

Lewis B Lane, Stanley E Asnis and John S Crombie

Introduction

In hand and wrist surgery compression of bone fragments is often achieved by the use of screws. After analysis of modern bone screw design and insertion technique, a number of problems were identified as being unresolved despite recent advances. A new compression screw was designed with the intention of addressing these problems, many of which are listed below.

Shearing of screw threads and loss of fixation in bone may occur with the lag screw technique due to overtightening. Penetration of a lag screw either into the soft tissues or into or across a joint can be problematic. Up to 40% of the compression can be lost when a fully threaded screw is lagged, because its threads partly engage both fragments, even when the near side is overdrilled.[1] Up to 85% of the torque used to insert a screw can be consumed overcoming metal-on-bone friction during screw insertion.[2] Fracture reduction can be lost if a screw, lagged across a fracture site, is changed. Loss of fixation can theoretically occur when a screw is used with a different thread pitch on each end because the threads advance at different rates during insertion.[3] Stripping of threads from bone will occur during the final stage of tightening a screw as the head engages the bone, if the head does not advance and the bone does not compress at a rate equal to the advancing bone thread (e. g. 3.5 mm per revolution).

In order to address these problems, a new concept in compression lag screw design was developed with the following goals:

(1) to generate more controlled compression
(2) to reduce the risk of stripping the screw's threads
(3) to have an adjustable length without advancing the screw tip
(4) not to require a jig for insertion or compression
(5) to reduce metal-on-bone friction
(6) to be simple to insert.

Technical aspects

Design

The screw (Universal Compression Screw, Howmedica Inc, USA) is a two-component single-unit lag screw manufactured from 316L stainless steel. The first component, the head and outer sleeve of the shaft, is hollow and has an internal 0.5 mm pitch machine thread. It engages, and cannot be separated from, the second solid component which has a 0.5 mm pitch external machine threaded shaft proximally and 3.5 mm European bone threads distally (Figure 1a,b). In addition, 4.5 mm and 6.5 mm screws were designed.

The two-part screwdriver can be locked together so that the two-component screw can be advanced as a single unit, or unlocked so that one component can be held stationary (typically, the distal piece with the bone threads) while the other component (typically, the head and outer sleeve) can be advanced, shortening the screw

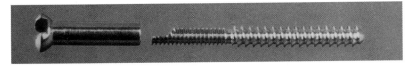

a

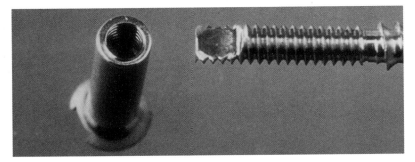

b

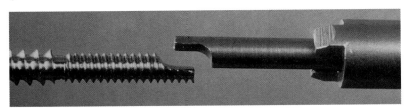

c

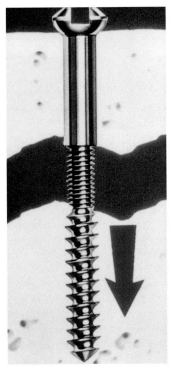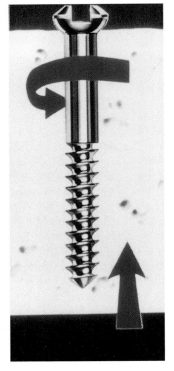

d

Figure 1

(a,b) Photographs of the screw, disassembled, to show the male machine thread on the shaft of the bone thread portion of the screw and the female machine thread on the head portion of the screw. (c) Photograph of the screwdriver tip near the tip of the bone thread portion of the screw showing how the surfaces mate. The outer driving shaft engages the screw head (not shown). (d) Drawings of the screw in bone. On the left: before tightening, with the screw in the open position. On the right: after tightening, with the screw shortened and the bone fragments compressed.

(Figure 1c). Fracture compression is generated as the screw shortens (Figure 1d).

Laboratory testing

The authors conducted two experiments testing 3.5 mm ASIF cortical screws and 3.5 mm Universal Compression Screws (UCS) across a fracture model. These revealed that the UCS screws demonstrated more axial compression and holding strength than the ASIF screws.

A study by Newport and associates compared the 3.5 mm UCS with the 2.7 mm and 3.5 mm ASIF cannulated screws, the Herbert screw, and the Herbert–Whipple screw in a scaphoid fixation model.[4] The UCS had the greatest compression for two-finger tightness and was equal to the 3.5 mm ASIF for greatest failure strength. For cantilever bending the authors concluded that the UCS was 'considerably stronger' in both the failure mode and in ultimate failure strength. Because of the large compression forces generated, the UCS had the highest rate of fracture of the scaphoid (catastrophic failure). In comparison, the Herbert screw was weaker in compression and resistance to bending but had a 0% catastrophic failure mode.

Surgical technique

The UCS should be used as a lag screw for compression. As with any other lag screw the two bone fragments are provisionally reduced. Compression is not required as the screw will create its own compression. The path for the screw is determined, the hole drilled and measured, the near end is overdrilled, and the far side tapped in routine fashion. Because the UCS can shorten, the next longer screw, closest to the length measured, is selected. The screw is inserted with the special UCS driver as a single-unit screw. Once the bone threads have been inserted to the correct depth, the latchpin on the driver is released to unlock the two components of the driver. The driver handle is held still to ensure that the bone threads do not advance. The knurled wheel is turned, advancing the screw head and the near end of the screw. This shortens the screw, and compresses the two bone fragments together.

Care must be exercised when the screw is removed in order not to separate the two pieces. The center shaft of the screwdriver must be fully engaged with the inner shaft of the screw before the screw is turned counterclockwise. It is best to engage the head also, but this is not critically important. If only the head portion is engaged, the head could be separated from the shaft of the screw. Although this is hard to do, it is theoretically possible. If separation occurs, the 'easy-out', the left-hand-threaded female machine thread removing tool included with the instrument set, should be placed over the end of the shaft of the screw and then turned counterclockwise to remove the shaft.

Pros and cons

The UCS functions as a lag screw. It has the capacity to create significant compression between two bone fragments. The UCS can generate more torque and compression than comparable screws. A second valuable attribute is that the depth of insertion of the far end of the screw can be controlled exactly. This is beneficial in intercarpal arthrodeses when the tip of the screw must remain intraosseous. Because the distal bone threads do not move as the head is tightened, it is theoretically less likely to cut out than other lag screws. Theoretically, this allows for an infinite number of lengths for any one screw within its compression range. For example, the 32 mm length screw can assume any length between 32 mm and 24 mm. This is beneficial, for example, if an inoperative radiograph were to show that a screw had been advanced too deeply. It is not necessary to remove the screw and exchange it for a shorter screw, rather the screw merely needs to be unscrewed sufficiently to adjust the bone thread depth to the desired position, and the head advanced, thus shortening the screw a comparable amount, to restore compression.

The UCS has other applications as well. It has been used for arthrodesis of the metacarpophalangeal joint of the thumb and for the distal radioulnar joint (Sauve–Kapanji procedure). It has shown usefulness in lagging across

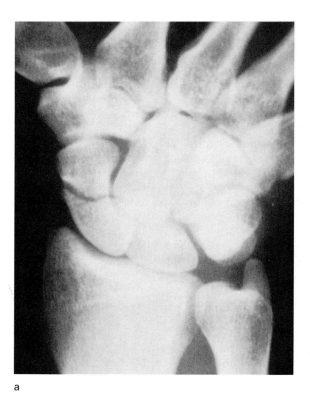
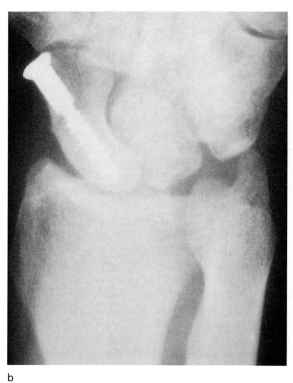

a   b

Figure 2

(a,b) Preoperative and postoperative radiographs of an acute scaphoid facture. The postoperative radiograph was taken at 8 weeks when the patient returned to full activities.

fractures, such as scaphoid and radial styloid fractures, and in treatment of scaphoid nonunions. In the scaphoid its advantage is in achieving considerable compression of both fractures and bone graft without the need for a jig for insertion or to gain compression.

In consideration of the disadvantages, the head of the UCS is similar to that of a ASIF 3.5 mm screw, and this size is too large for certain small bone applications. For example, the head is too large to be inserted antegrade through the proximal pole of a scaphoid. It cannot be buried beneath the surface of the scaphoid. It may be too large for a patient with an especially small scaphoid or with a 'cashew-shaped' scaphoid. A 3.5 mm UCS is too large for most metacarpal and essentially all phalangeal applications where 1.5 mm, 2.0 mm, and 2.7 mm size screws are more

appropriate. If tightened excessively, the UCS may fracture the bone[4] or the head may continue to compress, sinking into the bone, and thus require the use of a washer. Although the UCS achieves good compression and fixation, it, of course, cannot overcome a faulty construct and should not be overly relied upon.

Results

The UCS has been used in 31 cases in 28 patients since September 1991. The average age was 43 and ranged from 19 to 79. Patient diagnoses were rheumatoid arthritis in 8, posttraumatic reconstruction in 8, nonunion in 5, acute fracture in 4, and osteoarthritis in 3. The procedures performed were radiocarpal arthrodesis in 10, other arthrodesis in 12, scaphoid nonunion in 5, and open reduction internal fixation in 4. Patients were casted for an average of 4 weeks, with a range of 2–9 weeks, and then splinted for 2–6 more weeks.

The time to radiographic union ranged from 4 to 14 weeks; 29 of 31 cases healed uneventfully (Figure 2a,b) All but one patient achieved a level of functioning postoperatively that had been projected preoperatively.

Indications

The UCS can be used whenever a 3.5 mm lag screw is needed. However, it is especially indicated in situations where the precise placement of the distal end of the screw is important, such as for intercarpal arthrodeses, or fractures in or near joints. A second indication for use of the UCS is in those situations where a large amount of compression is needed. A third indication is for osteoporotic bone where risk of stripping of threads is greater. A fourth indication is for instances in which the precise length of the screw needed is uncertain, or might change in the process of insertion or tightening. For example, when a fragment which compresses excessively is lagged, the conventional screw will likely penetrate too deeply. Because the UCS can assume a variety of lengths, the position of the far end of the UCS can be controlled while compression is applied by tightening of the head of the screw; thus the screw will not advance any further than desired.

References

1   Tencer A, Asnis SE, Biomechanics of cannulated and non-cannulated screws. In: Asnis SE and Kyle R, eds, *Cannulated Screw Fixation: Mechanics, Operative Techniques, and Clinical Applications* (Springer Verlag: New York, 1996) 127–33.

2   Perren S, Klaue K, The limited contact dynamic compression plate (LC-DCP), *Arch Orthop Trauma Surg* (1990) **109**:304–10.

3   Davis M, Evans PD, Richards J, Laboratory comparison of the cannulated Herbert bone screw with ASIF cancellous lag screws, *J Bone Joint Surg* (1993) **75B**:89–92.

4   Newport ML, Williams CD, Bradley WD, Mechanical strength of scaphoid fixation, *J Hand Surg* (1996) **21B**:99–102.

15

Bone fixation with shape memory staples

Landino Cugola and Ruggero Testoni

Introduction

Due to the variety of fixation devices currently available, we can cope with any type of situation in which it is necessary to maintain the reduction of a fracture, osteotomy or arthrodesis. Advances in scientific and technological research, together with commercial considerations, have led to the development of more sophisticated surgical instruments; the shape memory staple (SMS) is one result of this research.[1] The staples are also called ACR, from the French 'agrafes à compression dynamique et retentive'. They are made from a nickel and titanium alloy, which is thermoplastic and biocompatible. Shape memory means the capacity to change and return to its original shape with contentive action and dynamic compression under the effect of particular stimulants.

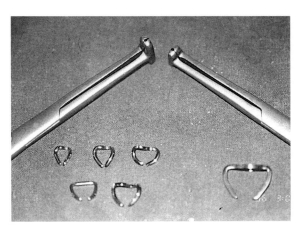

Figure 1

Various shapes and dimensions of shape memory staples.

Physical and chemical properties

- Fusion point 1200–1300°C.
- Density 6.5 g/cm³.
- Thermal dilation 10–10.61°C.
- Resistivity (20°) 50–100 Ω cm.
- Thermal conductivity 1.2 W/°C cm.
- Resistance to corrosion is better than titanium and stainless steel.

Mechanical properties

- Breakage point 150–180 ng/mm².
- Elasticity E = 90.000 MPa; G = 35 000 MPa.

- Hardness 300 HV.
- Deformability maximum 50%.
- Resistance excellent.

The SMS consists of a 'body' and two 'arms'; the body can be straight, curved, S or omega shaped, whereas the arms are slightly curved and convergent (Figure 1). The length and calibre of the SMS can vary. The force of compression varies from 2 to 5 kg, depending on the size of the staple.

We use the SMS in hand surgery, but its application extends to the whole of orthopaedic surgery.[2] In addition, orthoses for hand splinting have been developed with the same shape memory alloy.[3]

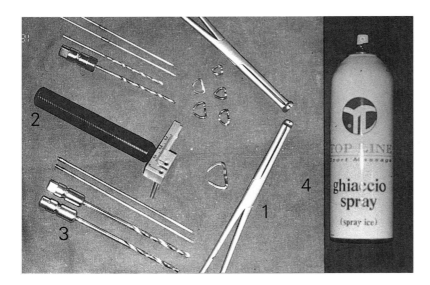

Figure 2

Surgical kit: (1) specific forceps, (2) drill bit guide, (3) drill bits of various diameters, (4) refrigerant spray.

Materials and methods

The surgical kit consists of forceps for handling the staples, a drill bit guide, drill bits of various diameters according to the size of the staples and a refrigerant spray (Figure 2). There are two main differences between SMS and classic staples:

(1) Classic staples are inserted by percussion with the accompanying risk of dislocating bone fragments, whereas the SMS are inserted into holes of the requisite size previously drilled into the bone.
(2) The SMS have a compressing action on fragments which reduces the risk of disassembling the fragments.

It is also necessary to compare the SMS with Kirschner pins and Herbert screws. The Kirschner pins are versatile, ubiquitous and easy to insert, but it is not possible to obtain compression and they may loosen and require removal. The Herbert screw assures excellent maintenance of reduction, but only in static compression and not in dynamic compression as is the case for SMS. Furthermore there is little margin for error and in certain cases the technique of applying the screw is difficult.

The shape of the staple may be varied by cooling, while heating restores the staple to its original shape (hence the name 'shape memory' staple); this results in a compression force on the bone fragments.

Surgical technique

The surgical approach is the same as for other osteosynthesis techniques. Once the bone fragments have been placed in the correct position (by an osteotomy or an arthrodesis, or in a fracture) two holes are drilled into the bone, with the help of the drill guide, at distances and diameters corresponding to the chosen SMS. When the reduction and synthesis are performed it is important that the axis of the two holes is perpendicular to the fracture line in order to obtain the best compressive forces and to avoid the risk that the two bone surfaces might shift with consequent displacement. The next step is to cool the SMS (held with the forceps); first the body is cooled, then the arms. The SMS can be frozen by any of the following means:

• sterile gas spray (freon, ethyl chloride);
• immersion in liquid nitrogen;

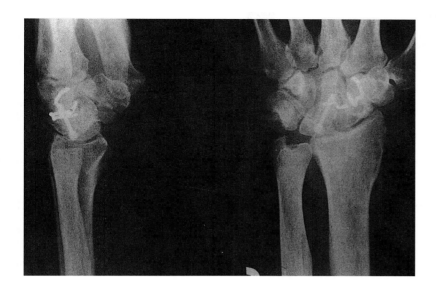

Figure 3

Rheumatoid wrist arthrodesis with an SMS and a Herbert screw.

- in the freezer: in this case the SMS is put in the freezer at least 2 hours before use, then taken out 10–15 minutes before application.

With progressive force on the forceps, the body is first straightened then, with a needle holder, the arms are modelled into the required shape. The SMS must be placed rapidly and without force; if resistance is met while the staple is applied it is necessary to verify that the two holes are completely free of debris, then the staple must be cooled again and the procedure repeated. Never try to bend or straighten the SMS if it has not been frozen first, otherwise it may break. It can be frozen whenever needed with no risk whatsoever.

Once introduced, the staple will return to its original shape within 3–4 minutes by absorbing heat from surrounding tissue, or within 1–2 minutes if a gauze soaked in physiological solution at 45°C is applied; or the staple can be made to return to its original shape immediately by use of the coagulation function of the electrocautery.

One or more SMS can be used according to the need, and in particular cases a supplementary fixation device or orthosis can be used (or may be necessary) (Figure 3). The staple can be removed if a scalpel is used as a lever or the body of the SMS may be cut and the two arms removed. This is rarely necessary because the SMS maintains the tendency to close over time, and adapts continuously to the remodelling surfaces of the bone—consequently it never moves.

Patients

Over a 5-year period we inserted 55 SMS. We used the SMS extensively in the first 2 years with the intention of being more selective in the indications for their use. Our experience includes:

(1) Fractures and osteotomies of the second phalanx: 4 cases.
(2) Fractures and osteotomies of the first phalanx: 6 cases (Figure 4).
(3) Fractures and osteotomies of the metacarpals: 15 cases (Figures 5–7).
(4) Arthrodesis of the carpal bones: 11 cases (Figure 8).
(5) Nonunion and fracture of the scaphoid: 8 cases (Figures 9 and 10)
(6) Fracture of the radius: 2 cases.
(7) Fracture of the ulna: 2 cases.
(8) SMS employed in addition to other synthesis devices: 7 cases.

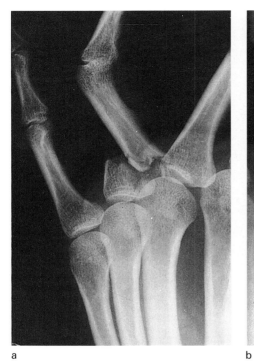
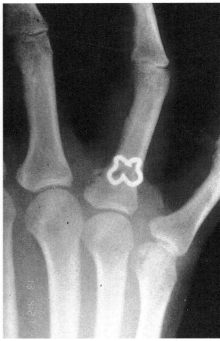

a

b

Figure 4

(a) Base of proximal phalanx of fourth finger fracture, (b) treated with two SMS after open reduction.

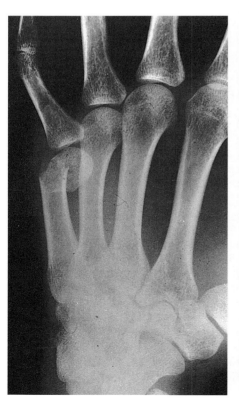
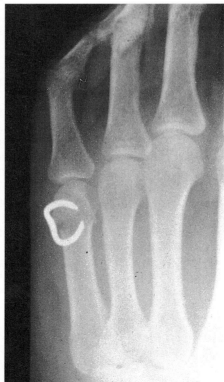

a

b

Figure 5

(a) Transverse fracture of a fifth metacarpal neck, (b) treated with one SMS and splint for 2 days.

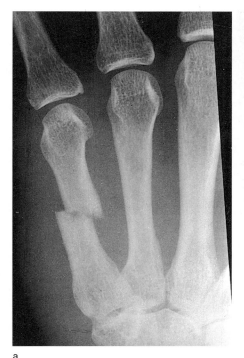

a

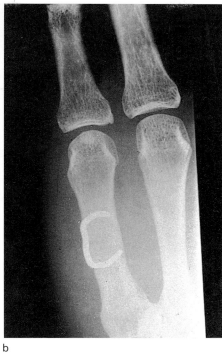

b

Figure 6

Fifth metacarpal shaft fracture. (a) Preoperative and (b) postoperative.

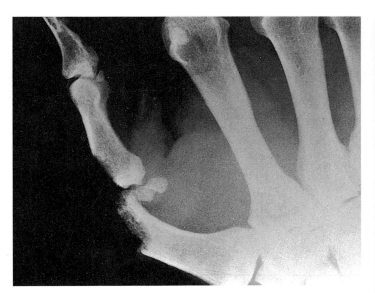

a

Figure 7

(a) Injury at the first MP joint with bone loss. (b) Arthrodesis with two SMS.

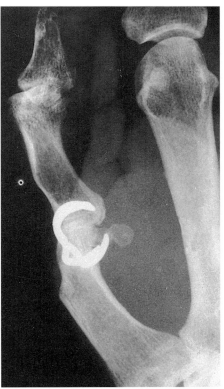

b

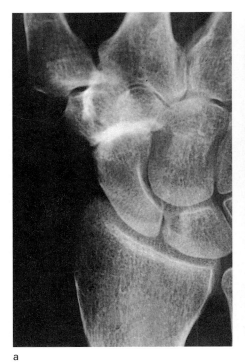
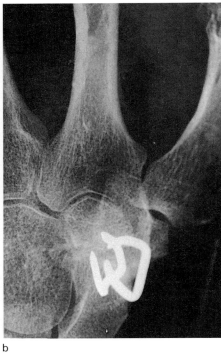

a   b

Figure 8

(a) Scaphoid–trapezium–trapezoid painful osteoarthritis. (b) Arthrodesis with two SMS.

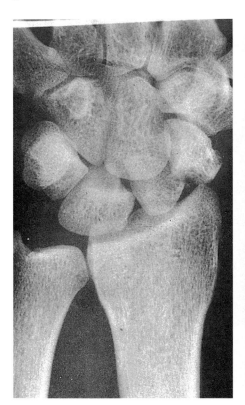
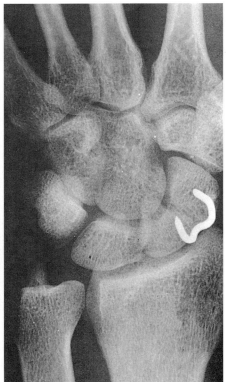

a   b

Figure 9

(a) Transverse scaphoid fracture, (b) treated with one SMS and immobilization for 1 month.

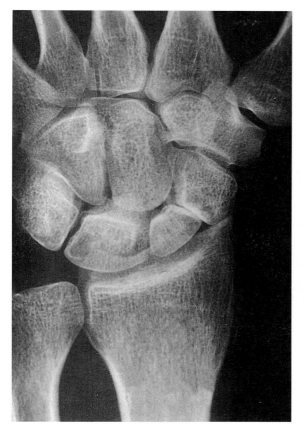

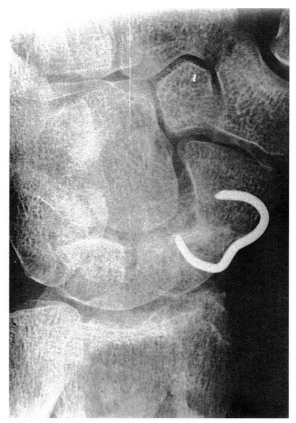

a

c

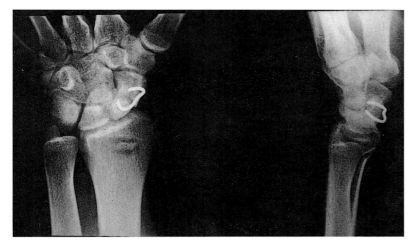

b

Figure 10

(a) Scaphoid nonunion (b) treated by cancellous graft and synthesis with SMS (volar approach). (c) Radiograph 2 months after surgery.

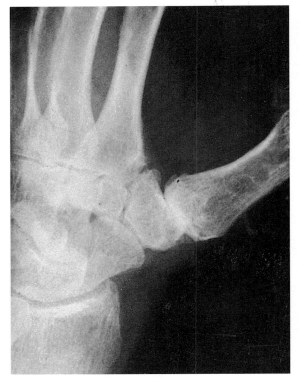

a

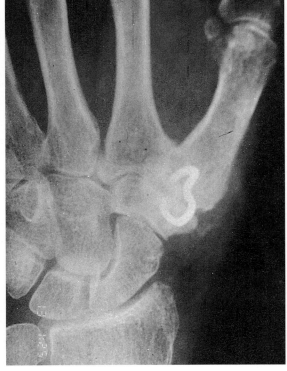

b

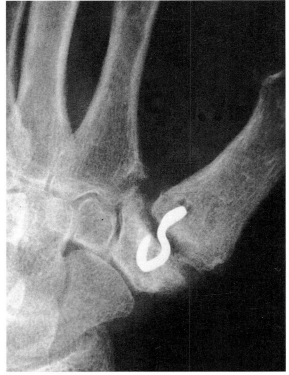

c

Figure 11

(a) Trapeziometacarpal painful osteoarthritis. (b) Immediately after surgery, arthrodesis with one SMS. (c) 2 months after surgery, pseudoarthrosis has developed. One staple was inadequate—in this case two SMS were beneficial.

Results

The average radiograph healing time (i.e. when signs of injury are no longer evident on radiograph) was 56 days for scaphoid nonunion, 42 days for scaphoid fractures, 32 days for metacarpal fractures and 39 for metacarpal osteotomies, 46 days for arthrodesis of the carpal bones, 36 days for fracture of the radius and 43 days for fracture of the ulna; these were similar to published reports.[4]

It is important to assess the dimensions of the staple accurately in relation to the force necessary to maintain the reduction of fracture, because an erroneous choice of size may incur a risk of displacement, nonunion or fracture.[4] We had three cases of erroneous staple dimension which caused displacement in one case (Figure 11) and pseudoarthrosis in two cases (the SMS was too small, with a subsequent inadequate compression force and poor fixation). Other complications included a case of infection which was resolved without the need to remove the staple (by antibiotic therapy) and one case of tendinitis due to interference with extensor tendon excursion (treated by immobilization and antiflogistic (anti-inflammatory) drugs for 15 days).

Discussion

There are technical and biomechanical advantages to SMS. The technical advantages are:

(1) A strong osteosynthesis.
(2) The wide choice of shapes and dimensions (for better outcome in specific situations).
(3) Easy placement with minimal surgical invasion.
(4) Reduction in the time in surgery.
(5) High resistance to corrosion.
(6) Easy removal (rarely necessary).

From the biomechanical point of view, there is stable reduction and fixation and long-lasting immobilization, which protects the newly-formed capillary system, enhancing and orienting the recovery process. Bone fusion is facilitated with minimum resorption of the fractured edges, no widening of the gap between fragments, minimal formation of periosteal callus and finally there is no inhibition of the endosteal callus. Furthermore, the continuous compression avoids mobilization of the osteosynthesis, reducing the need for removal. However, there are cases in which the use of SMS is not recommended: for instance, sometimes the staple is too large for the bone fragments; it may cause articular impingement (for instance at the proximal third of the scaphoid); where there is inadequate space (at the distal phalanx level) or where it may interfere with tendons gliding.

Conclusion

We have found the SMS to have an important role in hand surgery; it is a valid alternative to the traditional staples and other fixation devices, particularly when the cost is taken into consideration. We feel that the indications are the following: proximal third of the first phalanx fractures; metacarpal neck fractures; middle third of scaphoid fractures and nonunion; intercarpal, carpometacarpal and metacarpophalangeal arthrodeses; fractures and osteotomies of the distal third of the radius and ulna.

References

1   Bensamann G, Baumgart F, Hartwing J, et al, Untersuchungen der Memory-legierung Nickel-Titan und Uberlegungen zu ihrer Anwendung in Bereich der Medizin, *Tecn Mitt Krupp Forsc-Ber Band 37* (1979) **H1**:21–33.

2   Yang PJ, Zhang YF, Ge MZ, et al, Internal fixation with Ni-Ti shape memory alloy compressive staple in orthopedic surgery. A review of 51 cases, *Chin Med J (Engl) (China)* (1987) **100**:712–14.

3   Takami M, Fukui K, Saitou S, et al, Application of a shape memory alloy to hand splinting, *Prosthet Orthot Int (Denmark)* (1992) **16**:57–63.

4   Moretti F, Rossello MI, Cangemi F, et al, The use of ACR agraphes in hand surgery: consideration about a series of 75 cases. In: *Sixth Congress of the International Federation of Societies for Surgery of the Hand (IFSSH)* (abstracts) Helsinki, Finland, 3–7 July 1995.

16

Use of bone substitute for fracture fixation of the distal radius

Jesse B Jupiter and Edward D Wang

Introduction

Bone is a composite material made up of organic as well as inorganic components. The mineral phase of bone comprises approximately 60–70% of the total dry bone weight, while the remainder is composed of organic materials such as collagen. Bone mineral is an apatitic calcium phosphate termed dahllite which contains carbonate and small amounts of sodium, magnesium, and other trace compounds.

The most commonly used calcium phosphates for bony defects to date have been thermally processed hydroxyapatite and tricalcium phosphate. The production of these materials involves processing at high temperature which produces a preformed, highly crystalline, dense, bioinert ceramic. Because of their low fatigue properties, they have found limited application in orthopedics.

A new process for the in situ formation of the mineral phase of bone has been developed which allows for the operative implantation of a paste that hardens in minutes under physiologic conditions.[1] Monocalcium phosphate monohydrate [MCPM, $Ca_3(PO_4)2H_2O$], tricalcium phosphate [TCP $Ca_3(PO_4)_2$], and calcium carbonate (CC, $CaCO_3$) are dry mixed. A sodium phosphate solution is added, and with subsequent mixing a paste is formed in a few minutes. This paste is formable and injectable for about 5 minutes while maintaining physiologic temperature and pH. Upon implantation in a bony defect the paste hardens due to the crystallization of dahllite within about 10 minutes and attains an initial compressive strength of ~ 10 MPa. Within 12 hours, the material is about 85–90% dahllite

and the final strength is achieved, with the final maximum compressive strength being around 2.1 MPa. Relative to cancellous bone, the compressive strength of the new biomaterial is greater, while the tensile strength is about the same. In this way, fractured bones can be held in place while the native bone remodeling process replaces the implant with living bone, thus an implant–bone composite is created.[1,2]

Replacement of this biomaterial by living bone in animal studies appears to occur in a manner similar to bone remodeling, with osteoclasts and osteoblasts present at the interface of the new biomaterial within 2 weeks after implantation.

Given that fractures of the distal end of the radius are common injuries, particularly in patients with underlying osteopenia, manipulative realignment of the fracture will commonly result in a metaphyseal defect. When treated by a cast alone, loss of this realignment over the initial 6–12 weeks postinjury is commonplace. Alternative methods which have been utilized include external skeletal fixation alone or in conjunction with percutaneous pin fixation, autogenous or allogenic bone grafting, or in some cases operative realignment and support with late and screw fixation.[3] These alternative methods, while often successful, have had less optimal results in the osteopenic patient. Furthermore, the use of external pin fixation, or even formal internal fixation, exposes the elderly to further risks of infection and problems in wound healing, and in maintaining the stability of fixation at the pin–bone or screw–bone interface.

With these difficulties in mind, the potential for a bone substitute that can be injected percutaneously as a paste, yet which rapidly hardens

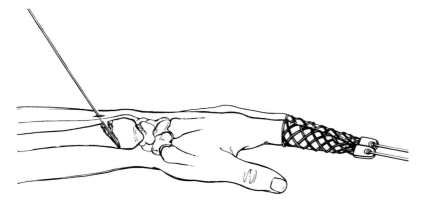

Figure 1

Guide wire placement. The guide wire is inserted percutaneously through the dorsal cortex of the fracture to the volar cortex.

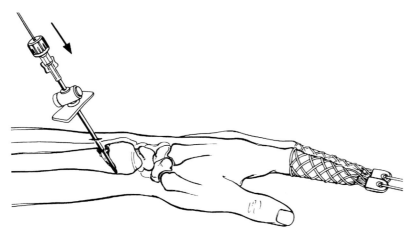

Figure 2

Cannula and dilator position. The cannula and dilator are placed over the guide wire and advanced to the volar cortex. The cannula is then withdrawn until the distal tip is within the dorsal cortex. The cannular seal is affixed to the skin.

and holds both the reduced fracture fragments in place while preventing loss of reduction, stimulated a prospective study designed to test the efficacy of the hypothesis in unstable extraarticular fractures of the distal radius.

Procedure

Under regional anesthesia the fracture is reduced by closed manipulation and stabilized on a fracture table with continuous traction of 5–15 lb (2–7 kg) with finger traps. The adequacy of the fracture reduction is controlled using image intensification. The site of introduction of the bone paste (Norian SRS™, Norian Corporation, Cupertino, California) is also determined by use of the image intensifier. A small stab wound is made on the dorsal surface over the fracture site and a guide wire is advanced into the fracture under fluoroscopic control (Figure 1). Care is taken to avoid penetration of the volar cortex with the guide wire. A cannula/dilator assembly system is advanced over the guide wire until the distal tip of the cannula reaches the volar cortex (Figure 2).

The cannula is then retracted until its distal tip is at the dorsal cortex, creating a pathway to introduce the bone paste within the cancellous bone. A plastic cannular border is then positioned with self-retaining paper strips or a single skin suture. The guide wire and dilator are then simultaneously removed while the distal tip

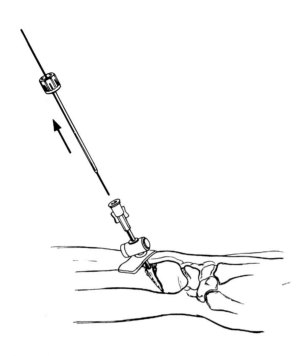

Figure 3

Guide wire and dilator removal with the cannula's distal tip maintained within the dorsal cortex. The guide wire and dilator are simultaneously removed.

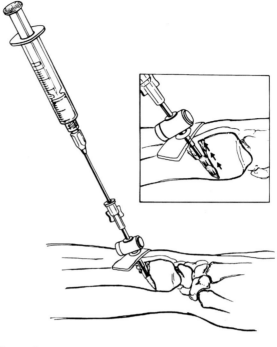

Figure 4

Bone paste implantation. With the cannular tip location in the dorsal cortex confirmed, the percutaneous delivery syringe is positioned at the volar aspect of the fracture. Retrograde injection of bone mineral substitute is performed to completely fill the defect.

of the cannula is maintained within the dorsal cortex (Figure 3). A syringe is inserted through the cannula and the fracture site flushed with sterile saline to dissolve any residual hematoma or blood clots within the fracture site.

The sterile calcium and phosphate source powders are manually mixed dry for 30 seconds. The solution is added to the dry components and mixed for 2 minutes to form a paste. The paste is transferred with a spatula into a percutaneous delivery system syringe. A working period of 3–5 minutes exists in which the SRS is injectable. The percutaneous delivery system syringe is inserted through the cannula to the volar cortex. The limb is maintained in traction and injection of the radiopaque bone mineral substitute is started at the volar cortex (Figure 4). The paste

is injected in an attempt to fill the entire defect. After administration the cannula is removed from the dorsal cortex and the limb stabilized without manipulation for 10 minutes.

In the initial clinical trial the limb was immobilized in a short-arm fiberglass cast for 6 weeks. Subsequent clinical experience has suggested that the duration of immobilization can be decreased to 2 weeks.

Pros and cons

The bone mineral substitute fixation of an unstable fracture of the distal radius has several distinct advantages. In the first place the

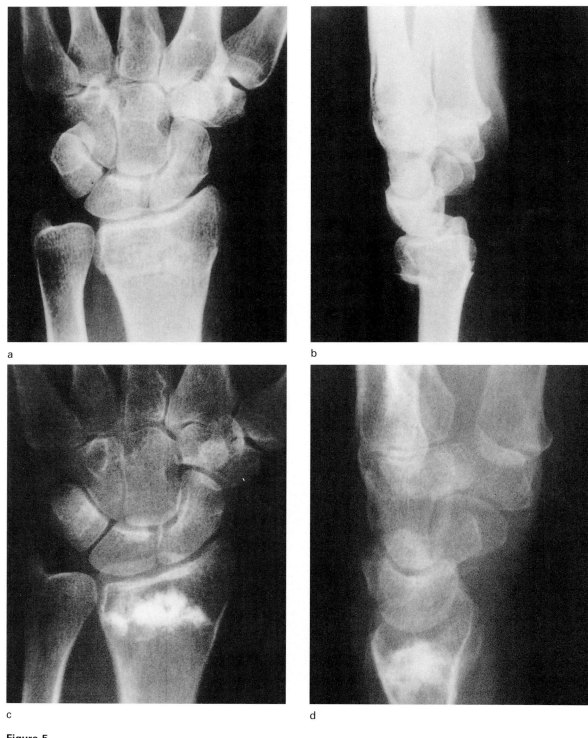

a

b

c

d

Figure 5

(a, b) Unstable distal radius fracture; (c, d) 3 months after injection of bone mineral substitute.

procedure is minimally invasive, the material is directed specifically to the zone of bony injury, the material has proven to be clinically safe and the material is well tolerated and relatively easy to apply. Second, the stability afforded by the material minimizes the need for external support, thereby enhancing functional use of the limb—of particular importance in the elderly. Third, and of equal importance, the bone mineral substitute is recognized by the host bone in a like manner to normal bone undergoing osteoclastic and osteoblastic bony turnover with the potential at some point of being completely replaced by host normal bone. The bone substitute has been seen to disappear over a 4–6 month period when it had extravasated into the soft tissues.

Arguments against this approach include the fact that it is invasive, presents only a limited period of time during which the material can effectively be injected, and would require an extensive operative approach if the material passed out the volar cortex threatening the median nerve or flexor tendons.

Results

A preliminary efficacy study of the technique has recently been completed.[4] Five patients with a comminuted displaced fracture of the distal end of the radius were treated with the bone mineral substitute and a short-arm cast. Three fractures were extraarticular, with two having nondisplaced fracture lines into the radioulnar joint and radiocarpal joint in one each. Posteroanterior and lateral radiographs were taken at 1 and 6 weeks and 3, 6, and 12 months. These were measured for radial length, radial angle, and volar angle and compared to the contralateral side. Hand function was assessed by measurement of the range of motion and grip strength. At 12 months follow-up the radial length was a mean of 9.9 mm, with an average loss of less than 1 mm from postoperative radiographs; the radial angle was maintained at a mean of 25.4°; the volar angle was within normal range (0–21°) in four patients, and one had a dorsal angle of 7°. The wrist range of motion improved 50% between 6 weeks and 3 months and improved further by 12 months when the grip strength reached a mean 88% of the contralateral side. These findings equaled or exceeded reported results for conventional fixation methods. There were no clinically significant adverse effects or complications of bone paste injection. Dorsal or volar extrusion of the injected material in four patients resolved over time.

Indications

At the present time the percutaneous administration of this bone mineral substitute is indicated for displaced, comminuted extraarticular fractures of the distal end of the radius (Figure 5). An ongoing multi-center clinical trial is currently investigating its use along with percutaneous Kirschner wires and/or external fixation in more complex intra- and extraarticular fractures.

References

1   Constantz BR, Ison IC, Fulmer MT, et al, Skeletal repair by in situ formation of the mineral phase of bone, *Science* (1995) **267**:1796–9.
2   Poole R, Coral chemistry leads to human repair, *Science* (1995) **267**:1772.
3   Fernandez DL, Jupiter JB, *Fractures of the Distal Radius. A Practical Approach to Management* (Springer-Verlag: New York, 1996) 1–52.
4   Jupiter JB, Winters S, Sigman S, et al, Repair of five distal radius fractures with an investigational bioremodelable bone mineral substitute. A preliminary report, *J Orthop Trauma* in press.

Commentary

Chapter 12

Although internal fixation is finding an increasing place in the tool kit of the hand surgeon, the most severe injuries are not often suitable for internal fixation. In such cases mini external fixation can play a major role in assisting in wound management and maintaining length and alignment of the digit. Doctor Cziffer, a world renowned expert in this area, here summarizes current knowledge and future directions in this area.

PCA

Chapter 13

Often hand surgeons must work in narrow confines, yet somehow achieve secure fixation of tendon or ligament to bone. Traditional techniques have included pull-out sutures and other types of suture through intraosseous tunnels. A newer option is the use of suture anchors in the hand and wrist. Doctors Griggs and Weiss here review the current state of this art.

PCA

Chapter 14

It is increasingly appreciated that the Herbert screw provides little, if any, compression. When compression is indicated, the surgeon is faced with the need to decide between lagging a cortical screw, or using a cancellous type screw as a lag screw. Both types of screws, however, have the disadvantage that further compression can only be achieved by driving the tip of the screw further into (or beyond) the bone. Doctor Lane has developed a compression screw which seats the distal portion of the screw exactly where the surgeon wishes, and then permits compression by telescoping the proximal portion of the screw within the distal portion of the screw. This seems a useful tool to have available for those circumstances where both compression and precise screw position are critical, and there is little if any margin for error.

PCA

Chapter 15

This is a fascinating application of metallurgical prowess to hand surgery. I am looking forward to trying these devices once they become approved for use in the United States.

PCA

Compression has always been one of the goals of bone fixation. It has been proved that compression lasts only 1 or 2 days with the usual devices and results in a good bone coaptation. Will the shape memory staples provide continuous compression? Very promising results for limited carpal arthrodeses and osteotomy fixation have been experienced with this new device. Fixation was good and healing was faster than usual.

PS

Chapter 16

Here is an example of something which is on the horizon and which seems quite promising—a substitute for autogenous bone grafting which does not pose a risk of disease transmission and which is eventually replaced by the patient's own bone. Furthermore, the substance apparently does not induce an allergic reaction, and provides instant stability. The substance seems ideal in many regards. It is only available for experimental use in the United States at present but one hopes that before long it will be available for wider distribution.

PCA

17
Proximal interphalangeal joint midlateral approach

Philippe Saffar

Introduction

The proximal interphalangeal (PIP) joint is surrounded by extensor and flexor tendons and it is very difficult to reach the appropriate elements of the joint without cutting the extensor tendon dorsally or opening the flexor sheath and the volar plate volarly. Different approaches have been described:

(1) The *posterior approach* has been recommended by several authors:
- transverse section of the extensor tendon[1]
- longitudinal section of the extensor tendon[2]
- elevation of a triangular flap of the extensor tendon[3] (Figure 1)

(2) The *anterior approach*:
- the A3 pulley is cut, the flexor tendons are retracted and the volar plate is elevated[4] (Figure 2).

Technique

The aim is to work on the PIP joint without opening the flexor sheath and without cutting

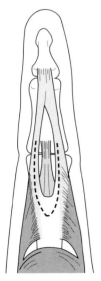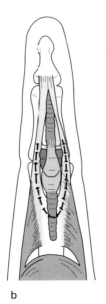

a   b

Figure 1

Chamay's dorsal PIP approach: (a) elevation of a distally based flap of the extensor tendon lateral bands; (b) suture of the extensor flap.

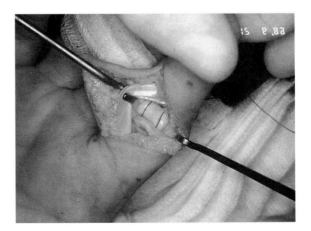

Figure 2

The volar PIP approach.

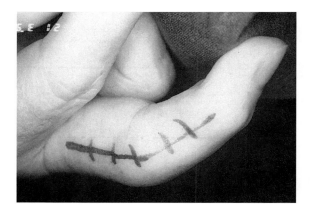

Figure 3

Anterolateral skin approach.

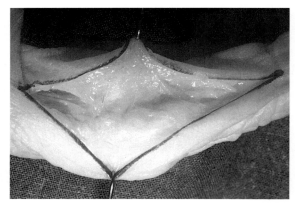

Figure 4

The neurovascular bundle is in the volar flap.

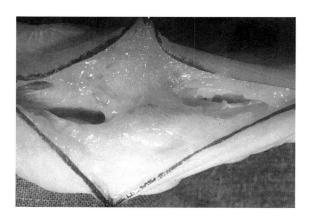

Figure 5

Subperiosteal elevation of the flexor sheath from the first and second phalanges.

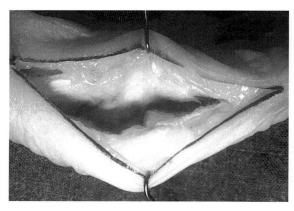

Figure 6

Elevation of the volar plate.

the extensor tendons. We now use a midlateral approach based on a technique called total anterior tenoarthrolysis, which we described in 1978 for the treatment of fixed flexed deformity of the PIP joint.[5] The technique is based on a subperiosteal dissection. We demonstrated that the periosteum of the first and second phalanges is in continuity with the volar plate and may be elevated together from the volar aspect of these phalanges.

A midlateral approach at the junction of the dorsal and volar skin is performed, extending from the middle of the proximal phalanx to the distal part of the second phalanx (Figure 3). This incision is located volarly to the extensor tendon and dorsally relative to the neurovascular bundle (Figure 4). No attempt is made to dissect upward and downward. The extensor tendon is retracted dorsally and the oblique fibers of the retinacular ligament are cut. Direct contact is made with the

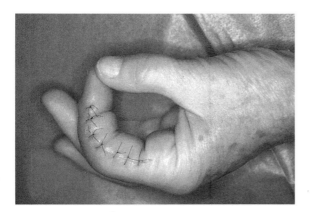

Figure 7

Early postoperative mobilization.

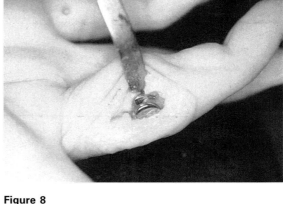

Figure 8

A prosthesis inserted by the volar approach.

lateral aspects of the phalanges. A periosteal incision is made on the lateral aspect of the first and second phalanges. A subperiosteal elevation of the periosteum is made volarly from the lateral aspect of the phalanx, then from the volar and opposite aspect of the first and second phalanges (Figure 5). This should be made with care, slowly, as it is one of the most important steps of the procedure. An elevator and a scalpel are used alternately to detach the periosteum without opening the flexor tendon sheath, and are always kept in contact with the bone. Two retractors are used to raise the periosteum separated from the bone, forming a bridge at the PIP joint. The volar plate which is in continuity with the periosteum is freed from its attachment to the bone with a scalpel and is then elevated when the accessory ligaments of the PIP joint are cut. The anterior aspect of the joint is then visible (Figure 6). If this joint was fixed in a flexed position, the anterior part of the lateral ligaments are cut to straighten the finger. If it is necessary in the course of the procedure, the lateral ligament on the side of the approach may be proximally detached.

It is then possible to perform a distal bone resection perpendicular to the axis of the first phalanx and to prepare the intramedullary canal for insertion of the stem of a prosthesis. No bone resection is performed at the base of the second phalanx, to prevent detachment of the central slip insertion of the extensor tendon. The intramedullary canal of the second phalanx is then prepared, and it is possible to insert a prosthesis.

The lateral ligament detached proximally may be sutured to the volar plate in an oblique direction. Closure of the skin should only be made with the finger in extension to prevent fixation in flexion of the joint.

Postoperative care

As no tendons have been cut, postoperative active mobilization may be initiated as early as the third day for arthrolysis or prosthesis insertion (Figure 7), although this depends on the type of procedure that has been performed.

Discussion

The vascular bundles and the transverse anastomosis between the two lateral arteries proximal to the PIP, which provides the vincula for flexor tendon vascularization, is contained in the volar flap elevated from the periosteum; this vascularization is not impaired.

It is not necessary to modify the incision in the presence of previous scars; it is, in fact, better to choose the side where scars already exist.

This approach should not be used if there is a particular procedure to perform on the extensor tendon, except for extensor tenolysis. Approaches that cut the extensor tendon do not usually allow early active mobilization. We had to perform secondary extensor tenolysis when we used a dorsal approach, even after early passive rehabilitation, and extensor tendon adhesions frequently arise.

Indications

(1) Insertion of implants and prostheses (Figure 8): the early mobilization allowed by an intact extensor gives better results in terms of the range of motion obtained.

(2) PIP arthrolysis: with the anterior approach, the cartilage status is completely checked and arthrolysis more easily performed.

(3) In acute intraarticular fractures and in malunions of the PIP joint, the midlateral approach is recommended.

(4) In long-standing fixed flexed deformity after tendon division, which may already have been operated on several times, the incision may be extended distally to elevate the DIP volar plate and perform total anterior tenoarthrolysis.[5]

References

1   Iselin F, Pradet G, Traitement des lésions enraidissantes des doigts par résection-arthroplastie IPP avec implant de Swanson. In: Tubiana R, ed, *Traité de Chirurgie de la Main* (Masson: Paris, 1984) 937–49.

2   Swanson AB, Maupin BK, Gajjar NV, et al, Flexible implant arthroplasty in the proximal interphalangeal joint of the hand, *J Hand Surg* (1985) **10A**:796–805.

3   Chamay A, A distally based dorsal and triangular flap for direct access to the proximal interphalangeal joint, *Ann Chir Main* (1988) **7**:179–83.

4   Lin HH, Wyrick JD, Stern PJ, Proximal interphalangeal joint silicone replacement arthroplasty: clinical results using an anterior approach, *J Hand Surg* (1995) **20A**:123–32.

5   Saffar Ph, Rengeval JP, Total anterior tenoarthrolysis. Treatment of the finger flexed deformity, *Ann Chir* (1978) **32**:579–82.

18

Treatment of the carpal boss by carpometacarpal arthrodesis

Timothy J Herbert, W Bruce Conolly and Andrew M Clarke

Introduction

The carpal boss is a relatively common lump occurring on the dorsum of the hand over the index and/or middle carpometacarpal (CMC) joints (Figure 1). It consists of a prominent bone spur often with an overlying ganglion (Figure 2).

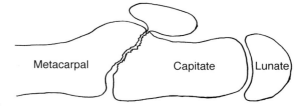

Figure 2

Schematized diagram of a carpal boss showing a bony lump and associated ganglion.

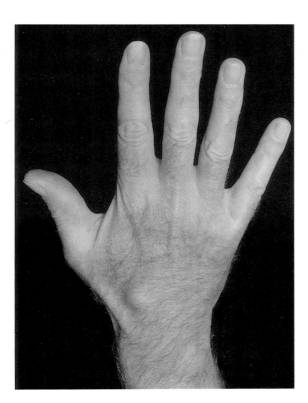

Figure 1

A large carpal boss.

The bone spur represents a local degenerative process involving the styloid process of the second or third metacarpals. In many of these patients the styloid process remains unfused, then being known as the os styloideum.

A carpal boss seldom causes sufficient trouble to require treatment. However, some patients do complain of significant pain and weakness associated with this condition. Surgery is indicated if these symptoms fail to respond to conservative treatment, as well as in cases where the site of the swelling interferes with hand function or provokes secondary effects such as radial neuralgia or tendinitis.

The most commonly recommended procedure involves excision of the swelling and all underlying prominent bone, back to healthy joint surface.[1] In spite of previous reports to the contrary,[1-6] it has become clear in recent years that this procedure often fails to relieve the problem. Under these circumstances arthrodesis of the joint is normally recommended.[7]

Unfortunately, the results of the CMC joint arthrodesis are also unpredictable, and it can be very difficult to achieve a solid fusion mass at this site. For these reasons, we now favour a more formal type of fusion, involving wide joint excision, bone grafting and internal fixation.

Technical aspects of the dowel technique

Either a transverse or longitudinal incision can be used and should be centred over the boss. The extensor carpi radialis brevis tendon is retracted radially or, alternatively, the area can be approached between the two wrist extensor tendons. All branches of the superficial radial nerve must always be gently retracted and protected throughout the procedure. The bony protuberance is then excised flush with the second or third metacarpal.

The principle of the technique is then to achieve a four-bone fusion between the bases of the second and third metacarpal, the trapezoid and capitate bones. Fluoroscopy is essential at this stage because the cylindrical core of bone (resembling a dowel) which has to be removed must incorporate a small part of each of the four bones mentioned above. Control by radiography allows for accurate siting of the trephine (Figure 3). The depth of the core should be approximately 75% of the depth of the metacarpal base. The precision bone graft system (Kaltec, Adelaide, South Australia) is an ideal bone trephine because of its ability to harvest a whole

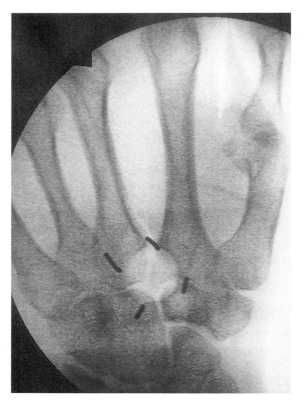

Figure 3

Intraoperative radiograph after excision of the second and third carpometacarpal joints using the dowel trephine.

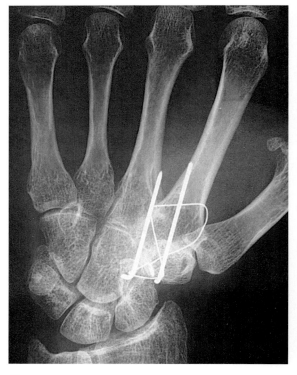

Figure 4

Posteroanterior radiograph demonstrating internal fixation of the dowel graft. This patient had a good result after three unsuccessful surgical interventions using other methods to treat the painful carpal boss.

series of different sizes of graft. A cortico-cancellous iliac crest bone graft, one size larger than that which has been removed from the hand, can now be tamped into place. The extra size of the graft ensures a good tight fit.

Internal fixation is then used to immobilize the fusion mass; Kirschner wires alone are usually inadequate and should be combined with the use of a tension band wire (Figure 4). Alternatively, a low-profile H or T plate may be used to fix the second or third metacarpals to the carpus. In any event, postoperative immobilization in plaster is required for at least 6 to 8 weeks, and the metal will almost certainly need to be removed once the fusion is sound.

Pros and cons compared to classical techniques

The dorsal slot inlay graft method is the most commonly used to achieve a CMC fusion. It remains a simple technique and the morbidity is small. However, our experience has been that pain and weakness persist in an unacceptably high proportion of these patients. We believe that the primary reason for this is that the fusion mass created with this technique is not large enough to create a solid arthrodesis. The dowel graft technique is a more extensive procedure and more elaborate instrumentation is needed. The surgical insult to the hand is greater and consequently patients may need more postoperative analgesia. However, the iliac crest donor site morbidity using the trephine graft system is minimal. The method of internal fixation is currently giving rise to the greatest debate within our unit. Although we favour tension band wiring, the rigidity of fixation is still not ideal and we are searching for other more satisfactory alternatives.

We believe that the overall success of the arthrodesis by this technique justifies the use of this procedure, although we concede that greater numbers are required for a fuller analysis.

Results

Our experience has shown that only 50% of patients who have local excision have a good

outcome. We have used CMC arthrodesis as both a primary and a secondary procedure and found that the outcomes are not different for the two groups. The success rate with standard CMC fusion is only 50%, but the dowel technique seems to give better results. More cases are needed to determine a true success rate, but our excellent early experience with this technique has made it the treatment of choice in our unit.

Indications

Our current rationale is to offer surgery for a carpal boss only if the patient's symptoms are severe enough to cause a functional loss in the hand. In our experience, a painless lump on the hand seldom justifies surgery. However, if surgery is necessary, we rely on the finding of a badly degenerating CMC joint to guide us toward CMC arthrodesis rather than a wide local excision. Two key features help us with this decision. If stressing the second and third CMC joints causes pain and an isotope bone scan is positive, then we feel that local excision will not be extensive enough to provide symptomatic relief. In our opinion, a primary CMC arthrodesis using the dowel graft method is then indicated. Secondary CMC arthrodesis can be used if an adequate local excision has been tried previously and symptoms persist.

References

1   Cuono CB, Watson HK, The carpal boss: surgical treatment and etiological considerations, *Plast Reconstr Surg* (1979) **63**:88–93.

2   Fusi S, Watson HK, Cuono CB, The carpal boss: a 20-year review of operative management, *J Hand Surg* (1995) **20B**:405–8.

3   Artz TD, Posch JL, The carpometacarpal boss, *J Bone J Surg* (1973) **55A**:747–52.

4   Hultgren T, Lugnegard H, Carpal boss, *Acta Orthop Scand* (1986) **57**:547–50.

5   Hazlett JW, The third metacarpal boss, *International Orthop* (1992) **16**:369–71.

6   Lenoble E, Foucher G, The carpal bump, *Ann Chir Main Memb Super* (1992) **11**:46–50.

7   Joseph RB, Linscheid RL, Dobyns JH, et al, Chronic sprains of the carpo-metacarpal joints, *J Hand Surg* (1981) **6**:172–80.

19
Proximal interphalangeal joint arthroplasty

Philippe Saffar

Introduction

Posttraumatic proximal interphalangeal (PIP) joint stiffness in young adults may be due to extra- or intraarticular causes. Extraarticular causes may be treated conservatively by rehabilitation and flexor and/or extensor splints. Extensor or flexor tenolyses combined with arthrolyses may be performed if articular contours are normal and stiffness is due to soft tissue adhesions or deficiencies.

If the joint is destroyed and, moreover, malaligned, three surgical possibilities exist: arthrodeses, prostheses and arthroplasties. Arthrodeses may be useful for the fourth and fifth fingers but may not be recommended for the index and third fingers. Prostheses are rarely indicated in young active adults because of frequent failures. Ruptures, infections, loosening and silicone synovitis have been reported. There is now a wide variety of new PIP devices but without any significant follow-up. Arthroplasties have not been frequently reported for the PIP joints. Different techniques have been described for metacarpophalangeal (MP) and PIP joints. In 1954, Carroll and Taber described 30 PIP arthroplasties without interposition and with Kirschner wire distraction by elastic bands through a plaster.[1] The tendons around the joint were not injured. Others reported various types of interposition for PIP joints: fascia lata,[2] fascia and periosteum,[3] extensor tendons,[4] perichondrium[5,6] and silastic sheet. The use of external fixation without interposition was also reported.[7]

Tupper (Figure 1a,b) described a volar plate interposition for the MP joint. The volar plate was detached proximally and interposed after

bone resection. Eaton and Malerich (Figure 2) reported a limited PIP arthroplasty by volar plate advancement and transosseous reattachment, which is indicated for dorsal PIP subluxation or

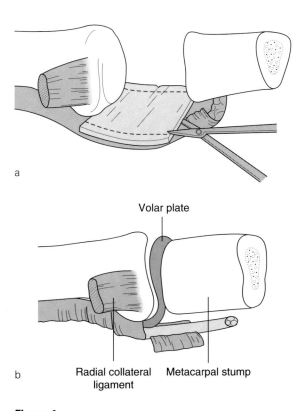

a

Volar plate

b

Radial collateral ligament   Metacarpal stump

Figure 1

(a,b) Tupper MP volar plate interposition arthroplasty.[8]

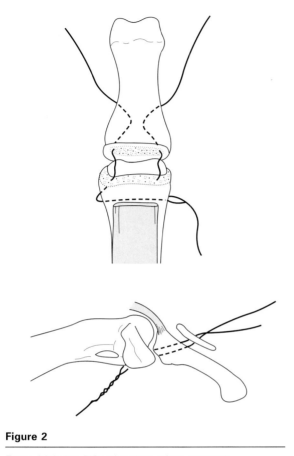

Figure 2

Eaton–Malerich PIP volar plate advancement.[9]

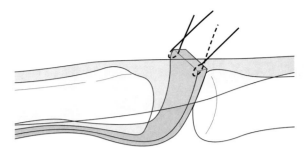

Figure 3

Modified Tupper's technique for PIP volar plate interposition arthroplasty.

dislocation associated with a fracture avulsion of the volar part of the base of the second phalanx.

The technique presented here is a volar plate interposition derived from Tupper's technique with a distal volar plate detachment derived from the Eaton–Malerich technique. The approach may be volar or dorsal.

Technique

The volar approach is of the Brunner type. The sheath and the A3 pulley are opened and the flexor tendons and neurovascular bundles are retracted, taking care to avoid injury to the flexor tendon vincula. The volar plate is detached distally from the bony insertion at the base of the second phalanx and from the lateral borders along the joint. A subperiosteal elevation is then performed at the first phalanx since the volar plate is in continuity with the periosteum of the first phalanx, as has been proved with total anterior tenoarthrolysis. This facilitates an easy advancement of the volar plate in order to perform the interposition. Resection of 1 cm of the distal bone of the first phalanx is performed and the bone ends are rounded off. In this process, lateral ligaments are usually detached and are too short to be reattached proximally. There is no resection of the base of the second phalanx, except if realignment of the finger is indicated which cannot be corrected by insertion of the first phalanx head. Osteotomy should be calculated and the proximal part of the second phalanx may be resected on a few millimeters. Two stitches are then passed at each lateral part of the distal volar plate. Volar plate advancement and interposition between the two phalanges is then possible. Each stitch is passed lateral to the lateral bands of the extensor tendon apparatus and through the dorsolateral skin. The two stitches are passed through a button and sutured to each other (Figure 3).

A dorsal approach may be used if there is an associated dorsal procedure to be performed. In this case, subperiosteum elevation should be carefully performed before bone resection and distal volar plate detachment. The stitches are passed, if possible, proximal to the extensor tendon repair.

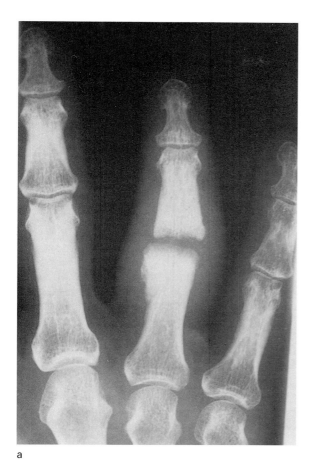

a

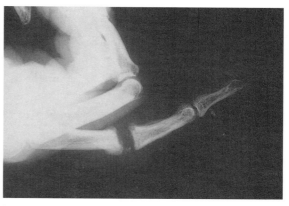

b

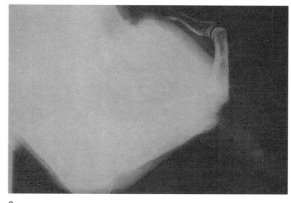

c

Figure 4

(a–c) Motion after 6 months.

Associated procedures: oblique pinning of the PIP joint may be necessary. An extensor tenolysis performed by the same approach may be necessary.

Postoperative rehabilitation is extremely important. Patient compliance is necessary because it may be painful and pain medication should be prescribed if necessary. The procedure is as follows:

- The finger is held on a splint in an extended position for 1 week and in the intervals between rehabilitation sessions.
- Careful passive flexion and extension are initiated after 1 week in a 0–45° arc of flexion,

extending to 70° at the end of the third week.
- Active motion in flexion and extension is allowed after 3 weeks during a 2-month period (Figure 4).

Continuous passive motion allows faster and better results and is usually not painful. Flexion and extension splints are another option.

Materials and methods

The technique was performed on eight patients (Table 1): six males and two females. The

Table 1   Results analysis.

Age	Sex	Finger	Side	Ext°	Flex°	Pain	Clino	Ext° (post)	Flex° (post)	Pain (post)	Clino (post)	Follow-up (months)
24	M	II	L	20	70	Y	Y	10	60	N	Y	11
25	F	IV	R	0	55	Y	Y	0	50	N	N	7
25	M	V	L	0	10	Y	Y	30	40	Y	Y	31
60	F	V	R	0	10	Y	Y	0	40	N	N	12
31	M	III	L	0	0	Y	N	50	60	N	N	13
44	M	IV	R	0	0	Y	N	30	80	N	N	15
23	M	V	L	0	0	N	N	0	50	N	N	5
18	M	V	R	0	55	Y	Y	15	60	N	Y	5

Clino = clinodactyly; Ext = extension; Flex = flexion; N = no; Y = yes

average age was 31 years. The fingers operated on were the ulnar ones (IV and V) in six out of the eight cases. The initial accident was a crush in four cases, a dorsal wound by a circular saw in one and an intraarticular fracture in three. Associated injuries were the rule with an extensor tendon severed in five cases. The aetiologies were the sequelae of joint wounds, posttraumatic postinfection joint destruction. Preoperative pain was present in six cases. The average preoperative range of motion was 22°. Clinodactyly was present in five cases.

Results

The results are shown in Table 1. Postoperative pain was absent or present for significant strains in two cases. The postoperative range of motion was 33°. According to Carroll's criteria (Table 2), range of motion was good in four cases (50° or more), fair in one (30°) and not improved in three (10°). Lateral stability was always obtained and clinodactyly was present in three cases (10–20°). One patient sustained a postoperative infection and was not improved.

Table 2   Carroll's criteria for range of motion.

Good	10–55°
Fair	less than 10° or clinodactyly
Failure	not improved

Global results and patient satisfaction were good due to pain relief. Follow-up was short (6–15 months). The final result was obtained in 3–6 months and maintained with time when the follow-up was sufficient to appreciate this feature. Failures were related mostly to noncompliance of patients in rehabilitation.

Indications

The indications are posttraumatic stiffness associated with pain and malalignment in young adults. This technique may sometimes be performed after prosthesis failure and idiopathic osteoarthritis. Patient motivation is essential.

References

1   Carroll RE, Taber TH, Digital arthroplasty of the proximal interphalangeal joint, *J Bone Joint Surg* (1954) **36A**:912–20.

2   Payr E, Weitere Erfahungen uber die operative Mobilisierung ankylosieter Gelenege mit Berucksichtigung des spateren Schicksals des Arthroplastik, *Dtsch Z Chir* (1914) **129**:341–463.

3   Hesse E, Beitrage zur Frage der operativen Mobilisierung versteifter Fingergelengke, *Arch Klin Chir* (1922) **119**:1–12.

4   Hellum C, Vainio K, Arthroplasty of the metacarpophalangeal joints in rheumatoid arthritis with transposition of the interosseous muscles, *Scand J Plast Reconstr Surg* (1968) **2**:139–43.

5   Engvist O, Johansson SH, Skoog T, Recon-
    struction of articular cartilage using autologous
    perichondrial grafts. A preliminary report, *Scand J
    Plast Reconstr Surg* (1954) **9**:203–6.

6   Skoog T, Johansson SH, The formation of carti-
    lage from free perichondrial grafts, *Plast Reconstr
    Surg* (1976) **57**:1–6.

7   Sokolow C, Les nécroses articulaires de l'inter-
    phalangienne proximale: traitement par résection-
    distraction à l'aide du fixateur multicentrique MS3,
    Ann Chir Main (1995) **14**:202–6.

8   Tupper JW, The metacarpophalangeal arthro-
    plasty, *J Hand Surg* (1989) **14A**:371–5.

9   Eaton RG, Malerich MM, Volar arthroplasty of the
    proximal interphalangeal joint: a review of ten
    years' experience, *J Hand Surg* (1980) **5**:260–8.

20

Conchal cartilage interposition arthroplasty for small joint reconstruction of the hand

Colin Song, George Psaras and Morris Ritz

Introduction

Injury to the joints of the hand can often render severe disability especially in the younger patient. In this age group the usual aetiological factors include inter alia gunshot wounds and severe crush injuries related to either industrial or motor vehicle accidents. The more insidious injury, namely rheumatoid arthritis, bears certain broad-based comparisons but is an additional consideration for reconstruction.

Severe joint injury to small joints of the hand often renders these patients sufferers of painful, unstable angulated or stiff joints. In particular the concomitant severe soft tissue damage of the surrounding area contributes considerably to the disablement. Loss of joint motion, particularly in the proximal interphalangeal (PIP) joint, compounds the problem considerably. It has often been stated that this joint is the key to hand function after these injuries.

Reconstruction of these joints has remained a major challenge given that the treatment objectives have to balance the intricacies of maintenance of joint integrity to achieve mobility, stability and pain-free excursion. Two surgical options are available as far as the reconstructive options are concerned.

Arthrodesis is indicated in situations in which the small joints of the hand are damaged to such a degree that a stable reconstruction with painless motion is impossible.[1] The general indications for arthrodesis are pain, instability, deformity and loss of muscles to control the joint mobility. Arthrodesis is almost always the major alternative to arthroplasty and is seen as a salvage procedure

with major limitations as far as mobility is concerned. The loss of joint mobility necessitated by arthrodesis is an obvious disadvantage, especially in the younger patient, whose hands often represent his ability as a breadwinner. It is particularly in this group of patients that the arthroplasty method is often the preferred one.

Many varied techniques of arthroplasty for small joints of the hand have been described. Broadly classified these comprise:

- Resectional arthroplasty.
- Interposition arthroplasty.
- Replacement arthroplasty.

Interposition arthroplasty is a concept apparently first utilized by Payr in 1914.[2] He is reported to have used a flap of fatty tissue in the PIP joints of two patients, with resultant painless joints with good motion. Other sources of autogenous tissue, including periosteum, fascia, tendon, dermis and joint capsule, have been described. Perichondrial grafting has been described by various authors.[3–7] The concept of resurfacing damaged articular surfaces with transplanted perichondrium in young patients with traumatic arthrosis in the presence of good bone stock has varied results, with the Louisville group voicing their concerns.[8] Problems arose particularly where both articular surfaces in a joint were replaced and a sheet of silicone rubber was used to prevent ankylosis. After removal of this sheeting, results in terms of mobility were noted to be less satisfactory. In the older age group the perichondrium showed the visual appearance of cases of chondromalacia.

Vainio utilized the extensor tendon in metacarpophalangeal (MP) joint arthroplasty.[9] This procedure is not, however, indicated in traumatic arthrosis and in general limits the use in long and ring fingers. It requires an extensor mechanism that is distended over the MP joint. Tupper utilized the volar plate as the interpositional material in MP joints after resection arthroplasty.[10] The use of alloplastic materials as interpositional agents remains with the use of silicone elastomer spacers as popularized by Swanson.[11] The procedure involved interposition of the silicone with insertion of stems of the prosthesis in the two articulating surfaces. The resultant incidence of loosening and fracture at 2 to 3 years after implantation prompted the response of strengthening the implants by cementing. Bone resorption is an additional problem related to the use of these alloplastic materials.[12]

The use of conchal cartilage grafts in interposition arthroplasty addresses the goals of arthroplasty:

(1) Pain-free motion of the reconstructed joint.
(2) Stability of the articulating surfaces.
(3) Facilitation of the repair of adjacent flexor and extensor tendon mechanisms.
(4) Stability of the joint and surrounding structures.

Materials and methods

Six patients, four males and two females, with ages ranging from 24 to 36 years, had conchal cartilage interposition arthroplasty of four PIP joints and two MP joints. Five patients had suffered gunshot wounds while the sixth patient fell from a motorcycle and sustained a crush injury of the nondominant hand.

All the injuries involved intraarticular fractures with some degree of comminution. At least one of the articular surfaces was involved in each joint. In addition, bone loss of the metaphysis adjacent to the articular surface was evident in two-thirds of the cases. Associated soft-tissue injuries included lacerations through the extensor mechanisms in all joints and incomplete lacerations of the flexor tendons in two cases.

Debridement

The initial management of these injuries involved aggressive debridement of all non-viable and contaminated tissue under tourniquet and blood perfusion assessed after release of the tourniquet. Interim cover utilized occlusive dressings consisting mainly of hydrogels contained by two overlying polyurethane adhesive sheets in which the finger or hand is sandwiched. This ensured viability of exposed vital structures such as blood vessels, nerves and tendons.

At the 48-hour observation under the tourniquet, tissue viability was re-assessed. Where further debridement was indicated this was effected. 'Sculpturing' of the damaged articular surface was performed using a bone rongeur where indicated. Where bone graft was a necessary part of the reconstruction, a reciprocal shape recipient bone stump was fashioned. The source of the bone graft included the distal radius or iliac crest.

Harvest of conchal cartilage

The conchal cartilage was harvested from the pinna through a posterior incision. By bimanual digital guidance (to ensure that the anterior pinna skin is not breached) the cartilage was scored with a number 15 surgical blade. An ellipse was scored roughly 1–1.5 cm in its widest distance (Figure 1). The posterior perichondrium was harvested with the cartilage, care being exercised to ensure that the anterior perichondrium was preserved. The wound was closed using a subcuticular absorbable suture.

The natural curvature of the conchal cartilage affords this an ideal material for interpositional placement (Figure 2). This shape facilitates fixation to the bone end of either the bone graft or the proximal bone end (Figure 3). One or two fine drill holes were effected to allow passage of a 5/0 clear nylon suture.

Where the original skin wound was not overlying the joint, access was usually gained through a dorsal straight incision. Extensor tendon splitting incision allowed access to the joint. The bone grafts were fixed with titanium plates and 1.7 mm screws (Leibinger, Germany). The collateral ligaments and volar plates of each joint were meticulously repaired.

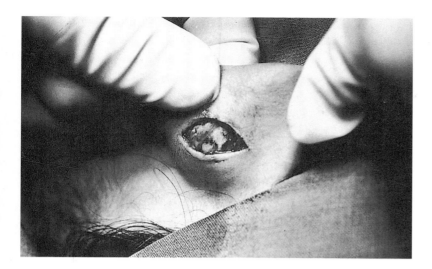

Figure 1

The conchal cartilage is readily accessible through a posterior approach. Care must be taken to preserve the anterior perichondrium.

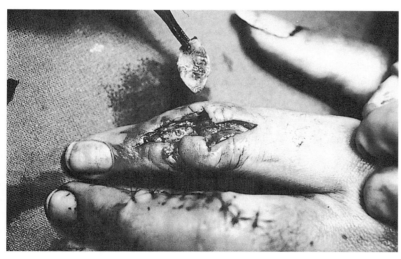

Figure 2

The cartilage has an ideal shape and configuration for use as an interpositional graft.

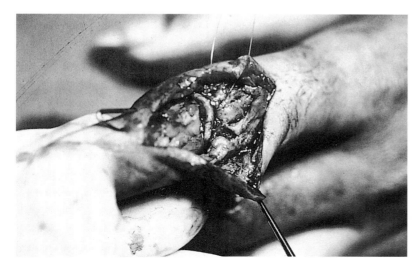

Figure 3

The cartilage has been placed between the two articular surfaces damaged by the initial trauma and matches well the presenting surfaces.

Postoperative care

Except where tendons were repaired, the initial 48 hours required splinting in the functional position, ensuring 15–20° dorsiflexion at the wrist and 70° flexion of the MP joints. The interphalangeal (IP) joints were maintained in extension. Thereafter, guarded active exercises were permitted under the supervision of a physiotherapist. Buddy splinting to adjacent fingers allowed continued guarded motion with the protection of the collateral ligaments.

Where flexor tendon injuries were repaired, the statutory programme of 18–21 days in a splint with the wrist in the neutral position, MP joints in 70° flexion and IP joints in extension was followed. Thereafter guarded but intensive active physiotherapy was administered. Buddy splinting was prescribed as well.

For extensor tendon repairs the functional splint was applied. When splitting of the extensor mechanism was all that was needed to gain access to the joint, guarded active mobility was begun in earnest after 24 hours. Buddy splinting was very useful to maintain the integrity of the collateral ligaments. The management of extensor lag consisted of night-time splinting in extension.

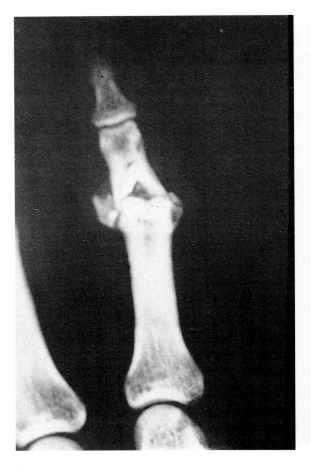

Figure 4

Case study one: preoperative radiograph of the hand of a 24-year-old electrician showing the extent of the intra-articular fracture involving the PIP joint.

Results

Table 1 illustrates the results obtained in this series. The assessment revolves mainly around

Table 1 The ranges of the reconstructed joints measured as the active range in degrees as opposed to the passive joint range. The longer the follow-up period the more acceptable the improvement in terms of mobility.

Patient	Age (years)	Sex	Joint	Injury	AM/PM (degrees)	Follow-up (months)	Comments
BP	24	M	R-IF PIP	GSW	90/90	26	—
DF	34	F	L-MF MP	GSW	70/90	16	DIP joint stiffness
AS	36	M	L-MF MP	GSW	80/90	14	Intrinsic tightness
AC	28	M	L-LF PIP	GSW	90/90	22	Extensor lag
RVDS	25	F	L-IF PIP	MVA	70/90	15	—
PN	32	M	R-RF PIP	GSW	40/90	4	—

AM=active motion; PM=passive motion; R=right; L=left; IF=index finger; MF=middle finger; RF=ring finger; MP=metacarpophalangeal; PIP=proximal interphalangeal; GSW=gunshot wound; MVA=motor vehicle accident.

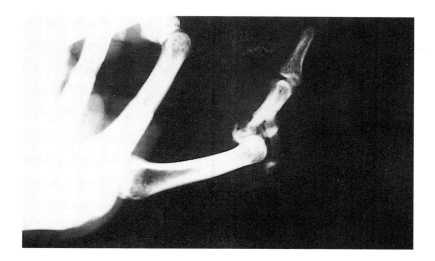

Figure 5

Case study one: lateral radiograph view of the extent of the fracture.

the degree of mobility of the reconstructed joints measured as the active motion in degrees against the measured passive range of the joint. It appears that the longer the patient follow-up, the more likely the range of motion will improve, indicative in most of the cases of the extent of soft tissue scarring, the recovery and the return to suppleness, which is a function of time.

Case study one, patient BP

This 24-year-old right-hand-dominant electrician suffered an accidental close range gunshot injury while cleaning his firearm and sustained severe comminution of the articular surface of the middle phalanx of the right index finger PIP joint (Figures 4 and 5). Bone graft and conchal cartilage graft with plate and interosseous wiring was used to achieve rigid fixation. The patient was mobilized after 48 hours of splinting. His 1-year follow-up range is illustrated in Figures 6 and 7.

Case study two, patient DF

This 34-year-old right-handed typist sustained an accidental close range gunshot to the left hand injuring the left middle finger MP joint. The

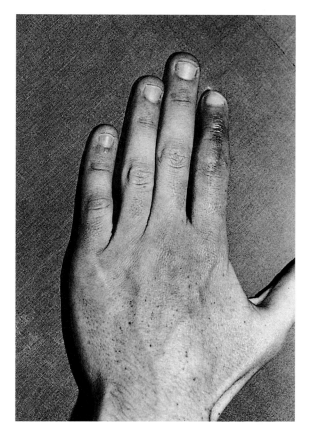

Figure 6

Case study one: 1-year follow-up photograph of the patient's hand.

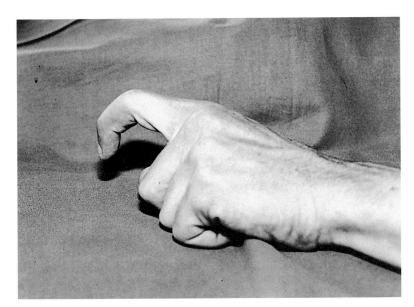

Figure 7

Case study one: active range of joint motion almost normal after 1 year.

radiograph (Figure 8) shows the extent of the damage to the articular surface of the metacarpal head. Bone graft harvested from the iliac crest and the conchal cartilage graft after fixation to the sculptured new metacarpal head was fixed to the third metacarpal shaft, (Figure 9), using an eight-holed Y-shaped titanium plate (Leibinger, Germany). Figure 10 shows this patient's range of motion at 16-month follow-up.

In one patient whose original injury was caused by gunshot, with consequential extensive flexor and extensor tenodesis requiring tenolysis, opportunity and patient consent allowed biopsy of the cartilage graft. Histological sections demonstrated incorporation of the cartilage graft to the bone stump, with evidence of chondrocytes to one side while osteoid was noted on the other.

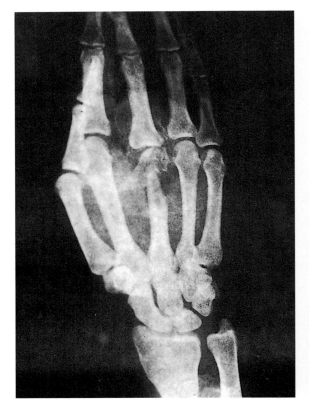

Figure 8

Case study two: prereduction radiograph of a 34-year-old woman who sustained gunshot injury to the left third metacarpal head.

Discussion

Hyaline or elastic cartilage of the concha is considered a morphologic cartilage with a fixed

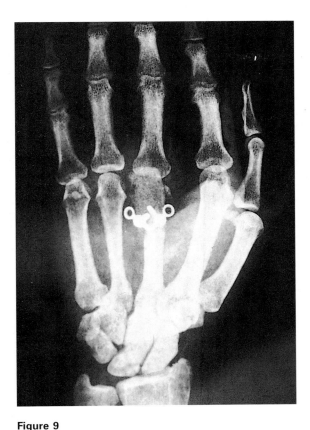

Figure 9

Case study two: postreduction radiograph showing plate internal rigid fixation. The conchal cartilage graft is fixed to the end of the bone graft.

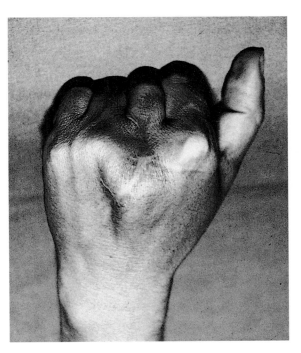

Figure 10

Case study two: at 16-month follow-up the patient has 70° flexion of the joint.

configuration recognizable as characteristic of the shape of the pinna. It is this configuration with a natural concave curvature that makes conchal cartilage ideal as an interposition graft for small joint arthroplasty of the hand.

We conducted an experiment on the rabbit forefoot to determine certain features of the graft which has been successful in restoring function to the reconstructed joints and we wished to know what actually became of the cartilage grafts. Five New Zealand white rabbits, each weighing 3.5 kg, had resection of one of the articular surfaces of the right elbow joint followed by a left pinna conchal cartilage interposition graft fixed to the bone stump. The left elbow joint served as the control.

Not only did we demonstrate in this pilot study that the cartilage grafts survived, but also that the hyaline cartilage thickened, indicating possible adaptation and modification of the structure of hyaline cartilage to the demands of a weight-bearing joint. The hyaline cartilage adapts and possibly even mimics the more demanding role of articular cartilage. The elbow joints retained full range of motion. In addition, regeneration of the auricular cartilage was evident given that we had ensured that the anterior perichondrium was preserved during harvest of the auricular cartilage.

This method of conchal cartilage arthroplasty is simple, effective and safe. This small series has shown benefit for the relatively young patients who have had traumatic arthroses. Benefit for patients suffering from degenerative and autoimmune arthritis remains to be assessed.

References

1   Brockman R, Weiland AJ, Small joint arthrodesis. In: Green DP, ed, *Operative Hand Surgery*, 3rd edn, Vol 1 (Churchill Livingstone: New York, 1993) 99–111.

2   Carroll RE, Taber TH, Digital arthroplasty of the proximal interphalangeal joint, *J Bone Joint Surg* (1954) **36A**:912–20.

3   Engkvist O, Johansson SH, Perichondrial arthroplasty: a clinical study in twenty-six patients, *Scand J Plast Reconstr Surg* (1980) **14**:71–87.

4   Engkvist O, Johansson SH, Ohlsen L, et al, Reconstruction of articular cartilage using autologous perichondrial grafts. A preliminary report, *Scand J Plast Reconstr Surg* (1975) **9**:203–6.

5   Ohlsen L, Nordin U, Tracheal reconstruction with perichondrial grafts: an experimental study, *Scand J Plast Reconstr Surg* (1976) **10**:135–45.

6   Skoog T, Johansson SH, The formation of articular cartilage from free perichondrial grafts, *Plast Reconstr Surg* (1976) **57**:1–6

7   Sully L, Jackson IT, Sommerlad BC, Perichondrial grafting in rheumatoid metacarpophalangeal joints, *Hand* (1980) **12**:137–48.

8   Seradge H, Kutz MD, Kleinert HE, et al, Perichondrial resurfacing arthroplasty in the hand, *J Hand Surg* (1984) **9A**:880–6.

9   Vainio K, Vainio arthroplasty of the metacarpophalangeal joints in rheumatoid arthritis, *J Hand Surg* (1989) **14A**:367–8.

10 Tupper JW, The metacarpophalangeal volar plate arthroplasty, *J Hand Surg* (1989) **14A**:371–5.

11 Swanson AB, Maupin BK, Gajjar NV, et al, Flexible implant arthroplasty in the proximal interphalangeal joint of the hand, *J Hand Surg* (1985) **10A**:796–805.

12 Beckenbaugh RD, Linscheid RL, Arthroplasty in the hand and wrist, In: Green DP, ed, *Operative Hand Surgery*, 3rd edn, Vol 1 (Churchill Livingstone: New York, 1993) 143–87.

Commentary

Chapter 17

Having used the total anterior teno-arthrolysis technique since Philippe Saffar described it, I can recommend this approach which derives from the original technique. Two pitfalls are worth mentioning: firstly, the approach of the opposite collateral ligament is quite limited, and secondly, if a previous midlateral incision has been used, it is safer to use the same side as a previous injury of the dorsal branch of the palmar collateral artery on both sides could jeopardize the vascularization of the dorsal skin of the second phalanx.

GF

Chapter 18

Although this technique may seem demanding, we share the opinion that carpometacarpal arthrodesis is indicated in young females with hypermobile carpometacarpal joints. Dorsal excision alone is a destabilizing procedure and pain often persists. We now favor the use of shape memory staples for fixation. Care should be taken not to detach extensor carpi radialis brevis and extensor carpi radialis longus insertions during the procedure and to maintain a gliding surface between extensor tendons and bone.

PS

Chapter 19

This is another interesting technique for resurfacing a very challenging joint. However, in young individuals with limited bone loss and two patent collateral arteries I continue to favour an homodigital island compound DIP to PIP transfer.

The range of motion obtained is more rewarding but at the price of a much more demanding procedure. The technique described here will find an indication for patients in their 40s.

GF

Chapter 20

This group of six patients presents the worst conditions for repair: emergency cases, gunshot injuries, open comminuted fractures, bone loss, associated soft-tissue injuries. Bone grafting was often associated with arthroplasty and one wonders how collateral ligament repair and volar plate reattachment may be performed. However, amazing results were obtained by the authors for these complex injuries. This technique should be tried by other emergency teams to assess its benefits.

PS

This is another interesting interposition technique presenting several original points: the authors use conchal cartilage and do not hesitate to use it to cover a bone block in case of bone loss. According to Table 1, the results are far superior to those of free vascularized joint transfer, at least in adult patients. However, it is a two-stage procedure: it seems to have been used only when one side of the joint was intact and preservation of conchal 'cartilage' on a long term basis remains a concern. I have experienced an initial good range of motion in perichondrial graft with progressive decrease with time. The follow-up of the short series is relatively limited and we are looking for a longer follow-up with a good X-ray of the joint and a good picture of the motion; the 'almost normal' active range of motion of Figure 7 is not convincing enough and the malunion visible on Figure 10 could explain some lack of extension.

GF

21

Recent advances in the treatment of congenital vascular anomalies

Joseph Upton and Patricia E Burrows

Introduction

What is new in the field of congenital vascular anomalies? During the past 5 years a new classification system has been validated following more than 10 years of experience, surgical indications and treatment have become more refined, technology has allowed the invasive radiologist to become an integral part of both the diagnostic and therapeutic team, and finally the field of angiogenesis research has developed a new treatment for hemangiomas. The specific advances include:

(1) The Mulliken–Glowacki biologic classification
(2) Magnetic resonance imaging (MRI)
(3) Sclerotherapy
(4) Embolotherapy
(4) Indications for surgery
(5) Alfa-2a interferon therapy.

Classification

The biologic classification of congenital vascular anomalies proposed in 1982 by Mulliken and Glowacki[1] separated these lesions into two major categories: hemangiomas and malformations. Hemangiomas are described as proliferative lesions with a biphasic growth curve exhibiting a rapid growth phase within the first 18 months of life and followed by a slow, spontaneous involution which is completed by 7–9 years of age. The endothelial cells are actively dividing, accompanied by many mast cells, and produce basic fibroblastic growth factor (b-FGF) during the growth phase.

In contrast, malformations are considered as developmental anomalies which are biologically quiescent. They grow commensurately with the patient and are classified by both their predominant vascular channel (capillary, arteriovenous, venous, lymphatic, or mixed) and by flow characteristics (slow-flow, fast-flow). During the past 14 years this system has been used in a large number of clinics and has proven to be extremely useful to the practising clinician. The initial diagnosis based on morphology and growth characteristic alone is very accurate.[2,3] Biopsy is rarely necessary as radiologic techniques (discussed below), can be used to confirm specific lesions. The first outcome studies using this classification have been able to more specifically define each lesion and consequently provide more specific information in regard to natural history and indications for nonsurgical and surgical treatment.[4]

Magnetic resonance imaging (MRI) and other techniques

Vascular lesions can be readily distinguished by MRI, CT, ultrasound and conventional angiography (Table 1). Of these, recent experiences with MRI imaging have been most dramatic.[5,6] The hallmark of a hemangioma is the presence of an enhancing parenchymal mass, with evidence of high flow. These lesions are typically isointense or hypointense to muscle on T1 weighted imaging, and moderately hyperintense on T2 weighted imaging, with a lobulated configuration. Flow voids are seen. Gradient imaging demonstrates high flow vessels, usually at the

Table 1 Imaging findings in vascular anomalies.

Lesion	Angiography	MRI T1	MRI + Contrast	MRI T2	MRI Gradient	Ultrasound	CT
Hemangioma							
Proliferating	Dil. feeding arts; cap. staining; dil. draining veins	STM; iso- or hypointense to muscle; flow voids	Uniform intense enhancement	Increased signal; lobulated STM; flow voids	HFV within and around STM	Discrete STM containing HFV; decreased art. resistance	Uniformly enhancing STM; dil. vessels
Involuting	As above	Variable fat content	As above	Variable fat	As above	As above	Variable fat content
Involuted	Avascular	High signal (fat)	No enhancement	Decreased signal (fat)	No HFV	Echogenic avascular STM	Fat density; no enhancement
Kasabach–Merritt phenomenon	Hypervascular; diffuse cap. staining	Diffuse STM; skin thickening	Diffuse enhancement	Diffuse increased signal; subcut. stranding	Mildly dil. vessels in and around STM	Diffuse STM with HFV	Diffuse enhancing STM; subcut. stranding
Vascular malformation							
Arteriovenous malformation	Dil. feeding arts, nidus, early opacification of draining veins	STT; flow voids	Diffuse enhancement	Variable increased signal; flow voids	HFV throughout abnormal tissue	HFV with low art. resistance; AV shunt; ±STT	Enhancing vessels and STT; bone sclerosis or destruction
Venous malformation	Contrast puddling on venous phase; sinusoidal spaces and varices on direct injection	Isointense to muscle on T1; ± high signal thrombi	Diffuse or inhomogeneous enhancement	Septated STM; high signal; signal voids (phleboliths)	No HFV; signal voids (phleboliths)	STM of mixed echogenicity; low velocity flow; compressible	STM; variable contrast enhancement; lamellated calcifications (phleboliths)
Lymphatic malformation; macrocystic	Avascular STM; Dil. or anom. veins	STM; low signal; septated	Rim or no enhancement	STM; high signal; fluid/fluid levels	No HFV	Cystic STM; ± vessels in septae	STM; low attenuation; no or rim enhancement
Lymphatic malformation; microcystic	Avascular or cap. staining	STT; hypo- or isointense to muscle	No enhancement	Diffuse increased signal; subcut. stranding	No HFV	STT; echogenic; avascular	Diffuse STT; nonenhancing; subcut. stranding

Abbreviations: anom. = anomalies; arts = arteries; cap. = capillaries; dil. = dilated; HFV = high flow vessels; STM = soft tissue mass; STT = soft tissue thickening; subcut. = subcutaneous. (Reproduced from Burrows et al.[6])

center or along the periphery of the lesion. Ultrasound, with Doppler interrogation, CT imaging, and angiography also provide specific findings (Table 1).

MRI studies have become the 'gold standard' for the evaluation of malformations.[5] Fast-flow malformations with arteriovenous fistuli (AVF) are characterized by dilated feeding arteries and draining veins. A parenchymal mass is not present and should not be confused with adjacent fibrofatty tissue or edema. In the slow-flow group, MRI findings in the capillary group are absent and positive findings should not be confused with another associated deep malformation. Venous malformations may contain phleboliths. Characteristic MRI findings include focal or diffuse collections of high T2 signal, often containing identifiable spaces of variable size separated by septations.[3,5] Small fluid levels may be visible. Flow sensitive images demonstrate no high flow vessels within or around the lesions, but may show evidence of an old thrombus. Contrast administration results in variable enhancement. Lymphatic malformations may be classified as macrocystic, usually found in the axilla, neck, and chest, or microcystic. Evidence of hemorrhage or thrombosis may be present. Microcystic malformations seen in the upper extremity appear typically as a diffuse sheet of bright signal on T2 weighted spin echo MRI, usually without contrast enhancement. CT scans best demonstrate any skeletal distortion.

injection is made, and recorded with serial imaging to document the cannula position within the malformation and the presence or absence of venous blood flow. In the presence of significant venous outflow, local compression is applied around the lesion and the contrast injection repeated until the venous outflow is no longer present. An estimation of the volume of the cannulated part of the malformation is also made from the contrast injection.

Contrast medium is then aspirated or expressed from the malformation and an appropriate quantity of sclerosant is injected. The total volume of injected ethanol should not exceed 1.0 ml per kg of body weight. The most common complications are soft tissue ecchymosis, blistering, and possibly full thickness skin loss. Cardiovascular complications including bradycardia, arrhythmias, and cardiac arrest have been reported. This mandates anesthesia and careful monitoring. Sclerotherapy is not usually curative but can be used to treat symptomatic areas and to significantly decrease the size and pain of large malformations. Small, well localized venous malformations or discrete regions of pain associated with thromboses are best treated with surgical excision.

Symptomatic lymphatic malformations are generally treated by surgical excision. Residual or recurrent cysts may be treated by sclerosant injections, including hypertonic glucose, ethanol, deoxycycline, Ethibloc and OK 432.[9,10]

Sclerotherapy

Sclerotherapy is an important adjunct in the management of slow-flow malformations. It has no role in the treatment of hemangiomas of the upper extremity, which by definition spontaneously involute, or for fast-flow lesions. For venous malformations on the dorsum of the hand, digits and forearm direct percutaneous cannulation of the malformation and contrast injection will specifically define the size and location of the lesion. Injection of sclerosants, most commonly sodium tetradecyl or 100% ethanol, typically results in localized thrombosis and gradual shrinkage. It has become a preferred treatment for large lesions in our center.[7-9] After confirmation of free blood return, a contrast

Embolotherapy

In the past embolization has been indicated after failure of medical therapy and only for the treatment of very complicated, life-endangering hemangiomas and malformations. More recently it has been utilized very effectively preoperatively prior to resection of fast-flow lesions in the head and neck region. Its use in the upper extremity has been quite restricted due to the risk of distal migration of embolized particles and resultant digital or hand loss. Embolization is usually used at the same time as diagnostic angiography.[7,11] Improvements in catheter design and cannulation techniques have enabled our invasive radiologists to become superselective (Figure 1). Our invasive radiologists are able to

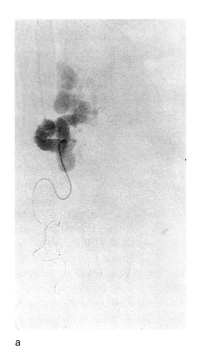

a

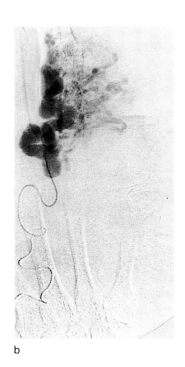

b

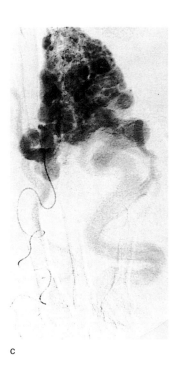

c

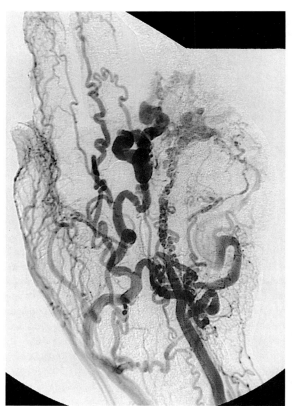

d

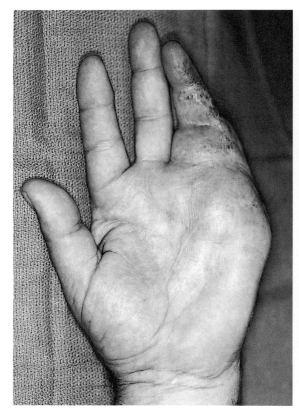

e

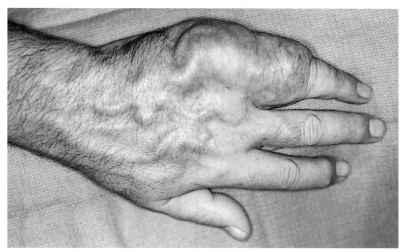

f

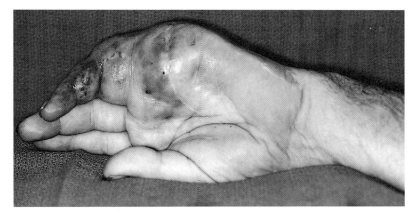

g

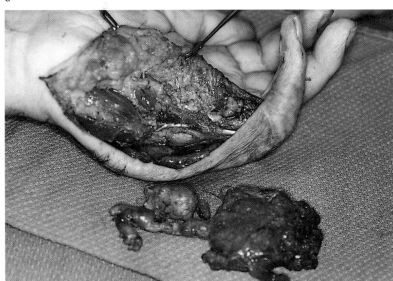

h

Figure 1

(a,b,c) Superselective catheterization of a specific shunt within a fast-flow malformation. (d) Postembolization angiogram. (e,f) Preembolization appearance of the hand in a 40-year-old person with a fast-flow lesion which had been present for 28 years. Pain and steal symptoms of the ring finger had become prominent. (g) Considerable ecchymosis developed postembolization. (h) Surgical resection of the major shunts was then performed with preservation of the ring finger. Healing was uncomplicated.

isolate specific shunts within a fast-flow lesion and to isolate a digital artery of a small child at the proximal interphalangeal joint level.[4] The embolization should result in occlusion of the fistula itself, not just the feeding artery, in order to prevent recurrence through collaterals. Effective devices include steel wire and platinum/fiber coils, detachable balloons, and tissue adhesives. Recently, embolization with 100% ethanol has been proposed as an ablative procedure.[12] Detachable balloons placed in the axillary artery and large associated shunts prior to major upper limb amputation have significantly decreased blood loss.

In general, arteriovenous malformations are impossible to cure with embolization alone and those fast-flow malformations of the upper extremity which are amenable to surgical excision can be effectively treated with presurgical embolization. Experience with these techniques in the upper extremity is very limited! Children with fast-flow, Type C malformations in the hand and forearm are presently being embolized, but their prognosis is poor due to the progressive natural history of these difficult lesions.[11,12] Most progress to amputation.[4]

Surgical resection

A recent review of 209 patients with malformations treated over a 25-year period of time indicated that surgery can be safely performed in certain slow-flow groups. Within the slow-flow group 131 procedures were performed in 51% of 152 venous, lymphatic, and combined malformations after failed conservative treatment. Most procedures were performed for relief of pain, mass effect, or functional impairment. Compression neuropathies were not common. Within the fast-flow group 45 procedures were performed in 18 of 25 total patients. Nine of these patients ultimately had amputations for uncontrollable progression of Type C fast-flow lesions. Embolization was used six times prior to a major resection and/or amputation. Types A and B fast-flow malformations, which were confined to specific regions of the hand and did not progress, were the most amenable to surgical resection. Microvascular revascularization and tissue replacement as needed were useful.[4]

Interferon therapy

Interferon is an FDA approved drug which was originally investigated for its antiviral effects in the treatment of those with the acquired immunodeficiency syndrome (AIDS). Anecdotal clinical reports and the observation that interferon inhibited the locomotion of capillary endothelium in vitro[13] indicated that alfa-2a interferon inhibited angiogenesis in mice[14]; this finding led to its first clinical uses.[15]

For the past 5 years it has been used for the treatment of life-threatening hemangiomas of infancy in the Boston Children's Hospital.[16] Children with life-threatening or vision-impairing lesions are treated with daily injections of up to 3.0×10^6 units per m^2 of body surface area per day with treatment courses lasting up to 12–18 months. There has been an 85% positive response rate in contrast to a 15% response rate from corticosteroids. Transient side effects of treatment with interferon alfa 2a include fever, neutropenia, and occasional skin necrosis with dramatic response of massive lesions. Spastic diplegia observed in one patient has been the only long-term toxic result after a mean follow-up of 20 months. Although there were some expressed reservations about the results of this study because it was not a randomized, double-blind study, the data have been scrutinized by the National Institutes of Health (NIH) and the Harvard Medical School and interpreted as valid. This drug appears to induce the early regression of hemangiomas of infancy. It has no effect upon malformations.

Future research and treatment of these difficult hemangiomas and malformations will be directed to specifically targeting the endothelial cell within each specific lesion for treatment. The fields of angiogenesis and gene-directed therapy offer tremendous promise for future management of the difficult vascular anomalies seen in children.

References

1   Mulliken JB, Glowacki J, Hemangiomas and vascular malformations of infants and children: a biological classification based on endothelial characteristics, *Plast Reconstr Surg* (1982) **69**:412.

2   Finn MC, Glowacki J, Mulliken JB, Congenital vascular lesions: clinical application of a new classification, *J Pediatr Surg* (1983) **18**:894.

3   Jackson IT, Carreno R, Potparic Z, et al, Hemangioma, vascular malformations, and lymphovenous malformations: classification and methods of treatment, *Plast Reconstr Surg* (1993) **91**:1216.

4   Coombs C, Upton J, Mulliken JB, et al, Vascular malformations of the upper limb: a review of 209 patients, *J Hand Surg* (1996) in press.

5   Meyer JS, Hoffer FA, Barnes PD, et al, MRI correlation with biological classification of soft tissue vascular anomalies, *Am J Radiol* (1991) **157**:559.

6   Burrows PE, Robertson RI, Barnes PD, Angiography and the evaluation of cerebrovascular disease of childhood, *Neuroimag Clin N Am* (1996) **6**:561.

7   Burrows PE, Fellows KE, Techniques for management of pediatric vascular anomalies. In: Cope C, ed, *Current Techniques in Interventional Radiology* (Current Medicine: Philadelphia, 1995) 12–27.

8   de Lorimer A, Sclerotherapy for venous malformations, *J Pediatr Surg* (1995) **30**:188.

9   Dubois JM, Sebag GH, De Prost Y, et al, Soft-tissue venous malformations in children: percutaneous sclerotherapy with Ethibloc, *Radiology* (1991) **180**:195.

10 Ojita S, Tsuto T, Deguchi P et al, OK-432 therapy for unresectable lymphantiomas in children, *J Pediatr Surg* (1991) **26**:263.

11 Lasjaunias P, Berenstein T, Craniofacial hemangiomas, vascular malformations and angiomatoses: specific aspects. In: *Surgical Neuroangiography*. Vol 2. *Endovascular Treatment of Craniofacial Lesions* (Springer-Verlag: Heidelberg, Berlin, 1987).

12 Gomes AS, Embolization therapy of congenital arteriovenous malformations: use of alternative approaches, *Radiology* (1994) **190**:191.

13 Brouty-Boye D, Zetter BR, Inhibition of cell motility by interferon, *Science* (1980) **208**:516.

14 Sidky YA, Borden EC, Inhibition of angiogenesis by interferons: effects on tumor and lymphocytic-induced vascular responses, *Cancer Res* (1987) **47**:5155.

15 White CW, Sondheimer HM, Crouch EC, et al, Treatment of pulmonary hemangiomatosis with recombinant interferon alfa-2a, *N Engl J Med* (1989) **320**:1197.

16 Ezekowitz RAB, Mulliken JB, Folkman J, Interferon alfa-2a therapy for life-threatening hemangiomas of infancy, *N Engl J Med* (1992) **326**:1456.

22

Treatment of vasospastic disease in the hand

Charles L Puckett, Joseph L Grzeskiewicz and Geoffrey J Yule

Introduction

There are few problems in hand surgery more difficult than vasospastic phenomena. Although the occasional patient will present with a localized or idiopathic form of vasospasm (Raynaud's phenomenon), the majority of patients will have some underlying disorder. Thus a superimposed component of local vasospasm may aggravate an occult or apparent collagen disease, Buerger's disease, or an even more obscure pathophysiology. Maurice Raynaud described with clarity the phenomenon of extremity vasospasm in his 1862 work *On Local Asphyxia and Symmetrical Gangrene of the Extremities.*[1] Temporary or more permanent relief of vasospasm is a worthwhile pursuit that can diminish the degree of ischemia despite the fact that the underlying disease may be untreatable and thus ultimately progressive.

While the precise pathophysiology of vasospasm remains obscure, two remediable influences are often involved. These are heightened sympathetic activity and a local response to nicotine. At present, alterations in the effects of these two entities are our major opportunities for improvement. There now appears to be sufficient experience to indicate that efficient interruption of sympathetic activity can be of at least palliative value in the relief of vasospasm and thus may be helpful in many collagen vascular disease patients and in some of those patients who might fit into the broad category of Buerger's disease.

Medical therapy

It is not our intent here to provide a comprehensive review of medical treatment for vasospastic disease of the hand. However, it would be inappropriate to fail to mention some cardinal tenets and therapeutic approaches that complement surgical treatment. All patients must avoid exposure of their hands to cold and must relinquish exposure to nicotine in any form. In those patients in whom vibration-induced occupational vasospasm is documented, cessation of that exposure will often lead to improvement. In our experience, the most valuable of these three entities is nicotine avoidance.

Systemic sympatholytic medications may offer some relief of symptomatology, but often at the cost of unacceptable side-effects. For this reason intraarterial injection has been employed to focus effect and minimize dosage. Reserpine has perhaps had the widest use in this form, but with results ranging from marked improvement to none. We have noted occasional improvement with intraarterial thorazine. Other systemic drugs which can effect relaxation of vascular smooth muscle have demonstrated varying improvement, but often with troublesome side-effects: these include nifedipine, captopril, prostaglandins PGE_1 and PGI_2, and ketanserin (a serotonin antagonist). Viscosity and rheology modifying drugs (aspirin, dextran, and pentoxifylline) are often employed as adjunctive therapy.

Freedman has demonstrated improvement utilizing biofeedback training in some Raynaud's disease patients.[2]

Surgical management of vasospasm

The following discussion on surgical management of vasospasm does not intend to be a comprehensive discussion of the overall management of such patients, but instead emphasizes principles and techniques, some new, some old, which we currently find to be of value. In addition to the techniques discussed, and depending on the degree of ischemia, these patients may also of course require care of ischemic wounds and, not infrequently, amputations of varying degree. Our discussion will be on the relief of vasoconstriction.

Historically, cervicothoracic sympathectomy was the standard therapy for sympathetic over activity in the upper extremity just as lumbosacral sympathectomy was at one time for the lower extremity. Poor response and cure rates initially and recurrence of vasospastic phenomena after apparent initial success have placed this operation in disfavor. The benefits of a more distal sympathectomy were probably first appreciated as vascular reconstruction was applied to patients with hypothenar hammer syndrome. With resection of the thrombosed segment of ulnar artery and arterial reconstruction, it became apparent that the sympathectomy thus accomplished might be as important an effect as the reestablishment of ulnar artery flow. Despite patency rates of only 50%, most patients noted relief of symptoms and this improvement was thought to reesult, in significant part, from the sympathectomy occasioned by the arterial resection.

In 1980 Flatt first reported on digital sympathectomy, a new method of reducing sympathetic tone at an even more peripheral level.[3] He noted that the routes of sympathetic nerve supply to the vascular tree in the hand were numerous, and that the blood vessels to the hand have a constant and identifiable sympathetic nerve supply from the major peripheral nerves. The distal third of the radial artery is innervated by one filament from the superficial branch of the radial nerve and by a total of eight additional branches from the lateral cutaneous nerve of the forearm. The distal third of the ulnar artery is supplied by three branches from the ulnar nerve and a branch from the medial cutaneous nerve of the forearm. Within the hand, the superficial palmar arch receives almost a dozen branches from the common digital nerves arising from the median and ulnar nerves. The deep palmar arch receives two branches from the deep branch of the ulnar nerve and an additional one from the median nerve. The digital arteries receive anywhere from three to twelve branches from the digital nerves. These nerves are readily identifiable at exploration (Figure 1). Their sympathetic fibers ramify in the adventitia of the digital arteries.

Flatt based his technique of a careful and tedious circumferential excision of the adventitia of the proper digital arteries on the knowledge of these anatomical points. He described an approach utilizing a transverse zig-zag incision at the level of the palmar crease to enable adventitial stripping of the digital vessels. Under magnification with loupes or a microscope, the adventitia was removed circumferentially from the proper digital artery for a longitudinal distance of at least 3–4 mm. He pointed out that the depth of the excision is a judgement area, as one must be careful not to perforate the vessel by being too aggressive, while at the same time recognizing that the more adventitia that is removed, the more likely it is that a therapeutic sympathectomy will be achieved. He reported on his series of eight patients treated with this procedure, and while he utilized finger temperature recording as his only objective measurement, he was able to demonstrate subjective improvement in a majority of his patients, a significant temperature elevation of between 1° and 4° in all of them, and healing of ulcers in all but one of the patients.

Wilgis subsequently modified the techniques of Flatt, surmising that because there exist sympathetic nerves in the distal peripheral nerves and the objective of treatment is pain relief in the digits, the sympathetic interruption should be performed as far distally as possible.[4] Using a similar transverse zig-zag incision to expose the vessels and with the aid of the microscope, he removed the adventitia from the

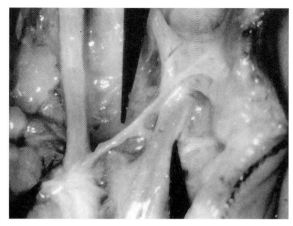

a

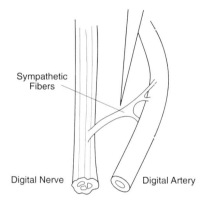

b

Figure 1

(a) Intraoperative view of a common digital neurovascular bundle demonstrating sympathetic fibers from the digital nerve joining the adventitia of the digital artery in the hand. (b) Diagram of the intraoperative view.

common and proper digital arteries for a distance of up to 2 cm, occasionally going as far distally as the proximal interphalangeal joint. He stressed patient selection, making the point that surgically correctable arterial lesions should be identified and addressed appropriately first. He only performed this procedure on those patients who demonstrated a change in digital response to cold provocative testing with bupivacaine digital nerve blockade.

Of the 10 patients included in Wilgis's series, 9 showed improved digital blood flow as measured clinically as well as with pulse volume recordings and radioisotope studies. Wound healing within 2 weeks occurred in all patients with ulcers, and all but one had a significant improvement in cold tolerance over a follow-up period of 4 years. He was careful to warn that the response to surgery may not be immediate due to residual sympathetic activity from circulating humoral factors. However, a response is usually seen within hours after operation, and within 24 hours the fingers are warmer. Egloff et al corroborated the results of Wilgis with their series of 13 patients in whom they performed digital sympathectomies extending well out in the proper digital arteries.[5]

The majority of the patients demonstrating therapeutic response to this type of procedure have been those suffering from chronic ischemia secondary to trauma and frostbite injuries, and as Jones points out,[6] the results have been less satisfying in those patients suffering from the connective tissue diseases, especially scleroderma. This led Jones to further modify the techniques of peripheral sympathectomy. Because he initially began exploring the palms of patients with connective tissue diseases to determine their candidacy for microvascular reconstruction, his technique of digital sympathectomy has evolved into a much more extensive procedure than that of either Flatt or Wilgis. He made the observation that patients with connective tissue diseases have a striking amount of periadventitial fibrosis around the neurovascular bundles of the fingers as well as the common digital arteries and the superficial palmar arch producing external compression of those vessels. Consequently, he has utilized an inverted J-shaped incision extending from the carpus distally with the transverse portion of the J paralleling the palmar arch in the distal palmar crease, allowing for extensions distally into the fingers by Bruner incisions as deemed necessary by the surgeon to gain access to the proper digital vessels out to the level of the proximal interphalangeal joint.

Through this approach the entire superficial arch system can be visualized from distal radial and ulnar arteries to the proximal interphalangeal joint and from the radialis indicis artery to the ulnar digital artery of the small finger.

Segmental occlusions can be identified and bypassed or resected and reconstructed, and extensive stripping of fibrosis and adventitia can be performed. Jones noted that intraoperatively vessels which initially appeared occluded, became supple and patent after resection of the fibrotic adventitia. He proposed that the ischemic symptoms of these patients may be caused by three different mechanisms:

(1) an exaggerated sympathetic vasoconstrictive response to cold,
(2) segmental occlusions of the small arteries in the hand due to intimal proliferation, and
(3) external compression of the common and proper digital arteries due to periadventitial fibrosis.

Consequently, Jones suggested that digital sympathectomy in these patients may function not only by removing the sympathetic fibers from the digital arteries, but also by alleviating the external compression caused by the pathological fibrosis. He reported short term success with this type of technique in that his patients have experienced relief from their chronic pain, healing of ulcers, and improvement in the degree of cold tolerance. He noted that long-term follow-up data are not available yet, and will be required to accurately assess the benefits of this procedure. It was his impression, however, that the immediate benefit may not be a lasting one, as the progressive occlusive small vessel disease is likely to recur and ultimately become the predominant factor in the patient's ischemia.

While presently the data reflecting long-term follow-up on digital sympathectomy are sparse, some studies have been performed revealing beneficial results from the procedure. Levine et al reported encouraging outcomes in their series of 33 patients, in whom digital sympathectomy was performed between 1981 and 1992, and of whom a 1 to 11 year follow-up period was recorded in 30.[7] Their procedure involved sharply removing the adventitia from the common digital arteries from the superficial arch to 3–5 mm past the bifurcation or a similar distance along an isolated proper digital artery. They reported that while all of their patients experienced immediate postoperative pain relief, only 60% were totally relieved of cold intolerance. However of those 40% still reporting cold intolerance, all but two reported their symptoms to be mild and none required any further narcotics for the long term. Complications of wound healing, stiffness, and recurrent ulceration appeared to be more problematic in those patients with scleroderma and other collagen vascular diseases.

Authors' preferred technique

Our method of digital sympathectomy is modified from that of Flatt[3] and Wilgis[4] and employs a J-shaped or curved incision through which the superficial arch can be exposed. Extensions from this curvilinear incision are directed toward each interdigital space as longitudinal limbs. Through these incisions, we can access the common digital vessels to each of the web spaces and expose the proper digital vessels for approximately 2 cm. We have settled on this incision because it creates no real flaps which might, in turn, be made ischemic by virtue of the underlying pathophysiology. The index radial digital vessel and the fifth ulnar digital vessel can be visualized through these incisions, although usually they are not. Separate incisions overlying the paths of these two vessels can be made if necessary. Although longitudinal incisions of the volar aspect of the hand are generally not favored, the compromise here is the avoidance of ischemic palmar skin and to date we have not encountered any significant flexion contracture with these incisions.

Sympathectomy is begun by selection of the common digital vessel and identification of its bifurcation. We then proceed with an extensive sharp removal of adventitia from approximately 2 cm proximal to the bifurcation to an equal distance beyond in the proper digital vessel. We believe that sharp excision of the adventitia is less likely to traumatize the vessel at the intimal and medial levels than would blunt adventitial stripping.[8] We generally do this under relatively low power magnification, with the operating microscope and microsurgical instruments. During the process of this adventitiectomy one commonly encounters nerve filaments traveling from the proximal segment of the digital nerves to intertwine with this adventitia. Adventitial excision can be fairly aggressive since there is adventitia remaining surrounding the medial layer even when fairly extensive fibroareolar tissue has been removed. Obviously, care must be taken to avoid injuring the vessel and punctate bleeding may be encountered which probably represents divided vasa vasorum. Careful hemostasis should be obtained and gentle and accurate skin approximation completed. A very light compressive dressing is applied often utilizing synthetic cotton (Surgistuff). A dorsal splint may discourage movement, although the position of the hand and fingers is probably not critical.

As observed by others, our expectation following digital sympathectomy is improvement, not cure. In most patients ulcers heal, cold tolerance is improved, and pain is diminished. Response is closely tied to the degree of underlying pathology, particularly to the presence of obstructive vascular disease. Clearly, isolated vasospasm patients fare best, while collagen vascular disease patients do less well. We believe that relief of vasospasm is of value in these patients and may provide tangible improvement. However, with disease progression this relief may be of limited duration.

While some patients suffering from chronic digital ischemia may find their way to the office of the hand surgeon primarily, most will already have a diagnosis of Raynaud's disease or some form of secondary vasospastic disorder as a result of a collagen vascular disease or other systemic illness. Hence, most will have received treatment in the form of medical or conservative management by an internist or rheumatologist. The hand surgeon must understand the various nonsurgical treatment modalities available as mentioned earlier in this section. Furthermore, since patient selection is the key to success with all of the available surgical procedures, it is imperative that the hand surgeon be facile in the complete evaluation of these disorders including history and physical exam, noninvasive studies, and angiography. When the decision to operate is made it should be based upon conclusive studies if at all possible. While digital sympathectomy is no panacea for these patients, the available reports on this procedure show it to be a treatment based on sound rationale with a significant majority of the patients obtaining beneficial results. However, it should be noted that, when possible, correctable obstructive lesions should be addressed with vascular reconstruction such that the relief of vasospasm is complemented with maximal perfusion pressure.

References

1 Raynaud M, *On Local Asphyxia and Symmetrical Gangrene of the Extremities. Selected Monographs.* (Translated by T. Barlow.) (New Syderham Society: London, 1888) **121**:1.
2 Freedman RR, Physiological mechanisms of temperature of biofeedback, *Biofeedback Self-Reg* (1991) **6**:95–115.
3 Flatt A, Digital artery sympathectomy, *J Hand Surg* (1980) **5**:550.
4 Wilgis EFS, Evaluation and treatment of chronic digital ischemia, *Ann Surg* (1981) **193**:693.
5 Egloff DV, Mifsud RP, Verdan CL, Superselective digital sympathectomy in Raynaud's phenomenon, *Hand* (1983) **15**:110.
6 Jones NF, Ischemia of the hand in systemic disease, *Clin Plast Surg* (1989) **16**:547.
7 Levine NS, Lipton JS, Brou JA, et al, A long term experience with digital sympathectomy. In preparation.
8 Lohman R, Sieminow M, Rockwell WB, et al, Acute adverse effects of blunt adventitial stripping, *Ann Plast Surg* (1995) **35**:60.

23

Temporary ectopic implantation of amputated parts

Donald C Sheridan and Michael B Wood

Introduction

In the several decades since the first successful replantation was performed, the field of replantation surgery has been at the forefront of innovation. Viktor Meyer states

> 'The essence of replantation is to avoid stereotyped procedures while being prepared to constantly reorganize the five basic tissues (bone, blood vessels, nerves, muscle–tendon, and skin) according to the biologic, functional, and technical dictates of the individual situation'.[1]

This essence of innovation is epitomized in the development of techniques for temporary ectopic implantation. Temporary ectopic implantation involves the banking of an amputated part in a remote location for later replantation when immediate replantation or revascularization is not possible because of the nature of the injury at the recipient site or when the medical condition of the injured patient mitigates a prolonged reconstructive procedure.

With only four reported cases,[2–5] there is a paucity of information in the literature, and therefore any discussion of this topic is necessarily anecdotal. However, the nature of ectopic replantation makes any significantly large series unlikely for some time to come. A summary of the apparent indications and recommended techniques will provide a basis of knowledge and understanding for the microsurgeon faced with these difficult clinical challenges.

Indications

Although the published case reports are detailed and demonstrate considerable technical expertise, they are limited in number and therefore any stated indications for temporary ectopic replantation should be considered apparent or relative indications. These include devastating, segmental injuries in which the distal part is relatively uninjured, but in which the wounds themselves are extensive, ill-defined, and badly contaminated, when the necessary radical debridement required for primary replantation would lead to loss of important structures that are critical for a good functional and aesthetic result, and when these borderline structures might be salvaged by good open wound management or early coverage. There should be a relatively uninjured amputated part that is critical to the restoration of upper limb function such as a thumb or more proximal limb amputation. Additionally, severe segmental injury with amputation of a distal part as well as more proximal injury requiring reconstruction may be considered for the technique. Such wounds might occur in agricultural accidents, industrial machine crush injuries, gunshot wounds, and high voltage electrical burns.

When faced with such an injury, the treatment options formerly included immediate replantation or revascularization, debridement and open wound management with or without soft tissue coverage procedures, amputation and preservation of as much length of the limb as possible. Delayed replantation with temporary ectopic implantation may also now be considered as an option in the surgeon's armamentarium. Certainly the treatment option should be individualized to both the patient (who is optimally motivated, compliant, otherwise healthy and will not accept amputation), and the specific reconstructive needs in an attempt to maximize functional outcome within the limits of expense and effort acceptable to both patient and surgeon.

Techniques

Once the surgeon has determined that temporary ectopic implantation is indicated, several technical points should be considered. These include surgical preparation of the amputated part and stump wound, selection and preparation of the ectopic implantation site and vascular pedicle, interval period care of the ectopically implanted part and extremity wound, and finally the timing and techniques of definitive replantation.

Since the determination to proceed with temporary ectopic implantation is often made in the operating room by the surgical replantation team, the initial primary replantation protocol of patient management, amputated part handling and a two-team surgical approach is readily adapted to allow for ectopic implantation. Ideally, preoperative discussion with patient and family would include all potential options and allow an ascertation of their desires, but realistically the peri-injury period is such an understandably overwhelming and difficult period that even the most well adjusted could be expected to have difficulty comprehending a procedure as complex as temporary ectopic replantation. Therefore the early establishment of a trusting relationship between surgeon, patient and family is critical to assist them through this difficult time.

Treatment of the wound site and amputated part ideally would occur simultaneously to expedite the procedure and minimize ischemia time. If necessary, the use of temporary heparinized silicone or plastic stents can be considered to provide temporary blood flow to the amputated part if ischemia time is a concern.[2,5] As with any open injury, careful debridement is vital to a successful outcome. Since ectopic implantation of the amputated part will be performed as a primary procedure, the debridement needs to be radical and thorough. However, the stump wound should be conservatively debrided since the goal of temporary ectopic implantation is preservation of borderline tissues at the stump site.

Proximal segmental injuries to the bone should be managed at this time in order to provide stability. Soft tissue management of the stump should consist of appropriate open wound techniques and serial debridements. The concept of early soft tissue coverage which has been shown to reduce infection, minimize edema and enhance function is now generally well accepted.[6] Vascular repair is indicated in the proximal limb when indicated for the preservation of important and relatively uninjured tissues. Vein grafts should be utilized when segmental vessel loss is present. Nerve repair should be performed primarily when it is possible to identify the zone of injury. This is frequently not possible, however, due to the extensive and often high energy nature of these wounds. If a primary tension-free repair cannot be achieved, then nerve grafting should optimally be performed in a delayed fashion.

Selection of an appropriate temporary ectopic host site and vascular pedicle is a crucial step. The potential options are protean, but the apparent preferred sites from the reported cases appear to be on the abdominal or chest wall.[2-4] The abdomen and chest wall appear to be convenient and readily accessible and allow for stable immobilization and facilitation of interval period physiotherapy, but practically any site which meets these requirements may be utilized. The inferior epigastic vessels in the lower quadrant of the abdomen satisfy these requirements and are utilized in three reports in the literature.[2,4,5] Another reported pedicle that appears reasonable is the thoracodorsal vessels from the axilla to the chest wall.[3] One potential advantage of this pedicle is flexibility in dealing with vessel size mismatch. The diameter of the proximal thoracodorsal artery roughly matches the radial and ulnar artery at the wrist and more distally, near the branch to serratus, the thoracodorsal vessels are equivalent to digital level diameters. The authors have utilized the femoral/saphenous vessels with success.

Securing the amputated part to the host site is also an important step to avoid the catastrophic complication of inadvertent avulsion.[3] The use of circumferential skin sutures can be augmented by the suturing of deep fascial layers to provide added security. Additionally, implanting the amputated part with the digits oriented in a cephalad direction may minimize edema by improving venous outflow and facilitate physiotherapy by allowing the hand to swing outward for passive joint motion.[2]

The period between temporary ectopic implantation and definitive replantation is termed the interval period. In addition to standard post-microvascular replantation patient management, there are several features of the interval period that are unique, including preparation of the stump wound and care of the ectopically implanted amputated part. The stump wound should be treated aggressively with open wound management, serial debridements and early soft tissue coverage where indicated. The amputated part should be carefully monitored for any signs of vascular compromise, infection, or soft tissue necrosis. Splinting of the implanted part is not only important to prevent possible avulsion of the microvascular pedicle, but should also facilitate joint mobilization. Owing to the unique nature of this procedure, splint fabrication is not routine and the surgeon and splint technician must be both creative and cooperative to achieve the desired goals. The importance of interval period intensive physiotherapy cannot be understated. Anti-edema measures and passive joint range of motion are critical to preservation and eventual restoration of function of the amputated part following definitive replantation.

The timing of definitive replantation must be carefully planned. The patient should be medically stable and physiologically able to undergo the procedure. The wound must be free of any remaining necrotic tissue and contamination to avoid potential complications related to infection. The zone of injury should be clearly delineated particularly with respect to the vascular structures to be used for anastomosis. This will allow planning for the use of vein grafts where needed to avoid the use of any vessel with potential intimal injury. The techniques of bone fixation are similar to those used in replantation surgery and the method of osteosynthesis chosen depends on the individual reconstructive

needs and surgeon preference.[7] Nerve reconstruction may be considered at this point or delayed to a future date as can any additional soft tissue coverage or grafting as indicated. Although the interval periods in the two reported successful cases in the literature were both approximately 10 weeks, definitive replantation may be performed at any time when the above criteria are met.

Illustrative case

A previously unreported case of temporary ectopic replantation performed by the senior author illustrates the application of the above principles. A 37-year-old, otherwise healthy, right-hand-dominant female sustained a left trans-elbow amputation in an industrial conveyor belt accident, resulting in severe soft tissue injury. The proximal stump was essentially degloved from the mid-humerus with long skin flaps on the relatively uninjured distal part (Figure 1). The median, ulnar, and radial nerves were avulsed with a resulting long zone of injury. The joint surfaces on both the proximal and the distal part were pristine.

Both the proximal stump and distal amputated part were explored, irrigated and debrided simultaneously. Owing to the extensive soft tissue injury of the proximal stump, preservation of upper limb function required temporary banking until fear of sepsis and necrotic material had passed. An incision was made from the groin to the medial aspect of the distal thigh with exposure of the greater saphenous vein and superficial femoral artery. Anastomosis of the superficial femoral artery to the brachial artery was performed with a reverse vein graft segment. A branched segment of the greater saphenous vein was anastomosed to two veins of the forearm. This restored vascularity in the amputated part with excellent capillary refill. Total hypothermic ischemia time was 7 hours. A forearm fasciotomy was performed and the skin edges at both the amputation and fasciotomy sites were coapted to the long wound on the medial aspect of the thigh with sutures and skin staples (Figure 2). The patient was transferred to the intensive care unit for hemodynamic monitoring.

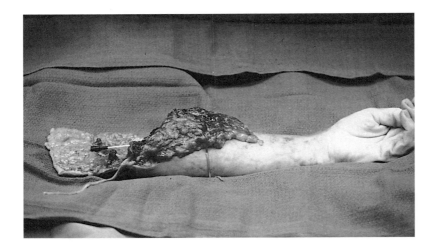

Figure 1

Trans-elbow level amputation sustained in a conveyor belt accident resulted in severe soft tissue injury at the amputation site, while the distal part is relatively uninjured.

At repeat debridement 2 days later it was noted that the proximal brachial artery was thrombosed for a distance of 15 cm proximal to the elbow. It is likely that use of this vessel for a primary replantation would have led to failure due to the extensive zone of injury. Identification of the problem allowed for the planning of the use of vein grafting at the time of definitive replantation. Over the course of the next 2 weeks passive physiotherapy was instituted on the ectopically implanted part and serial debridements of the stump were performed every other day (a total of five debridements were required to prepare the stump to accept implantation of the distal part). After this, the stump wound appeared clean with good granulation tissue and without the presence of necrotic material or frank infection (Figure 3).

Two weeks after injury definitive replantation was performed. The forearm was detached from its ectopic site and the femoral arteriotomy site repaired with a vein graft patch. Vein grafts were also used to anastomose the brachial artery and vein following stabilization of the elbow with two Steinman pins, tension band wiring of the olecranon and elbow ligament reconstruction with free tendon graft. Direct coaptation of the proximal median nerve to the distal ulnar nerve was performed with interfascicular grafting of the radial nerve utilizing a sural nerve graft. A latissimus dorsi myocutaneous flap was raised on its thoracodorsal pedicle and rotated to provide additional soft tissue coverage at the amputation site along with split-thickness skin grafting.

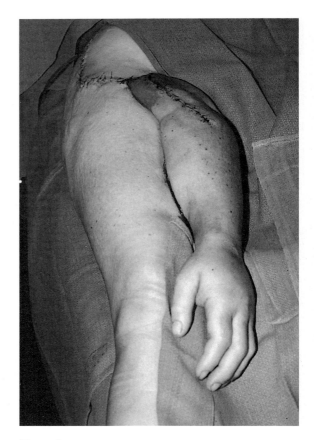

Figure 2

The amputated forearm was ectopically implanted on the medial aspect of the thigh with anastomosis to the superficial femoral artery and greater saphenous vein.

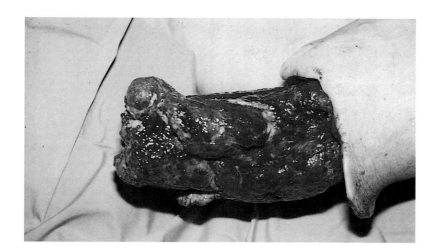

Figure 3

Immediately prior to definitive replantation the proximal stump wound was clean, had no evidence of necrotic tissue or infection, and was covered with good granulation tissue.

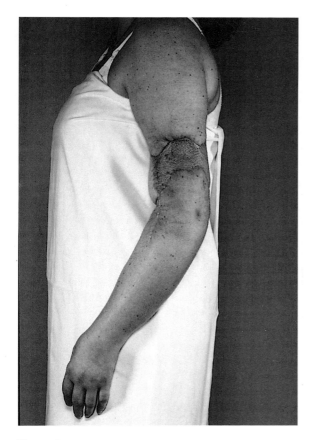

Figure 4

The final appearance of the upper extremity demonstrates a good overall cosmetic result that was acceptable to both surgeon and patient.

One week later additional split-thickness skin grafting was performed to cover the remaining areas of open granulation tissue. At 4 weeks following replantation the Steinman pins were removed allowing controlled passive elbow motion. At 6 months after replantation, bipolar advancement of the latissimus flap using a free plantaris graft distally was performed in order to restore active elbow flexion. At the same time sural nerve grafting was performed to the median–ulnar neurorraphy site along with flap resculpturing to improve cosmesis (Figure 4).

One year later, residual elbow stiffness was addressed with an elbow capsulotomy, triceps tenolysis, and heterotopic bone excision. Two years later, however, a total elbow arthroplasty was performed in an attempt to provide stable range of motion. At her last clinical follow-up approximately 4 years after initial injury, the elbow had passive range of motion from 20° to 110°. Active elbow extension was excellent, but active elbow flexion was possible only with gravity eliminated. Intrinsic motor recovery occurred including the interossei and adductor pollicis. Radial nerve recovery was also evident with active wrist extension of approximately 10°. Gross sensation was present in the median nerve distribution. Bipolar pectoralis major transfer was discussed in an attempt to improve elbow flexion but the patient was emotionally exhausted and refused further surgical intervention. At the last follow-up, questionnaire responses indicated that the patient had limited use of the replanted extremity and did not use it for activities of daily living but overall preferred the limb salvage procedure to amputation and was satisfied with the cosmetic result.

Conclusion

Temporary ectopic implantation of amputated parts is an innovative procedure that may be used in an attempt to restore function and preserve the appearance of a severely injured limb. Although the results in terms of functional outcome have been modest, which likely reflects the nature of the initial injury, temporary ectopic implantation is a viable option in a surgeon's armamentarium as an alternative to limb amputation. In the face of these difficult clinical challenges, the treatment options should be carefully reviewed and the option chosen individualized to both the patient and the specific reconstructive needs in an attempt to maximize functional outcome within the limits of expense and effort acceptable to both patient and surgeon.

References

1   Meyer V, Zhong-Wei C, Beasley R, Basic technical considerations in reattachment surgery, *Orthop Clin North Am* (1981) **12**:871–95.

2   Chernofsky M, Sauer P, Temporary ectopic implantation, *J Hand Surg* (1990) **15A**:910–14.

3   Godina M, Bajec J, Baraga A, Salvage of the mutilated upper extremity with temporary ectopic implantation of the undamaged part, *Plast Reconstr Surg* (1986) **78**:295–9.

4   Hallock G, Transient single-digit ectopic implantation, *J Reconstr Microsurg* (1992) **8**:309–11.

5   Mangus D, Ectopic vascularization using the inferior epigastric system, *Plast Reconstr Surg* (1987) **79**:495.

6   Godina M, Early microsurgical reconstruction of complex trauma of the extremities, *Plast Reconstr Surg* (1986) **78**:285–92.

7   Brown M, Wood M, Techniques of bone fixation in replantation surgery, *Microsurgery* (1990) **11**:255–60.

24

Fingertip reconstruction by free tissue transfer

Tsu-Min Tsai and Huey-Yuan Tien

Introduction

The goal in the treatment of fingertip injuries is to restore function and cosmetic appearance and to prevent complications. Besides return of fine sensibility and durable soft tissue cover, it is particularly important to restore the maximum length in critically opposing digits. Each treatment option should be evaluated according to the characteristics of the injury and the age, sex, vocation, and needs of the patient. Some people, such as guitarists and piano players, need finger pulps of normal sensitivity. Others, such as lawyers and politicians, typically desire fingers of near normal appearance because of their roles in public life. All factors should be taken into consideration when the treatment plan for a particular patient is chosen.

Selection of a treatment for a fingertip injury depends on the amount of soft tissue involved, the presence of bone and tendon exposure, and the function to be reconstructed. The simplest method of treatment is healing by secondary intention. A small pulp defect without exposed bone can be treated by either split- or full-thickness skin grafts. Fingertip injuries with exposed bone can be treated by various local flaps. Distally located flaps can also be harvested from the chest, abdomen, groin or contralateral arm.

The first toe-to-hand transfer was performed by Nicoladoni in 1898 (with a pedicle graft). In 1973, the American Replantation Mission to Red China reported that Yang had performed the first clinical transfer of second toe to thumb in 1966. The clinical feasibility of the venous flap from the foot was reported by Honda et al in 1984.[1] In

1987, we reported the clinical application of venous flaps from the adjacent finger, which was modified later with an arterialized pattern.[2] Free vascularized nail grafts have also been proposed by various methods. Improvements in microsurgical equipment and techniques have allowed replantation of amputated fingertips and free tissue transfers to become routine procedures for fingertip injuries. The next section focuses mainly on the field of free tissue transfer. Some major techniques, indications, and comparisons with classic techniques will be discussed.

Technical aspects

Various techniques are used to meet different reconstructive requirements. The following cases demonstrate the techniques used to fulfil specific demands.

Case 1: free toe-to-hand transfer to regain length and cosmetic appearance

A 37-year-old right-handed male radiologist sustained a lawn mower injury which resulted in traumatic amputations over the right index finger at the level of the mid-distal phalanx through the nailbed and middle finger at the distal interphalangeal (DIP) joint. Replantation was performed immediately after injury. The middle

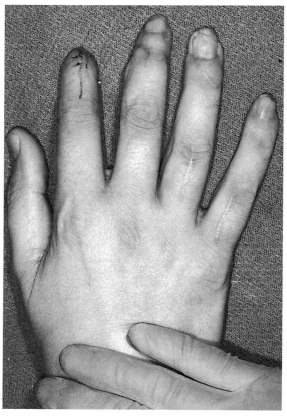

a

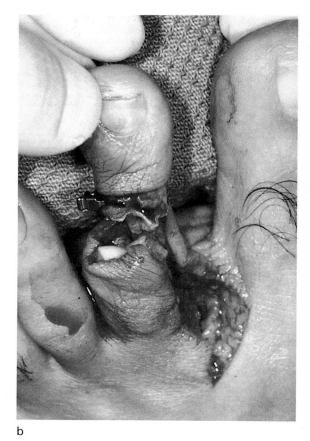

b

Figure 1

(a) Preoperative defect, which shows amputation just proximal to DIP joint. (b) Harvesting a flap from the left second toe. (c) Harvested flap. (d) The appearance of the index finger 6 years after operation.

finger survived, but necrosis was noted over the replanted part of the index finger. Five months after replantation, revision of the index finger tip was done to excise the nail remnant and necrotic stump up to the middle phalanx just proximal to the DIP joint (Figure 1a).

Due to the patient's strong desire to have a normal length and aesthetically pleasing index finger, a second toe transfer was performed 12 days after revision. A zig-zag volar skin incision and a longitudinal skin incision were made over the index finger to dissect the bilateral digital arteries and nerves. Two palmar and two dorsal veins were also dissected. A flap was designed

over the left second toe with the transverse skin incision about 2.4 cm from the tip of the toe (a length equal to the shortened index finger, Figure 1b). Bilateral digital arteries and plantar digital nerves were harvested with the medial pedicle 1 cm longer than the flap. Two plantar and two dorsal veins and extensor and flexor tendons were harvested at the same time. The bone was resected at the base of the middle phalanx (Figure 1c). The flap was then transferred to the index finger, and the bone was fixed with an interosseous wire and two crossed Kirschner wires. The extensor and flexor tendons were repaired with three 4-0 and 3-0 Ticron loop

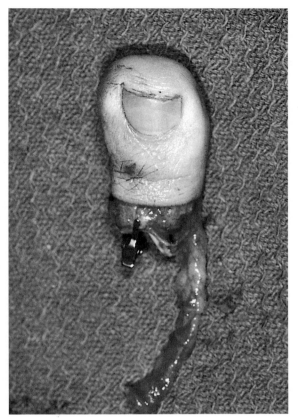

c

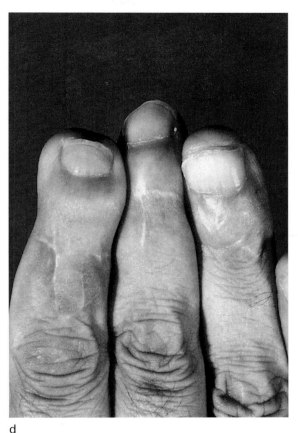

d

sutures (Davis and Geck, USA), respectively. The arteries, veins and nerve were anastomosed with 10-0 nylon sutures. The skin was closed with 6-0 nylon sutures.

The bone united and the original length of the index finger was regained. Six years after the operation, two-point discrimination was 6 mm. Decreased range of motion (ROM) with mild lag of extension was noted over the DIP joint. This may have been due to mild adhesion of the extensor tendon and the nature of the DIP joint of the toe. However, the patient was satisfied with the result and did not wish to undergo any further operations (Figure 1d).

Case 2: free toe pulp transfer to regain a durable and sensitive finger pulp

A 34-year-old male coal miner suffered a severe roller crushing injury over his right hand that resulted in partial amputations at the DIP joint level of the index and middle fingers and volar pulp of the ring finger with flexor tendon exposure (Figure 2a). Replantations of the index and middle fingers were performed. The pulp was crushed beyond repair, and so a free neurovascular pulp transfer was performed from

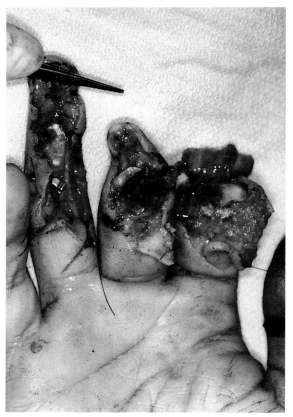
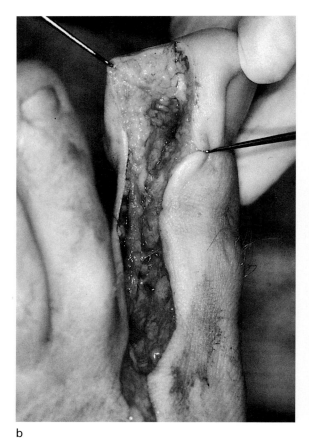

a   b

Figure 2

(a) Preoperative picture, which shows the pulp defect of the right ring finger with exposed flexor tendon. (b) Harvesting a toe flap from the lateral aspect of the left great toe. (c) Appearance of the pulp of the ring finger at 1 year after operation. (d) Appearance of the right hand when making a fist.

the left great toe to the right ring finger on the day of injury (Figure 2b). The lateral neurovascular bundle from the toe was harvested and anastomosed to the ring finger (first metatarsal artery to ulnar digital artery, plantar digital nerve to radial digital nerve, two veins from venae comitantes to dorsal veins). The defect over the toe and the dorsal aspect of the ring finger was covered with a split-thickness skin graft.

Venous congestion in the replanted index and middle fingers was noted after operation. Although leeches were applied, the replanted parts still necrosed, and amputation was performed 3 weeks later. The transferred pulp

survived, but scarring was noted at the edge of the flap, which led to breakdown at 4 months and mild widened claw deformity of the nail at 6 months. Z-plasty, partial ablation of the nail and nail bed, shortening of the distal phalanx and advancement of the volar pulp were performed. At 1 year after the initial operation, the patient had a durable, painless pulp over his ring finger (Figure 2c). However, ROM of the ring finger was moderately decreased (88° in the PIP joint and 30° in the DIP joint with 40° of extension lag) (Figure 2d). Two-point discrimination was 15 mm. Grip strength was 45% compared with the opposite hand.

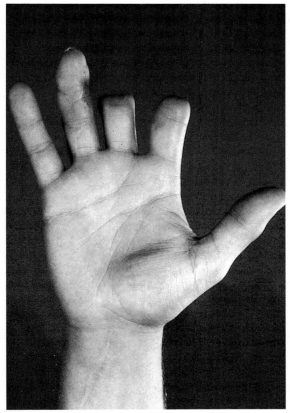

c

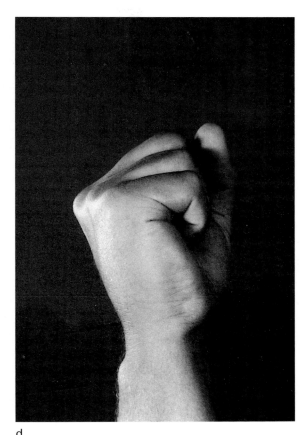

d

Pros and cons compared to classic techniques

Conservative treatment should always be considered first for fingertip injuries, especially in children. Good results can be achieved with healing by secondary intention, but only in minor soft tissue defects without bony exposure. Although conservative treatment avoids the need for surgical intervention, sequelae can include cold intolerance, hypesthesia and a poor cosmetic outcome; in addition, shortness of the finger is unavoidable.

Split- or full-thickness skin grafts to cover fingertip injuries are traditional methods but will prevent granulation tissue from replacing the lost tissue. In addition, undesirable characteristics of such grafts include poor sensation, mismatched skin pigmentation and poor overall appearance.

Local flaps are widely used but sometimes have limitations in that they are incapable of covering defects larger than 2 cm². Traditional V-Y flaps and various modifications are useful procedures if performed with meticulous techniques. The appearance is quite acceptable although common sequelae include cold intolerance, numbness, tenderness and hypersensitivity (but some reports have shown good quality of sensation). A thenar flap is a simple procedure used to cover pulp defects with bone or tendon exposure. It provides glabrous skin over the pulp but requires a two-stage operation. Notable disadvantages include an unpredictable return of sensitivity, painful scarring at the donor site within the palm and joint stiffness as a result of the immobilization required for the flap (which makes this flap undesirable in older patients). The cross-finger flap is a good option when a major loss of volar skin and subcutaneous tissue has occurred, especially when bone or tendon is exposed. Like the thenar flap, drawbacks of this technique include the variable quality of sensory return to the transferred tissue, the need for a two-stage operation and donor site appearance. A modification of techniques—a combination of the cross-finger flap with the transfer of the dorsal sensory branch of the digital nerve—was reported to have a two-point discrimination of 4.6 mm.

The local neurovascular island flap is a useful method to prevent most of the drawbacks and complications mentioned above. The fingertip can be resurfaced so that the finger skin and pad are virtually the same in appearance, texture and sensitivity to the original. The need for multiple operations and awkward positioning of an affected digit are thus avoided. However, problems related to cortical reorientation should be considered. The reverse vascular island flap has the advantages of simplicity, a one-stage procedure, a short hospitalization and minimal disability time. However, most of the reverse vascular island flap does not combine with nerve transfer, so the sensory recovery is rather unpredictable. Some procedures combined with the transfer of a dorsal branch of the digital nerve may have satisfactory sensory recovery.

Only free tissue transfer can reconstruct the shortened fingertip, especially when the fingernail or nailbed is to be reconstructed at the same time. A toe transfer and wrap-around flap are used to regain the length of the shortened fingertips, together with reconstruction of the fingernails. They have the same advantages of a single operation, good sensation, acceptable cosmetic appearance, glabrous skin and nail support. However, they also have the disadvantages of requiring microvascular expertise and a lengthy operation. A great toe-to-hand transfer can achieve good mobility and strength and, when used in children, has growth potential. The metatarsal can be included in the second toe-to-hand transfer, and the appearance of the donor site and finger is more readily accepted by the patient than when it is from the great toe. But the reconstructed finger is not as strong as it is from the great toe, and mallet deformity of the distal joint sometimes occurs. The wrap-around procedure has the most acceptable appearance with little donor site morbidity, but is not suitable for children because it has no growth potential. There is also no joint mobility and bone resorption sometimes occurs.

Venous flaps can be used in a dorsal skin defect when a vein graft is needed. This technique provides simultaneous venous drainage and flap coverage and thus avoids those complications often seen when skin is grafted over a venous anastomosis, such as vessel occlusion or haematoma formation. When venous drainage is not required for distal revascularization, a venous flap can still be used to cover the dorsal skin defect with an arterialized pattern.

No traditional method can reconstruct a fingernail or nailbed if it is destroyed. A free tissue transfer is particularly useful in these cases to build a normal nail appearance and prevent complications such as nail plate dehiscence and claw nail.

Results

In 1979, Buncke and Rose[3] reported six cases of fingertip injuries treated with free toe-to-fingertip neurovascular flaps. Four of the six flaps survived and two-point discrimination was 3–7 mm, which approaches that of the normal contralateral digits. None of these patients complained of pain in the recipient area or in the donor site.

Indications

No single procedure is appropriate for all cases of fingertip injuries. Final permanent residual disabilities are diminished with retained digital length, improved aesthetic appearance and less sensory impairment. When a treatment method is planned, a series of factors should be taken into consideration. These include the extent of the injury, age and medical condition of the patient, and the functional and cosmetic requirements of the patient. Traditional techniques should be considered in less severe injuries before more complicated procedures are contemplated.

However, with the improvements in microsurgical equipment and techniques, free tissue transfer has become a standard procedure in the treatment of fingertip injuries, especially when the above requirements are to be fulfilled. A toe-to-hand transfer and wrap-around flap are indicated for partial or total finger defects, particularly in the thumb, to regain normal digital length and good opposition. This is especially true when good sensation of the pulp and normal appearance of the nail or nailbed are to be provided. Toe pulp transfer is a good choice when adequate soft tissue padding and sensation are needed to rebuild the digital pulp defect, especially when bone or tendon is exposed. When the fingernail or nailbed is totally absent, free vascularized nail grafts using either a wraparound flap or an arterialized venous flap can achieve an acceptable cosmetic appearance.

References

1   Honda T, Nomura S, Yamauchi S, et al, The possible applications of a composite skin and subcutaneous vein graft in the replantation of amputated digits, *Br J Plast Surg* (1984) **37**:607–12.

2   Tsai TM, Matiko JO, Breidenbach W, et al, Venous flaps in digital revascularization and replantation, *J Reconstr Microsurg* (1987) **3**:113–19.

3   Buncke HJ, Rose EH, Free toe-to-fingertip neurovascular flaps, *Plast Reconstr Surg* (1979) **63**:607–12.

Commentary

Chapter 21

Congenital vascular anomalies are a difficult and extremely challenging problem for the hand surgeon. A systematic approach to these anomalies is necessary in order to provide the optimum treatment to an individual patient. In this chapter Doctors Upton and Burrows review the Mulliken Glowacki Classification and how this helps guide surgical and non-surgical treatment. This is an excellent summary of the current state of knowledge in this area.

PCA

Chapter 22

Vasospastic disease remains a difficult area where there is not much new and there is not even much that works. This review does an excellent job of putting the topic into perspective.

PCA

Chapter 23

Staged replantation is not often needed but in some circumstances can permit salvage of useful function, when the state of the initial wound does not permit direct replantation but the surgeon can foresee a time in the near future where the recipient site can be restored to a point where replantation will be possible. Here Doctors Sheridan and Wood elaborate on the initial experience of Marko Godina. This would seem to be a good example of a procedure which is no longer new but is still occasionally useful.

PCA

Chapter 24

It is certainly true that that which is possible, will be done. In this case, microsurgical techniques and free tissue transfer are possible; Drs Tsai and Tien review possible indications for their use to reconstruct fingertips. As this chapter indicates (and illustrates) there are some indications, but these are limited. For the most part, fingertips can be reconstructed satisfactorily by much simpler means, ranging from simple healing by second intention to closure with local tissues.

PCA

25
New trends in spasticity of the hand

Ann E Van Heest and James H House

Introduction

Spasticity causes muscle imbalance. The function of the hand, to interface and interact with the environment, is compromised by muscle imbalance. The goal of treatment for spasticity in the hand remains: to improve muscle balance in order to maximize hand function.

There are several new trends in the treatment of hand spasticity. First, in cerebral palsy, evaluation of the functional use of the hand is becoming more extensive. Evaluation may include assessment of dynamic deformity through videotaping of ADL (activities of daily living) functions and/or investigational use of the simultaneous electromyography (EMG)/video taping in the motion analysis laboratory. Second, more attention is now paid to individualizing treatment goals. After careful assessment of degree of involvement of mentation, sensation, static deformity, dynamic deformity, and timed testing, each child serves as their own benchmark for improvement of functional use after a treatment intervention. Third, botulinum toxin as a treatment modality is used with increasing frequency to reversibly reduce spasticity in the growing child. Its role continues to be defined. Lastly, spasticity is increasingly recognized in the tetraplegic hand. Its role in creating imbalance needs to be addressed in both the intrinsic and extrinsic reconstruction of the tetraplegic hand.

This chapter will focus on new trends in the treatment of hand spasticity by discussing recent developments in our evaluation and treatment of the hand in cerebral palsy, followed by a brief discussion of treatment of intrinsic imbalance in the tetraplegic hand.

Cerebral palsy

Cerebral palsy is the most common etiology treated for muscle spasticity. Cerebral palsy is due to a nonprogressive central nervous system injury resulting in peripheral motor deficit. Evaluation of the extent of the central nervous system insult is imperative in individualizing treatment for the spastic cerebral palsied hand.

By definition, a child's motor system is affected in cerebral palsy. However, impairment of sensation, coordination, and intelligence varies. Each of these areas affects motor function and needs evaluation as part of integrating care for the child with cerebral palsy.

Patient evaluation

Our evaluation of children with cerebral palsy has evolved to an integration of our assessment for each aspect of manifestation of cerebral palsy (see Table 1). Generalized groups based on the child's degree of involvement can be made in three levels: level I (severe), level II (moderate), and level III (mild).

Mentation

In evaluation of a patient's baseline function, in formulating realistic treatment goals, and in measurement of treatment outcomes, it is important to establish the degree of generalized central involvement. Mentation can be measured by IQ testing or, for the higher functioning child, by school performance. Motivation assessment is

Table 1 Cerebral palsy spastic[1] hemiplegia assessment.

Functional use (House classification)	Mentation/motivation	Sensation[2]
Level I a Nonfunctional b Paper weight c Fair passive assist	**Level I** • Severe retardation	**Level I** • 0–6/12 objects • 2 pt >1 cm
Level II a Good passive assist b Poor active assist c Fair active assist	**Level II** • Mild retardation or • Poor motivation	**Level II** • 7–9/12 objects • 2 pt 5–10 mm
Level III a Good active assist b Partial spontaneous c Complete spontaneous	**Level III** • Normal mentation • High motivation	**Level III** • 10–12/12 objects • 2 pt <6 mm

Static contracture/deformity	Dynamic deformity[2] (video evaluation)
Elbow Level I >90° flexion contracture Level II 45–90° flexion contracture Level III 0–45° flexion contracture	**Elbow (gait)** Level I Flex >90° Level II Flex 45–90° Level III Flex 0–45°
Forearm Level I < 0° supination Level II 0–45° supination Level III 45–90° supination	**Forearm** Level I No active supination Level II Supination 0–45° Level III Supination 45–90°
Wrist Level I >60° flexion contracture Level II 30–60° flexion contracture Level III 0–30° flexion contracture	**Wrist** Level I Flexion >60° 　　　　　　a UD >15° 　　　　　　b UD <15° Level II Flexion 0–30° 　　　　　　a UD >15° 　　　　　　b UD <15° Level III Flexion 0–30° 　　　　　　a UD >15° b UD <15°
Fingers Level I Fingers extended until >60° wrist flexion Level II Fingers extended until 30–60° wrist flexion Level III Fingers extended until <30° wrist flexion	**Fingers (grasp/release)** Level I Clenched fist Level II 'Poor' active Level III 'Good' active
Thumb (House) Type I MC adduction Type II MC adduction and PP flexion Type III MC adduction and MCP hyperextension Type IV MC adduction/PP and DP flexion	**Thumb (pinch)** Level I In palm—ineffective Level I In palm—ineffective Level III Effective at level of index finger

[1]Athetoid excluded.
[2]Stereognosis and static two-point discrimination.
DP, distal phalangeal; FCU, flexor carpi ulnaris; MC, metacarpal; MCP, metacarpophalangeal; PP, proximal phalangeal; UD, ulnar drift.

Table 2 Functional classification system (House[2]).

Class	Designation	Activity level
0	Does not use	Does not use
1	Poor passive assist	Uses as stabilizing weight only
2	Fair passive assist	Can hold onto object placed in hand
3	Good passive assist	Can hold onto object and stabilize it for use by other hand
4	Poor active assist	Can actively grasp object and hold it weakly
5	Fair active assist	Can actively grasp object and stabilize it well
6	Good active assist	Can actively grasp object and then manipulate it against other hand
7	Spontaneous use, partial	Can perform bimanual activities easily and occasionally uses the hand spontaneously
8	Spontaneous use, complete	Uses hand completely independently without reference to the other hand

important for the higher functioning child, particularly with tendon transfers which may require a highly motivated child to participate with postoperative therapy.

Functional use

We also ask the family to self-rate the child's functional use of the hand using House's functional use scale (Table 2). This provides a baseline that can be used to help the physician communicate the functional goals of the surgery with the parents. The functional use can then be reassessed postoperatively with the same scale to assess for improvement.

Sensation

Sensation can be evaluated by stereognosis, two-point discrimination, and proprioception. In our review of 40 children with spastic hemiplegia,[1] we have found that stereognosis is the most sensitive discriminator of degree of sensibility impairment, as shown in Table 3. We found that 97% had a stereognosis impairment using the 12 objects shown in Table 4. The six objects listed on the left discriminate gross motor function, and the six objects listed on the right discriminate fine motor function. The 40 children tested correctly identified all 12 objects on their unaffected side, verifying their understanding of the test. Furthermore, we found that those children with severe sensibility impairment had a significant size discrepancy when compared to the unaffected side. The shortened limb can be a useful clue to underlying sensibility deficiency, particularly in the child too young or too retarded to reliably perform a sensibility assessment.

Table 3 Sensibility deficiencies in 40 children with spastic hemiplegia.

Test	Percentage of children
12 object stereognosis:	
12 objects	3
8–11 objects	22
5–8 objects	40
0–4 objects	35
Two-point discrimination:	
Intact	10
Impaired	70
Absent	20
Proprioception	
Intact	54
Impaired	38
Absent	8

Table 4 Twelve objects tested for stereognosis function.

Gross discrimination	Fine discrimination
Wooden cube	Paper clip
Key	Safety pin
Pencil	Button
Marble	Penny
Balloon	Rubber band
Spoon	String

Deformity

The affected limb is then evaluated for static deformity. Static deformity is categorized as shown in Table 1 for degree of joint contracture for the elbow, forearm, wrist, and fingers. We continue to categorize thumb-in-palm deformities

Table 5 Classification of thumb deformities.

Type	Description
Type I	'Simple' metacarpal adduction contracture
Type II	Metacarpal adduction contracture and metacarpophalangeal flexion deformity
Type III	Metacarpal adduction contracture combined with a metacarpophalangeal hyperextension deformity or instability
Type IV	Metacarpal adduction contracture combined with metacarpophalangeal and interphalangeal flexion deformities

by the classification described by House et al[2] and shown in Table 5.

Evaluation of dynamic deformity now routinely involves use of videotaping the child for ADL activities. By videorecording the child during a therapy session, we have found this more accurately shows the child's spasticity present. Videotaping allows assessment of the spasticity encountered during routine ADLs and eliminates the stress of performance on demand in the physician's office. Furthermore, the videotape serves as a record for comparison after treatment intervention. Identification of the specific spastic muscle can be determined by the joint position; for example, excessive wrist flexion with ulnar deviation identifies the flexor carpi ulnaris as the spastic deforming force. Palpation of specific spastic muscles is also important in localizing the source of the dynamic imbalance. Voluntary control of the muscle also needs assessment. Additionally, spasticity versus dystonia should be noted. Dynamic imbalance of the elbow, forearm, wrist, fingers, and thumb are graded for severity as shown in Table 1.

The higher functioning child is also evaluated for motor function using the pediatric Jebson hand test. This test provides an age-matched control. Comparison to an age-matched control allows for longitudinal assessment of the child and allows evaluation of both their 'affected' and 'unaffected' sides to assess coordination and mentation as well.

Motion analysis

Most recently, we have begun using the motion analysis laboratory with EMG fine needle electrodes recorded and displayed simultaneously with video-input data. Our work in this area is preliminary, but shows definite differences in the phasic activity of the various spastic muscles. The children have tolerated the placement of the fine needle electrodes through use of topical anesthetic cream for one hour prior to electrode placement. In our experience, children need to be at least seven years of age to appropriately cooperate with the motion laboratory analysis.

By evaluating the degree of involvement of mentation, motivation, sensation, static deformity, dynamic deformity, timed testing, and functional use, we then integrate these data together to formulate an individualized treatment plan. Discussion with the parents and the child is imperative in formulating the individualized treatment plan and its expected outcome. The treatment can then be monitored and adjusted by periodic re-evaluation using the same evaluation measures.

Formulating a treatment plan

Because of the complexity of combinations of degree of involvement for each individual child, an exact 'algorithm' of treatment is not easily or specifically outlined. The cornerstone to treatment is first to evaluate and accurately diagnose the areas of impairment present for that particular child. By accurately characterizing the pattern of involvement, the different 'tools of the trade' (Table 6) can then be used to address the specific functional impairment present. Each child then serves as their own benchmark. The goal of treatment intervention is not normalcy. The goal of treatment is functional improvement for those areas in deficit.

Part of the integration of the individualized treatment plan is education of the child and parents. At present, we do not have treatment options to change mentation or sensibility deficiencies. The parents and child need to be informed as to the deficiencies of mentation and sensibilities as permanent parts of the child's disability. Treatment is thus aimed at the motor system, particularly in spastic imbalance which causes functional impairment.

It has been written that children with sensibility or mentation deficiencies do not deserve treatment intervention. To the contrary, we would

Table 6 Tools of the trade.

Procedure	Deformity:				
	Elbow flexion	Forearm pronation	Wrist flexion/ulnar deviation	Thumb-in-palm	Finger deformities
Joint stabilization			Wrist fusion ± proximal row carpectomy[6]	CMC fusion MCP fusion MCP capsulodesis[9] IP fusion	PIP fusion (rare)
Tendon releases	Biceps lengthening Brachialis release[3]	Pronator teres release[4] Biceps aponeurosis release	Flexor pronator slide[7] FCU tenotomy/lengthening[8]	Adductor release[2] FPL lengthening FDI release	Flexor pronator slide[7]
Tendon transfers		Pronator teres re-routing[5]	FCU to ECRB[9] FCU to EDC ECU centralization	PL to AbPL, EPB, or EPL[2] AbPL tenodesis[2] EPL re-routing Abduction-plasty[10] BR to AbPL, EPB, or EPL[2]	Lateral band re-routing (swan neck)[11] FDS tenodesis (swan neck)[12] Superficialis to profundus[13]

AbPL, abductor pollicis longus; ECRB, extensor carpi radialis brevis; ECU, extensor carpi ulnaris; EDC, extensor digitorum communis; EPB, extensor pollicus brevis; EPL, extensor pollicus longus; FCU, flexor carpi ulnaris; FDI, first dorsal interosseous; FPL, flexor pollicus longus; MCP, metacarpal phalangeal; PIP, proximal interphalangeal; CMC, carpometacarpal; BR, brachoradialis; FDS, flexor digitorum superficialis.

advocate that the sensibility and mentation deficiencies are fixed and need to be diagnosed. Children with sensibility or mentation deficiencies may be significantly functionally improved by an individualized treatment plan. For example, a child with poor sensibility or severe retardation may be improved from nonfunctional (House level 0), to paperweight function (House level 1), by wrist arthrodesis with wrist flexor tenotomies and superficialis-to-profundus transfers. The physician, therapist, parents, and child simply need to clearly understand the treatment goals preoperatively, and agree that the degree of expected improvement is worthwhile.

Patients with static deformity are initially treated with night-time splinting and daily range-of-motion exercises. Patients with dynamic deformity occasionally will see functional improvement with daytime splinting using a dorsal ring splint for severe wrist flexion, a neoprene splint for thumb-in-palm, or silver ring splints for dynamic finger swan neck deformities. If functionally helpful, the daytime splints will be gladly worn by the patient. Daytime splints should not be cumbersome and should stay out of the palm and off the fingers so that maximal use of the hand is possible.

Surgical treatment is indicated in those patients with static deformity not responsive to splints and causing impairment, and in those patients with dynamic deformity with functional impairment which could be improved by better joint positioning. In general, patients with severe involvement (level I) are best candidates for pre-positioning arthrodesis, tenotomies, and tenodeses which do not require postoperative dynamic control. Those patients with moderate and mild involvement (levels II and III) are best candidates for balancing operations using tenotomies or lengthenings of spastic muscles, along with appropriate augmentation of the antagonist muscles through tendon transfers. Simpler procedures are more predictable for moderately involved patients, while more sophisticated procedures can be performed for mildly involved patients who have better selective control. The reader is referred to the references for specific indications and techniques for these reconstructions.[2–13]

Treatment using botulinum toxin

The role of botulinum toxin injections for treatment of cerebral palsy continues to be defined.

Several facts of botulinum toxin injections are known. First, botulinum toxin type A acts as a reversible neuromuscular blockade to produce localized partial denervation. Botulinum toxin is injected directly into the muscle to locally block the release of acetylcholine, producing a chemical denervation with diminished muscle spasticity. Second, current research has shown botulinum toxin is effective in reversibly reducing spasticity due to cerebral palsy by both physician and patient rating of function.[14–20] In children with cerebral palsy, studies controlled by placebo injections have shown that botulinum toxin effectively reduces muscle spasticity with little or no side-effects. Third, laboratory evidence has shown that in the spastic mouse, local administration of botulinum toxin has effectively reduced spasticity, and allowed permanent muscle sarcomere lengthening with reduced secondary joint contracture.[21]

If botulinum toxin injections reduce spasticity, can passive stretch during this period produce permanent muscular lengthening in children? Can antagonist muscles be stretched? Can co-ordination be learned with less spasticity present? Can the muscle be stretched enough to keep up with skeletal growth? Many questions remain. Through careful selection of patients in further clinical trials, the role of this medication in the treatment of spasticity in cerebral palsy can be further defined. At present, we use botulinum toxin injections in conjunction with night-time splinting and passive muscle stretching for children with static isolated wrist and forearm deformities unresponsive to nighttime splinting alone; and for children with dynamic deformities which are mild enough to not require surgical intervention, but severe enough to cause functional impairment. Our use of botulinum toxin injections is part of ongoing prospective research.

Tetraplegia

Upper extremity paralysis due to spinal cord injury is commonly complicated by muscle spasticity. In the past, reconstruction of the tetraplegic hand has centered on tendon transfers to treat muscle paralysis. Tetraplegic deformities can involve not only muscle paralysis, but also muscle spasticity, which can create dysfunction and imbalance. Our recent review of tetraplegic hand reconstruction has focused not only on the extrinsic reconstruction of the paralytic muscles, but also on intrinsic reconstruction to provide balance in the tetraplegic hand.[22] Chronic spasticity in the tetraplegic hand produces further muscle imbalance and deformity. Spasticity needs to be addressed as part of the reconstruction of the paralytic deformity.

Most commonly, muscle spasticity is present in the superficial finger flexors. Flexor digitorum superficialis (FDS) spasticity in the paralytic hand causes proximal interphalangeal (PIP) flexion deformity. If this is present, reconstruction can include the FDS lasso procedure to eliminate the PIP flexion deformity and to transfer the spastic 'tone' to the metacarpophalangeal level. In combination with an extrinsic reconstruction restoring flexor digitorum profundus function, the FDS lasso prevents early digital roll-up and improves grasp function and grip strength. If the patient has central slip deficiencies due to prolonged FDS spasticity, an intrinsic tenodesis procedure may be necessary as well to provide optimum balance of the PIP joint.

Conclusion

Spasticity in the hand causes muscle imbalance that can interfere with functional use of the hand. Accurate diagnosis and appropriate treatment of hand spasticity is important for attaining improved muscle balance and, consequently, improved hand function.

In cerebral palsy, patient evaluation needs to encompass an integration of assessment of mentation, sensation, static and dynamic deformity. Dynamic deformity may be evaluated through analysis of videotaping of ADL functions or of simultaneous EMG/video motion analysis studies. Treatment goals are individualized and each child serves as their own benchmark for improvement of functional use after treatment intervention. The role of botulinum toxin as a treatment modality to reversibly reduce spasticity in the growing child continues to be defined. Lastly, spasticity is increasingly recognized in the tetraplegic hand. Spasticity in the paralyzed hand can create imbalance and needs to be addressed in both the intrinsic and extrinsic reconstruction of the tetraplegic hand.

References

1   Van Heest A, House J, Putnam M, Sensibility deficiencies in the hands of children with spastic hemiplegia, *J Hand Surg* (1993) **18A**:278–81.
2   House J, Gwathmey F, Fidler M, A dynamic approach to the thumb-in-palm deformity in cerebral palsy, *J Bone Joint Surg* (1981) **63A**:216–25.
3   Mital MA, Lengthening of the elbow flexors in cerebral palsy, *J Bone Joint Surg* (1979) **61A**:515–22.
4   Strecker WB, Emanuel JP, Dailey L, Manske PR, Comparison of pronator tenotomy and pronator rerouting in children with spastic cerebral palsy, *J Hand Surg* (1988) **13A**:540–3.
5   Sakellarides HT, Mital MA, Lenzi WD, Treatment of pronation contractures of the forearm in cerebral palsy by changing the insertion of the pronator radii teres, *J Bone Joint Surg* (1981) **63A**:645–52.
6   Omer GE, Capen DA, Proximal row carpectomy with muscle transfers for spastic paralysis, *J Hand Surg* (1976) **1**:197–204.
7   White WF, Flexor muscle slide in the spastic hand, *J Bone Joint Surg* (1972) **54B**:453–9.
8   Zancolli E, *Structural and Dynamic Bases of Hand Surgery*, 2nd edn (JB Lippincott: Philadelphia, 1968).
9   Filler BC, Stark HH, Boyes JH, Capsulodesis of the metacarpophalangeal joint of the thumb in children with cerebral palsy, *J Bone Joint Surg* (1976) **58A**:667–70.
10 Smith RJ, Flexor pollicus longus abductor-plasty for spastic thumb-in-palm deformity, *J Hand Surg* (1982) **7A**:327–34.
11 Tonkin MA, Hughes J, Smith KL, Lateral band translation for swan-neck deformity, *J Hand Surg* (1992) **17A**:260.
12 Swanson AB, Surgery of the hand in cerebral palsy and the swan neck deformity, *J Bone Joint Surg* (1960) **42A**:951–64.
13 Braun RM, Vise GT, Roper B, Sublimas to profundus transfers in the hemiplegic upper extremity, *J Bone Joint Surg* (1974) **56A**:466–72.
14 Corry IS, Cosgrove AP, Duffy CM, et al, Botulinum toxin A as an alternative to serial casting in the conservative management of equinus in cerebral palsy, *Dev Med Child Neurol* (1995) **37**(8):17–18, suppl 73.

15 Cosgrove AP, Corry IS, Graham HK, Botulinum toxin in the management of lower limb in cerebral palsy, *Dev Med Child Neurol* (1994) **36**:386.

16 Das TK, Park DM, Botulinum toxin in treating spasticity, *Br J Clin Pract* (1989) **43**:401–3.

17 Koman LA, Mooney JF, Smity BP, et al, Management of spasticity in cerebral palsy with botulinum-A toxin: report of a preliminary randomized double-blind trial, *J Pediatr Orthop* (1994) **14**:299.

18 Koman LA, Mooney FJ III, Smith BP, The use of botulinum toxin in the management of cerebral palsy in pediatric patients. In: Das Gupta BR, ed, *Botulinum and Tetanus Neurotoxins* (Plenum Press: New York, 1993).

19 Koman LA, Ferrari E, Mubarak S, et al, Botulinum toxin type A (TBA) in the treatment of lower limb spasticity associated with cerebral palsy, *Dev Med Child Neurol* (1995) **37**(8):17–18, supp 73.

20 Wall SA, Chait LA, Temlett JA, et al, Botulinum A chemodenervation: a new modality in cerebral palsied hands, *Br J Plast Surg* (1993) **46**:703.

21 Cosgrove AP, Graham HK, Botulinum toxin A prevents the development of contractures in the hereditary spastic mouse, *Dev Med Child Neurol* (1994) **35**:379.

22 McCarthy C, House JH, Van Heest A, et al, Intrinsic balancing in reconstruction of the tetraplegic hand, *J Hand Surg* in press.

26
Tubular repair of nerves

Göran Lundborg

Introduction

Injuries to major nerve trunks in the upper extremity still constitute difficult and challenging reconstructive problems. The functional result from repair of such nerves is often disappointing with inferior recovery of discriminative sensibility as well as motor function of the hand. Several factors may help to explain the incomplete functional recovery. First, the injury in itself may result in cell death in sensory ganglia.[1,2] Second, due to slow regeneration of axons, atrophy of distal targets may occur before axons reach their innervation territory. Third, there is considerable malorientation of regenerating axons, resulting in reinnervation of incorrect targets. This is associated with a functional reorganization at spinal cord level,[3] as well as in the somatosensory cortical area, resulting in problems with correct interpretation of the pattern of afferent signals from the hand.[4–7]

The surgeon can influence some of these factors by using an atraumatic technique and by being precise in performing the surgery. The development of microsurgical techniques has made it easier to surgically match and adapt functional subunits of a severed nerve. However, there is little evidence that such technical refinements in general result in superior functional recovery.[8] Such techniques may enable a perfect adaptation of the perineurial and epineurial layers, but it is still impossible to fully control the behavior of the regenerating fibers in the endoneurial space inside fascicles.

Nerve injuries with segmental defects introduce special problems. At present such injuries are best treated by the use of autologous nerve grafts,[9,10] but because it is necessary to sacrifice healthy nerves there is a need for alternatives. Freeze-thawed muscle may provide basal laminas supporting axonal growth,[11,12] but this principle has definite limitations in clinical use.[13]

With increasing insight into the occurrence and role of neurotrophic factors in nerve regeneration there has been optimism that new and better principles for nerve repair may develop. Following nerve transection there is a local synthesis and release of neurotrophic factors.[14–16] Among such factors are nerve growth factor (NGF),[17] brain-derived neurotrophic factor (BDNF),[18] and ciliary neurotrophic factor (CNTF).[19,20] Experimental studies have shown that such neurotrophic factors may accumulate inside a tube, encasing both ends of a cut nerve.[19–23] Over the last decade there has therefore been an increasing interest in utilizing tubes for primary nerve repair as well as bridging defects in nerve continuity.

The purpose of this chapter is to review current clinical experience of the use of tubes in clinical nerve repair, with special reference to major nerve trunks in the human forearm. A brief historical background will also be given regarding the evolution of the concept with reference to past and present experimental work.

Experimental background

In 1979 we published the first papers describing the use of 'mesothelial tubes' for bridging defects in rat sciatic nerve.[24,25] The principle was based on the idea that neurotrophic factors might be synthetized in a damaged nerve and that it would be an advantage if such factors were allowed to accumulate in a closed space. The mesothelial tube was created by leaving a silicone rod, surrounded by a metal spiral, subcutaneously for 3 weeks. A mesothelial-like cellular lining formed around the silicone rod and, because of the metal spiral, this tube did not

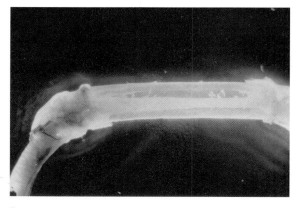

a

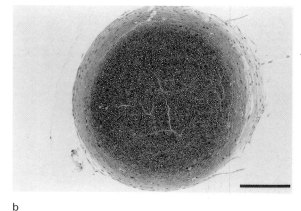

b

Figure 1

Experimental basis for the tubular repair concept. A short defect in rat sciatic nerve is bridged by a silicone tube; (a) 4 weeks later:the gap is bridged by a new nerve structure; (b,c) the regenerated nerve structure has a normal appearance with numerous myelinated axons. Bar = 100 μm (B) and 50 μm (c).

c

collapse after removal of the rod. When a 10 mm defect in rat sciatic nerve was bridged by such a tube it was found that, within 4 weeks, the space inside the tube was bridged by a spontaneously regenerated nerve structure with structural and functional properties of a peripheral nerve. Dellon and MacKinnon later demonstrated that the same principle can be used for successful bridging of a gap as great as 3 cm in the ulnar nerve of primates.[26] In their experiments it was found that at 12 months after surgery no significant electrophysiological difference could be found between the mesothelial (pseudosheath) tube group and control groups treated with autologous nerve grafts.

The mesothelial tube is a physiological, permeable, and well vascularized tubular structure

which, however, requires a complicated two-stage procedure for its use. Since we believed that the permeability and vascularization of the tube wall was essential, we wanted to demonstrate that the use of impermeable silicone tubes for the same purpose would not be successful. However, to our surprise, we found that a 10 mm gap in a rat sciatic nerve, bridged by a silicone tube, was successfully bridged within 4 weeks by a nerve structure of more or less normal appearance (Figure 1).[8,27] This finding was followed by a rapid further development of the silicone tube model as an experimental tool for studying the physiology of nerve regeneration. It was found that short gaps were successfully bridged by well developed new nerve structures, but the diameter of the nerve structure decreased with increasing gap length. A critical limit of 10–15 mm could be defined beyond which no or very inferior regeneration occurred.[8,28]

The structural and biochemical phenomena occurring inside the silicone regeneration tube have been well described. At first there is a fibrin cloth which becomes invaded by cellular elements and capillaries from the proximal as well as distal segment. Schwann cells and axons migrate into the matrix from the proximal site. Fibronectin and laminin can, at an early stage, be demonstrated in the matrix, and neurotrophic factors addressing sensory, motor, and sympathetic neurons accumulate in the chamber. The tissue fluid that accumulates in the chamber contains at least two types of neurotrophic activities, namely NGF and CNTF. It has recently been demonstrated that there is one major peak of neurotrophic activity early, about 3–6 hours after nerve injury.[19]

The tube model has been widely used for experimental purposes and its regeneration potential has been increased by various modifications, for example by varying its size or filling it with dialysed plasma,[29] laminin/testosterone/gangliosides,[30] collagen-glucosaminoglycan,[31,32] laminin and/or collagen,[33–38] Schwann cells,[39,40] or hyaluron.[41] Various types of biodegradable tubes have also been used, such as polyglycolic acid and associated substances.[26,42–45]

Experimental neuromas

It was noticed early on that with extension of the gap length the regenerated nerve structure inside a mesothelial or silicone tube became very thin. With a 15 mm gap there was usually only a thin tissue strand being formed in the tube containing no or very few axons.[28,46,47] The proximal nerve end in such cases tapered off over the first few millimeters of the tube without forming any classical neuroma (Figure 2). It was suggested that this model might be used for treating painful neuromas—not by preventing axonal outgrowth by a silicone cap,[48–51] but rather by achieving cessation of axonal growth by using a long tube with no distal nerve end. Experiments were performed in which the proximal cut end of the sciatic nerve was introduced in a 15 mm long mesothelial tube with no distal

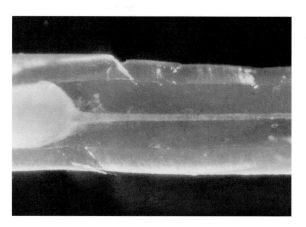

Figure 2

Proximal end of rat sciatic nerve introduced into a 20 mm long silicone tube. There is no regeneration. The nerve tapers off into a tiny tissue strand.

nerve segment.[52] Inside such tubes the nerve structure progressively thinned out and finally terminated in a thin tissue strand. Recordings from dorsal root filaments showed that fibres arising from such 'open' mesothelial chambers did not show any ongoing activity, they responded minimally to local mechanical stimulation, and noradrenalin had no effect on their activity. On the other hand fibres from experimental painful neuromas developed in control rats by ligation and capsulating of nerve ends showed ongoing spontaneous activity enhanced by mechanical stimulation and intravenous infusion of noradrenalin.

Clinical use of tubes

Use of tubes in primary nerve repair

Our experience of tubular repair of median and ulnar nerves of the human forearm dates back to 1988 and includes altogether 18 cases. The procedure is technically simple. We use sterile silicone tubes of appropriate length, usually 1.5–2 cm, and of a diameter exceeding the nerve diameter by

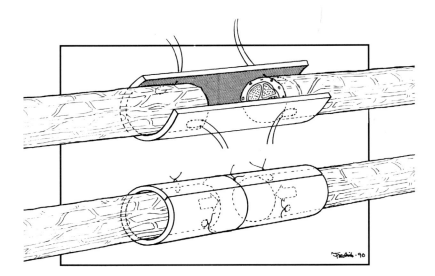

Figure 3

Clinical use of silicone tubes—
surgical procedure. The nerve ends
are left 3–4 mm apart inside the
tube. (Reproduced with permission
from Lundborg et al.[53])

about 30% to allow for swelling of the nerve ends without causing compression. To ensure an optimal orientation of the nerve ends we open the tube by splicing it longitudinally (Figure 3). The nerve ends are carefully pulled towards each other and fixed to the wall of the silicone tube with single stitches of fine suture material (9-0 Ethilon®, Ethicon). A gap measuring 3–4 mm is always left between the nerve ends. The tube is allowed to close and one or two sutures are wrapped around it to secure the closed position. The empty space inside the tube is filled with saline.

Our first case was a transected ulnar nerve, repaired at wrist level on an 21-year-old male patient.[53] He was initially lost for follow-up, but he appeared after 3 years complaining about a slightly disturbing contour from the tube protruding under the skin. He had no pain and no local discomfort. The clinical result was excellent with static two-point discrimination 6 mm in the little finger and normal abduction force in the first dorsal interosseus muscle. At exploration the tube was surrounded by thin mesothelial-like membranes without any obvious scar formation. Inside the tube the former empty space between both nerve ends was now occupied by a nerve-like structure in smooth continuity with the proximal and distal nerve ends without any signs of neuroma formation (Figure 4).

In another case report we described two cases of tubular repair of the median nerve in the human forearm in two male patients of 12 and 21 years age.[54] At 3-year follow-up there was in both cases excellent motor recovery of the thenar muscles. Outgrowth of sensory fibres was remarkably fast, and ultimate two-point discrimination was <6 mm and 8–10 mm respectively.

In one of the cases the tube was re-explored after 2 years because of slight local discomfort due to a disturbing contour of the tube under the skin. There was no local tenderness at the site of repair. At exploration the median nerve was in smooth continuity across the previous 4 mm space (Figure 5). There were no signs of neuroma formation. The tube was surrounded by a thin mesothelial-like membrane showing no evidence of inflammation or excessive fibrosis.

Encouraged by these individual cases we initiated a prospective, randomized, clinical study in order to compare tubular and conventional microsurgical repair of median and ulnar nerves in the human forearm. The study was approved by the Ethical Committee at Lund University. In total the study included 18 patients (14 males and 4 females) with a mean age of 29.5 (range 12–72) years. Inclusion criteria were transection of the ulnar or median nerve at wrist level or less than 10 cm proximal to the wrist level. The cases

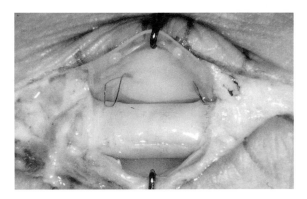

Figure 4

Appearance of regenerated ulnar nerve inside a silicone tube at wrist level after 3 years. The tube is opened. The former empty space (between sutures) is now occupied by a regenerated nerve structure in smooth continuity with proximal and distal segments. (Reproduced with permission from Lundborg et al.[53])

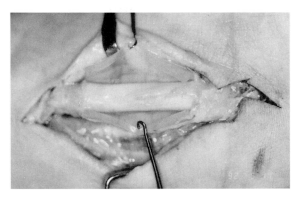

Figure 5

Exploration of a silicone tube 2 year after median nerve repair. The former gap inside the tube is bridged by a continuous nerve structure with no sign of neuroma formation. (Reproduced with permission from Lundborg et al 1994.[54])

were randomized to either tubulization (11 cases) or conventional microsurgical repair (7 cases). In the tubulization group there were five median and six ulnar nerve repairs. In the microsurgical repair group there were three median and four ulnar nerve repairs. The design of the study and the results at a 1-year follow-up were presented at the annual meeting of the American Society for Surgery of the Hand in San Francisco 1995.[55]

The patients were evaluated by a blind tester at regular intervals up to 12 months. The examinations included tests for Tinel's sign, tactilometry, Semmes–Weinstein monofilaments, tactil gnosis as assessed by static moving two-point discrimination,[56] and a shape-identification test.[57,58] Occurrence of neuroma at the repair site, hyperesthesia in the autonomous zone of the nerve, and cold intolerance were quantified in a ranking system. The test also included strength in palmar abduction of the thumb or abduction of the index finger.

On the basis of these tests there was no statistically significant difference between both techniques at 1-year follow-up. However, at the 3-month check-up there was a significant difference in perception of touch (Semmes–Weinstein monofilament) in favour of the tubulization technique. In one case the silicone tube was removed after 1 year because of local

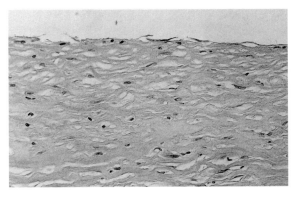

Figure 6

Histological appearance of the tissue surrounding the silicone tube at re-exploration at 12 months following implantation. There is a fibrous layer with few cells and few blood vessels. There are no signs of inflammation and no giant cells. ×300

discomfort when the wrist was extended and when local pressure was applied. The appearance of the contents was the same as described above, i.e. a nerve structure occupied the former gap in smooth continuity between the proximal and distal nerve segments with no signs of neuroma formation. Histopathological analysis of the thin mesothelium-like membrane surrounding the silicone tube showed connective tissue with few cells containing some blood vessels but no inflammatory elements or giant cells (Figure 6).

Tubes for bridging segmental defects

In our hands the silicone tube technique has been used only as an alternative to conventional microsurgical techniques for primary repair of transected nerves. In its present form this principle should not be used for bridging extended gaps in nerve continuity. In such situations permeable tubes allowing a more rapid vascularization of the central parts of the tubes may be expected to work better, provided the permeable material will not disturb the regeneration process. MacKinnon and Dellon have reported successful results from the use of resorbable polyglycolic acid (PGA) tubes for bridging digital nerve defects ranging from 0.5 to 3.0 (mean 1.7) cm.[45] Their material included 15 patients. The procedure was in all cases carried out as a secondary procedure. At follow-up at 11–32 months (mean 22 months) it was found that excellent functional sensation (moving two-point discrimination ≤3 mm and/or static two-point discrimination ≤6 mm) was present in 33% and good functional sensation (moving two-point discrimination 4–7 mm and/or static two point discrimination of 7–15 mm) in 53% of the digital nerve reconstructions. The authors concluded that reconstruction of nerve gaps of up to 3.0 cm with bioabsorbable PGA tubes gives clinical results at least comparable to the classic nerve graft technique while avoiding donor-site morbidity. Their concept has been further stressed in a case report describing successful use of a PGA tube to reconstruct a 25 mm defect in the right inferior alveolar nerve.[59] Two years following nerve reconstruction pain relief remained excellent and perception of pressure and vibration was similar to the thresholds for these perceptions on the contralateral lip.

Treatment of painful neuromas

Experimental studies have demonstrated that when a proximal nerve end is introduced into a silicone tube exceeding a critical length no or very limited axonal regeneration will occur inside the tube. Instead the proximal nerve end will extend only a few millimeters into the tube, forming a cone-shaped structure which extends into a tiny tissue strand and contains no axons (Figure 2). No true neuroma is being formed, and such nerve structures do not show the typical functional characteristics of a painful neuroma (see above).

Inspired by these observations we have applied the silicone tube principle to the treatment of painful neuromas in clinical cases. Our material consists of painful neuromas occurring after (1) resection of segments of sural nerves for grafting; (2) accidental transection of cutaneous nerve branches from the radial nerve at wrist level; and (3) accidental transection of the palmar branch of the median nerve at wrist level. In all cases silicone tubes of at least 20 mm length were used. The tube was opened at both ends, the proximal nerve end being introduced 2 mm into the proximal opening and secured in place with two epineurial sutures through the wall of the tube. When possible, the nerve branch and associated tubes were transposed and covered by muscle tissue or subcutaneous fat.

No prospective randomized study has so far been carried out to compare this technique with other available techniques for the treatment of painful neuromas. Hard data are therefore lacking. However, the majority of the patients describe much improvement or total relief from neuroma pain. No patient has deteriorated.

Conclusion

Tubular repair represents an attractive biological approach to nerve injuries.[21] Our experience in the use of silicone tubes as an alternative to conventional techniques for primary treatment of median and ulnar nerve transections shows that this technique is at least as good as conventional techniques with respect to recovery of sensibility and motor functions in the hand.[55] As more clinical cases occur, the technique will be better evaluated.

It has been reported that the use of silicone tubes or sheaths might induce unfavourable fibrosis around nerves.[60] However, we have not encountered such problems. As silicone tubes can be used experimentally as a model for nerve compression,[61-64] we are aware of the importance of using a tube whose inner diameter exceeds the thickness of the nerve by at least 30% to allow for swelling of the nerve ends. The histological appearance of the thin connective tissue sheath surrounding the silicone tube in one of our re-explored cases did not indicate inflammation or severe foreign body response (Figure 6). In the treatment of painful neuromas we do not believe in using silicone caps to inhibit the outgrowing axons. On the contrary our approach is to introduce the proximal nerve end into a free space of such a length that there is a cessation in axonal growth after a few millimeters.

For bridging extended gaps in nerve continuity, silicone tubes do not represent a solution since the impermeable silicone material does not allow vascular supply by ingrowing vessels along the segment. Other tube materials may prove more useful for this purpose. Bioartificial nerve grafts, where multiple longitudinal synthetic filaments serve as guidelines for regenerating axons, may prove an attractive solution for the future.[65]

References

1 Liss AG, af Ekenstam FW, Wiberg M, Cell loss in sensory ganglia following peripheral nerve injury. An anatomical study in the cat, *Scand J Plast Reconstr Surg Hand Surg* (1994) **28**:177–87.

2 Liss AG, af Ekenstam FW, Wiberg M, Loss of neurons in the dorsal root ganglia after transection of a sensory peripheral nerve. An anatomical study in monkeys, *Scand J Plast Reconstr Hand Surg* (1995) **30**:1–6.

3 Liss AG, af Ekenstram FW, Wiberg M, Changes in the spinal terminal pattern of the superficial radial nerve after a peripheral nerve injury. An anatomical study in cats, *Scand J Plast Reconstr Hand Surg* (1995) **29**:117–31.

4 Jenkins WM, Merzenich NM, Recanzona G, Neocortical representational dynamics in adult primates: implications for neurophysiology, *Neuropsychologia* (1990) **28**:573–84.

5 Jenkins WM, Merzenich NM, Ochs MT, et al, Functional reorganization of primary somato-sensory cortex in adult owl monkeys after behaviorally controlled tactile stimulation, *J Neurophysiol* (1990) **63**:82–104.

6 Wall JT, Kaas JH, Sur M, et al, Functional reorganization in somatosensory cortical areas 3b and 1 of adult monkeys after median nerve repair: possible relationships to sensory recovery in humans, *J Neurosci* (1986) **6**:218–33.

7 Wall JT, Kaas JH, Long-term cortical consequences of reinnervation errors after nerve regeneration in monkeys, *Brain Res* (1986) **372**:400–4.

8 Lundborg G, *Nerve Injury and Repair* (Churchill Livingstone: Edinburgh, 1988) 1–222.

9 Millesi H, Meissl G, Berger A, The interfascicular nerve grafting of the median and ulnar nerve, *J Bone Joint Surg* (1972) **54A**:727–50.

10 Millesi H, Meissl G, Berger A, Further experience with interfascicular grafting of the median, ulnar and radial nerves, *J Bone Joint Surg* (1976) **58A**:209–17.

11 Calder JS, Norris RW, Repair of mixed peripheral nerves using muscle autografts: a preliminary communication, *Br J Plast Surg* (1993) **46**:557–64.

12 Glasby MA, Hitchcock RJI, Huang CL-H, Effect of muscle basement membrane on regeneration of rat sciatic nerve, *J Bone Joint Surg* (1986) **68**:829–33.

13 Hems TEJ, Glasby MA, The limit of graft length in the experimental use of muscle grafts for nerve repair, *J Hand Surg* (1993) **18B**:165–70.

14 Varon S, Bunge RP, Trophic mechanisms in the peripheral nervous system, *Ann Rev Neurosci* (1978) **1**:327–61.

15 Lundborg G, Dahlin L, Danielsen N, et al, Trophism, tropism and specificity in nerve regeneration, *J Reconstr Microsurg* (1994) **5**:345–54.

16 Bates DJ, Ranford JA, Mangelsdorf DC, Blot and culture analysis of neuronotrophic factors in nerve regeneration chamber fluids, *Neurochem Res* (1991) **16**:621.

17 Heumann R, Korsching S, Brandtlow C, et al, Changes of nerve growth factor synthesis in nonneuronal cells in response to sciatic nerve transection, *J Cell Biol* (1987) **104**:1623–31.

18 Meyer M, Matsuoka I, Wetrose C, et al, Enhanced synthesis of brain-derived neurotropic factor in the lesioned peripheral nerve: different mechanisms are responsible for the regulation of BDNF and NGFmRNA, *J Cell Biol* (1992) **119**:45–54.

19 Danielsen N, Varon S, Characterization of neurotrophic activity in the silicone chamber model for nerve regeneration, *J Reconstr Microsurg* (1995) **11**:231–5.

20 Williams LR, Manthorpe M, Barbin G, et al, High ciliary neuronotrophic specific activity in rat peripheral nerve, *Int J Dev Neurosci* (1984) **2**:177–80.

21 Lundborg G, Dahlin LB, Danielsen N, et al, Nerve regeneration across an extended gap: a neurobiological view of nerve repair and the possible involvement of neuronotrophic factors, *J Hand Surg* (1982) **7A**:580–7.

22 Longo FM, Skaper SD, Manthorpe M, et al, Temporal changes of neuronotrophic activities accumulating in vivo within nerve regeneration chambers, *Exp Neurol* (1983) **81**:756.

23 Bates DJ, Mangelsdorf DC, Ridings JA, Multiple neurotrophic factors including NGF-like activity in nerve regeneration chamber fluids, *Neurochem Int* (1995) **26**:281–93.

24 Lundborg G, Hansson HA, Regeneration of peripheral nerve through a preformed tissue space. Preliminary observations on the reorganization of regenerating nerve fibres and perineurium, *Brain Res* (1979) **178**:573–6.

25 Lundborg G, Hansson HA, Nerve regeneration through preformed pseudosynovial tubes: a preliminary report of a new experimental model for studying the regeneration and reorganization capacity of peripheral nerve tissue, *J Hand Surg* (1980) **5A**:35–8.

26 Dellon AL, MacKinnon SE, An alternative to the classical nerve graft for the management of the short nerve gap, *Plast Reconstr Surg* (1988) **82**:849–56.

27 Lundborg G, Longo FM, Varon S, Nerve regeneration model and trophic factors in vivo, *Brain Res* (1982) **232**:157–61.

28 Lundborg G, Dahlin LB, Danielsen N, et al, Nerve regeneration in silicone chambers: influence of gap length and of distal stump components, *Exp Neurol* (1982) **76**:361–75.

29 Williams LR, Exogenous fibrin matrix precursors stimulate the temporal progress of nerve regeneration within a silicone chamber, *Neurochem Res* (1987) **12**:851–60.

30 Müller HW, Williams LR, Varon S, Nerve regeneration chamber: evaluation of exogenous agents applied by multiple injections, *Brain Res* (1987) **413**:320–6.

31 Yannas IV, Skin and nerve regeneration phenomena induced by polymeric templates. In: *Transactions of the 5th European Conference on Biomaterials* (Paris, 1985) 159–63.

32 Yannas IV, Orgill DP, Silver J, et al, Polymeric template facilitates regeneration of sciatic nerve across 15 mm gap. In: *Transactions of the 5th European Conference on Biomaterials* (Paris, 1985) 163.

33 da Silva C, Madison R, Dikkes P, et al, An in vivo model to quantify motor and sensory peripheral nerve regeneration using bioresorbable nerve guide tubes, *Brain Res* (1985) **342**:307–15.

34 Madison RD, Da Silva CF, Dikkes P, et al, Increased rate of peripheral nerve regeneration using bioresorbable nerve guides and a laminin-containing gel, *Exp Neurol* (1985) **88**:767.

35 Kljavin IJ, Madison RD, Peripheral nerve regeneration within tubular prostheses: effects of laminin and collagen matrices on cellular ingrowth, *Cells Mat* (1991) **1**:17–28.

36 Madison RD, DaSilva CF, Dikkes P, Entubulation repair with protein additives increases the maximum nerve gap distance successfully bridged with tubular prostheses, *Brain Res* (1988) **447**:325–34.

37 Valentini RF, Aebischer P, Winn SR, et al, Collagen- and laminin-containing gels impede peripheral nerve regeneration through semipermeable nerve guidance channels, *Exp Neurol* (1987) **98**:350–6.

38 Zeng L, Worseg A, Albrecht G, et al, Bridging of peripheral nerve defects with exogenous laminin-fibrin matrix in silicone tubes in a rat model, *Rest Neurol Neurosci* (1995) **8**:107–11.

39 Shine HD, Harcourt PG, Sidman RL, Tubular implants containing Schwann cells support PNS axonal regeneration, *American Society for Neurochemistry, 17th Annual Meeting*. Montreal, 1986.

40 Guénard V, Kleitman N, Morrissey TK, et al, Syngeneic Schwann cells derived from adult nerves seeded in semipermeable guidance channels enhance peripheral nerve regeneration, *J Neurosci* (1992) **12**:3310–20.

41 Seckel BR, Jones D, Hekimian KJ, et al, Hyaluronic acid through a new injectable nerve guide delivery system enhances peripheral nerve regeneration in the rat, *J Neurosci Res* (1995) **40**:318–24.

42 Molander H, Olsson Y, Engkvist O, et al, Regeneration of peripheral nerve through a polyglactin tube, *Muscle Nerve* (1982) **5**:54–7.

43 Molander H, Engkvist O, Hägglund J, et al, Nerve repair using a polyglactin tube and nerve graft: an experimental study in the rabbit, *Biomaterials* (1983) **4**:276–80.

44 Reid RI, Cutright DE, Garrison JS, Biodegradable cuff. An adjunct to peripheral nerve repair: a study in dogs, *Hand* (1978) **10**:259–66.

45 MacKinnon SE, Dellon LE, Clinical nerve reconstruction with a bioabsorbable polyglycolic acid tube, *Plast Reconstr Surg* (1990) **85**:419–24.

46 Danielsen N, Dahlin LB, Lee YF, et al, Axonal growth in mesothelial chambers: the role of the distal nerve segment, *Scand J Plast Reconstr Surg* (1983) **17**:119–25.

47 Williams LR, Danielsen N, Müller H, et al, Exogenous matrix precursors promote functional nerve regeneration across a 15-mm gap within a silicone chamber in the rat, *J Comp Neurol* (1987) **26**:284–90.

48 Tupper JW, Booth DM, Treatment of painful neuromas of sensory nerves in the hand: a comparison of traditional and newer methods, *J Hand Surg* (1976) **1A**:144–51.

49 Burke BR, A preliminary report in the use of silastic nerve caps in conjunction with neuroma surgery, *J Foot Surg* (1978) **17**:53–7.

50 Williams HB, The painful stump neuroma and its treatment, *Clin Plast Surg* (1984) **11**:79–84.

51 Midenberg ML, Kirschenbaum SE, Utilization of silastic nerve caps for the treatment of amputation neuromas, *J Foot Surg* (1986) **25**:489–94.

52 Danielsen N, Shyu BC, Dahlin LB, et al, Absence of ongoing activity in fibres arising from proximal nerve ends regenerating into mesothelial chambers, *Pain* (1986) **26**:93–104.

53 Lundborg G, Dahlin LB, Danielsen N, Ulnar nerve repair by the silicone chamber technique: case report, *Scand J Plast Reconstr Hand Surg* (1991) **25**:79–82.

54 Lundborg G, Rosen B, Abrahamsson SO, et al, Tubular repair of the median nerve in the human forearm. Preliminary findings, *J Hand Surg* (1994) **19B**:273–6.

55 Lundborg G, Rosén B, Dahlin LB, et al, Tubular vs. conventional repair of median and ulnar nerves in the human forearm. *J Hand Surg* (1996) in press.

56 Moberg E, Two-point discrimination test, a valuable part of hand surgical rehabilitation in tetraplegia, *Scand J Rehab Med* (1990) **22**:127–34.

57 Rosén B, Lundborg G, Dahlin LB, et al, Nerve repair: correlation of restitution of functional sensibility with specific cognitive capacities, *J Hand Surg* (1994) **19B**:452–8.

58 Lundborg G, Rosén B, Rationale for quantitative sensory tests in hand surgery. In: Boivie J, Hansson P, Lindblom U, eds, *Touch, Temperature and Pain in Health and Disease: Mechanisms and Assessments*, Vol 3 (IASP Press: Seattle, 1995) 151–62.

59 Crawley WA, Dellon AL, Inferior alveolar nerve reconstruction with a polyglycolic acid bioabsorbable nerve conduit, *Plast Reconstr Surg* (1992) **90**:300–2.

60 Merle M, Dellon A, Campbell YN, et al, Complications from silicon-polymer intubulation of nerves, *Microsurgery* (1989) **10**:130.

61 MacKinnon SE, Dellon AL, Hudson AR, et al, Chronic nerve compression. An experimental model in the rat, *Ann Plast Surg* (1984) **13**:112–20.

62 MacKinnon SE, Dellon AL, Hudson AR, et al, A primate model for chronic nerve compression, *J Reconstr Microsurg* (1985) **1**:185–95.

63 MacKinnon SE, O'Brien JP, Dellon AL, et al, An assessment of the effects of internal neurolysis on a chronically compressed rat sciatic nerve, *Plast Reconstr Surg* (1988) **81**:251–6.

64 MacKinnon SE, Dellon LE, Evaluation of microsurgical internal neurolysis in a primate median nerve model of chronic nerve compression, *J Hand Surg* (1988) **13A**:357–63.

65 Lundborg G, Kanje M, Bioartificial nerve grafts—a prototype, *Scand J Plast Reconstr Hand Surg* (1996) **30**:105–10.

Commentary

Chapter 25

This excellent chapter provides a useful guide for a better approach and a better pre- and post-operative assessment of the spastic upper extremity. We would like to add three points according to our experience. Firstly, botulinum toxin injection is a quite expensive technique, a concern in a cost-conscious era. Secondly, botulinum toxin injections are frequently of transitory effect but could allow the patient to better appreciate the possibility of surgery such as tenotomy or tendon lengthening procedures. Thirdly, the injections could be combined with reinforcement of antagonist muscles by electrical stimulation providing, without further surgery, a definite functional improvement.

GF

Chapter 26

This is a new, simple and attractive technique for mixed nerve repair. I have no experience of silicone tubes but I have been impressed by the clinical results of vein grafts (reverse) for collateral nerve repair in moderated losses (less than a centimetre). In acute cases, when a vein graft is harvested for arterial repair, a longer segment could be harvested to bridge the collateral nerve loss. We have used this technique in 11 clinical cases on the less relevant side of fingers (such as the ulnar side of the middle finger), with results comparable to conventional nerve grafts. Several technical problems remain, such as the choice of material to fill the vein graft in order to avoid collapse.

GF

Arthroscopic reduction with percutaneous fixation of Bennett's fractures

Richard A Berger

Introduction

In 1885, Edward Hallaran Bennett described an intraarticular fracture pattern involving the proximal end of the first metacarpal.[1] Substantial controversy has evolved regarding the optimal treatment for these fractures. It is well recognized that posttraumatic degenerative changes develop predictably in proportion to the degree of intraarticular incongruity, and are presumably influenced by the state of integrity of the surrounding soft tissue envelope. What remains unclear is the degree of impairment as it relates to the presence or absence of degenerative changes in the joint.

Gedda and Moberg were the first to strongly advocate attempts to restore the congruency of the joint surface via open reduction and internal fixation, noting substantial disability from degenerative arthritis.[2] Although there is a substantial tendency to develop radiographic signs of degenerative changes following displaced or comminuted fractures of the base of the first metacarpal, most authors report relatively mild symptoms following an adequate recovery period. In spite of this, the tendency to take patients with displaced intraarticular fractures of the base of the first metacarpal to surgery for open reduction and internal fixation has steadily increased. Recently, evidence has been collected which suggests that indeed patients with restoration of congruity of the articular surface in Bennett's fractures have improved chances of a more favorable outcome.[3-7] Because of the wide exposure necessary to expose the fracture site, and because of the limited visibility even with a wide exposure,

the concept of arthroscopically-assisted reduction of Bennett's fractures was developed.[8]

Conventional treatment options

The number of reported treatment options for Bennett's fractures is substantial.[2,5,6,7] Although the proponents of each technique claim significant advantages for that particular technique, there are potential disadvantages to each technique. For example, closed reduction, with or without pin fixation, relies on radiographic imaging to judge the adequacy of reduction. However, radiographs are often difficult to interpret. Because of the oblique nature of the fracture plane and the overlap of bony images in the plane best suited for imaging the fracture fragment, a potential exists for substantial displacement, in spite of apparent reduction by radiographic criteria. Additionally, radiographic imaging alone will not allow estimation of soft tissue injury or damage to the articular surface. On the other hand, open reduction carries potential morbidity due to the obligatory wide capsulotomy necessary to visualize the reduction of the small ulnar fragment from a radial perspective.

Arthroscopic examination of the first carpometacarpal joint was developed as a reliable technique approximately 2 years ago as a means of inspecting the joint surface in early degenerative joint disease.[8] The technique provides unparalleled visualization of the entire first carpometacarpal joint, including the proximal surface of the first metacarpal and the distal surface of the trapezium. Additionally, the articular ligaments[9,10] are generally clearly identifiable. These images are obtained through small skin and capsular incisions of no more than 2 mm width, resulting in a substantial potential reduction in morbidity due to the surgical approach. Arthroscopic reduction of Bennett's fractures seemed to be a logical 'next step' in the evolution of this technique.

Indications

The indications for arthroscopic reduction of Bennett's fracture are essentially the same as for open reduction. These include a classic Bennett's fracture with displacement, generally exceeding 1 mm step-off and/or 1 mm gap (Figure 1). This is generally accompanied by some degree of subluxation of the larger fragment; however, the degree of subluxation may be subtle. Another indication is to evaluate suspected substantial soft tissue injury, independent of fracture displacement. Finally, any desire to evaluate and document damage imparted to the articular surface, or to define the presence of pre-injury degenerative disease, is an ideal indication for arthroscopic examination.

Contraindications

Absolute contraindications for first carpometacarpal joint arthroscopy include gross contamination of the surrounding soft tissue envelope, substantial comminution of the fracture (such as a Rolando fracture) and coexisting hand compartment syndrome, especially involving the thenar compartment. Relative contraindications include an impacted fracture. This condition is determined radiographically following induction of anesthesia, where the major metacarpal fragment is manipulated in an attempt to achieve a provisional reduction. If the two fracture fragments do not exhibit motion tending toward reduction with this simple maneuver, it is unlikely that arthroscopic reduction will achieve any improvement. Any other condition which makes the patient a less ideal candidate for any surgical procedure must be weighed as a relative contraindication for this procedure.

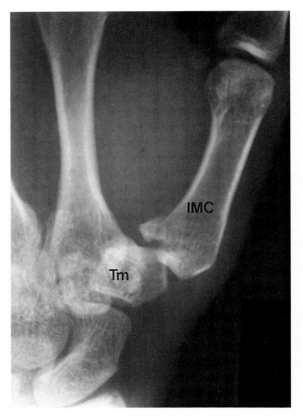

Figure 1

Radiographic appearance of a typical displaced Bennett's fracture. IMC = first metacarpal; Tm = trapezium.

Equipment

Standard arthroscopic support equipment will be required, including light source, video camera/video cassette recorder, sheaths, tapered trocars, and inflow/outflow tubing for either a 1.9 mm (preferred) or 2.7 mm obtuse viewing angle fiberoptic arthroscope. A 2.0 mm radial side shaver, small probe, and a set of small grabbers are preferred. Longitudinal traction will be required, and I prefer a portable traction tower with a single finger trap applied to the thumb. Fluid requirements are minimal, and I often have an assistant advance fluid through a 20 ml syringe through an extension tube attached to the arthroscope sheath. Outflow is optional. For fracture management, a small fluoroscopic system is recommended, as well as equipment for placement of Kirschner wires. Access to standard screws is recommended if conversion to open reduction is encountered.

Surgical technique

With the patient supine, the upper extremity is prepared and draped over a pneumatic tourniquet applied to the arm. A single finger trap is applied to the level of the proximal phalanx of the thumb, and between 5 and 8 lb (2.5 and 3.6 kg) of longitudinal traction is applied (Figure 2). Under fluoroscopic guidance, a single 0.035 or 0.045 inch (0.89 or 1.14 mm) Kirschner wire is

advanced through the base of the large fragment until it almost reaches the fracture, parallel to the joint surface, oriented in such a way that if it is advanced across the fracture the smaller fragment will be captured after reduction is achieved. Generally, this is achieved with an ulnar and slightly anterior orientation to the pin.

The landmarks for the arthroscopic portals are the extrinsic tendons of extensor pollicis brevis and abductor pollicis longus (Figure 3). The 1-R portal is developed just anterior to the abductor pollicis longus tendon, and will ultimately pass just posterior and lateral to the anterior oblique ligament of the trapeziometacarpal (TMC) joint. The 1-U portal is developed just posterior to the extensor pollicis brevis tendon, and will ultimately pass between the dorsal radial and posterior oblique ligaments of the TMC joint. Confirmation of the location of the portals can

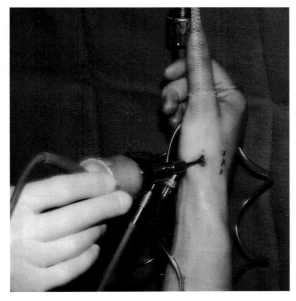

Figure 2

Intraoperative photograph of an arthroscopic reduction of a Bennett's fracture. The thumb is suspended by a single finger trap with approximately 5 lb (2.5 kg) of longitudinal traction. By use of the traction tower, there is easy access to the operative site for additional equipment necessary for the procedure, such as a powered drill, fluoroscopy, and a shaver.

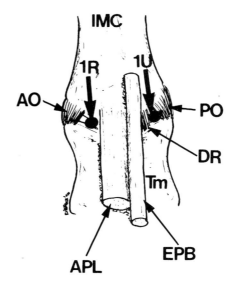

Figure 3

Drawing of the first carpometacarpal joint region from a lateral perspective, illustrating the location of the arthroscopic portals used for arthroscopic reduction of Bennett's fracture. 1-R = radial portal; 1-U = ulnar portal; IMC = first metacarpal; Tm = trapezium; APL = tendon of abductor pollicis longus; EPB = tendon of extensor pollicis brevis; AO = anterior oblique ligament; DR = dorsoradial ligament; PO = posterior oblique ligament.

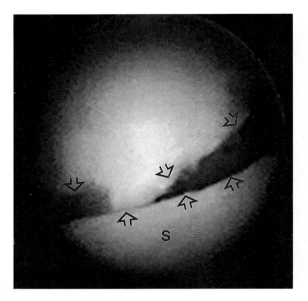

Figure 4

Arthroscopic view of the first carpometacarpal joint from the 1-R portal, illustrating the fractured articular surface of the base of a first metacarpal with a Bennett's fracture (arrow heads). Note the displacement of the fracture, with the smaller fragment (S) located near the bottom of the image.

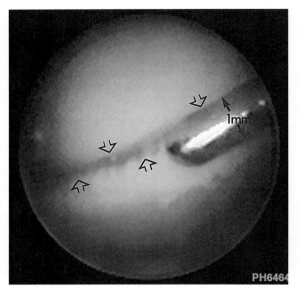

Figure 5

Arthroscopic view of the first carpometacarpal joint following reduction of the fracture. Note the restoration of congruency of the articular surface (arrow heads). A small probe is placed with the 1 mm angled tip parallel to the joint surface, indicating that no step-off is present.

be made fluoroscopically or by passing a small hypodermic needle (22 gauge) obliquely into the TMC joint. Two parallel longitudinally oriented incisions, each 2–3 mm in length, are made over the portal locations. Using longitudinally directed blunt dissection, the joint capsule is approached. Portals are established using a tapered trocar and the sheath for a 1.9 mm arthroscope is placed in either the 1-R or 1-U portal. A probe is advanced into the opposite portal. If visualization is obscured by blood or debris, the probe may be exchanged for the 2.0 mm shaver connected to low power suction, and the joint is debrided until visualization is clear.

The arthroscope is telescoped gently 1–3 mm to allow a complete survey of the joint, and the portal sites are liberally exchanged to allow for a complete assessment of the joint. By convention, I prefer to orient the image of the base of the metacarpal superiorly and the distal surface

of the trapezium inferiorly on the video screen. Soft tissue assessment includes a survey of the anterior oblique, posterior oblique, dorsal radial and ulnar collateral ligaments. Notations on the condition of the articular surfaces are carefully made.

The fracture fragment is identified near the anterior and ulnar extent of the joint (Figure 4). It is generally depressed distal to the lane of the large fragment joint surface. Under arthroscopic visualization, the thumb is maneuvered to reduce the large fragment to the small fragment. The manipulation should follow whatever pathway is necessary to reduce the particular fracture pattern present, but typically involves a combination of pronation, abduction, and palmar flexion (Figure 5). It may be necessary to dis-impact the fracture site with the probe to mobilize the fracture fragments, and occasional loose osteochondral fragments may be removed

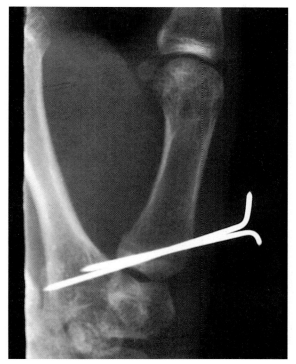

a

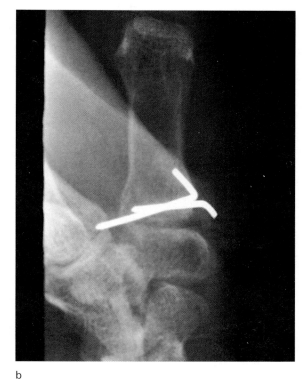

b

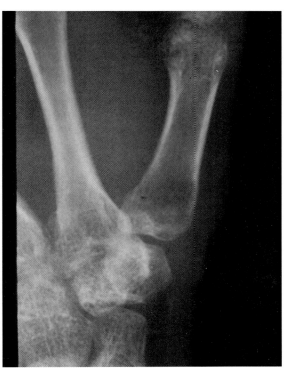

c

Figure 6

Posterior–anterior (a) and lateral (b) radiographs of the Bennett's fracture shown in Figures 1, 4 and 5 following arthroscopic reduction and percutaneous fixation. Two 0.045 inch (1.14 mm) Kirschner wires have been advanced through the fracture site, maintaining accurate reduction of the articular surface as well as restoring stability of the first metacarpal to the trapezium (c). The fracture healed with no obvious deformity and there were no perioperative complications. Within 6 weeks following removal of the pins, the patient had regained full range of motion compared to the contralateral thumb and had resumed full activities without difficulty.

arthroscopically. Once joint congruency is achieved by arthroscopic criteria, the fluoroscope is activated to confirm extraarticular reduction. The Kirschner wire is advanced across the fracture into the smaller fragment (Figure 6). If this fixation is inadequate, additional fixation may be achieved by cross-pinning the first metacarpal to the second metacarpal, or by lacing a transarticular in across the TMC joint. Final plain radiographs should be obtained in the operating room.

Postoperative management

The pin(s) is generally removed between 6 and 8 weeks postoperatively. A removable orthoplast splint is fabricated, and the patient undergoes rehabilitation which includes graduated range of motion and strengthening programs until full functional recovery is achieved.

Conclusions

Arthroscopic reduction combined with percutaneous fixation provides a safe alternative to open reduction of Bennett's fractures. It is felt that the arthroscope allows adequate, possibly superior visualization of the fracture site and the capsular soft tissues, while only minimally disturbing the joint capsule. This may enhance postoperative function by minimizing scar formation. After inducing appropriate anesthesia, the thumb is distracted with approximately 5 lb (2.5 kg) through a single finger trap. By the use of arthroscopic portals established on either side of the abductor pollicis longus/extensor pollicis brevis tendon group passing across the first carpometacarpal joint, a 1.9 mm arthroscope is used to visualize the fracture while standard reduction methods are employed. It is also possible to use a shaver, probe, or other arthroscopic instrument through these portals. Care must be exercised during placement of the portals to avoid injury to the branches of the superficial radial nerve passing near by. The surgeon must also be prepared to abort the arthroscopic procedure and proceed with an arthrotomy if an adequate reduction is not possible using the arthroscope.

References

1   Bennett EH, Injuries of the skeleton: value of the accumulation of specimens, *BMJ* (1885) **ii**:199.
2   Gedda KO, Moberg E, Open reduction and osteosynthesis of the so-called Bennett's fracture in the carpometacarpal joint of the thumb, *Acta Orthop Scand* (1953) **22**:249.
3   Cannon S, Dowd G, Williams D, et al, A long-term study following Bennett's fracture, *J Hand Surg* (1986) **11B**:426.
4   Howard FM, Fractures of the basal joint of the thumb, *Clin Orthop Rel Res* (1987) **220**:46–51.
5   Kjaer-Petersen K, Langhoff O, Andersen K, Bennett's fracture, *J Hand Surg* (1990) **15B**:58–61.
6   Moutet F, Lebrun C, Bellon-Champel P, et al, Les lesions articulaires de la premiere colonne du pouce, *Ann de Chir* (1989) **43**:491–502.
7   van Niewkerk JL, Ouwens R, Fractures of the base of the first metacarpal bone: results of surgical treatment, *Injury* (1989) **20**:359–62.
8   Berger RA, Arthroscopy of the first carpometacarpal joint, *J Hand Surg* (in press).
9   Imeada T, An K-N, Cooney WP, et al, Anatomy of trapeziometacarpal ligaments, *J Hand Surg* (1993) **18A**:226–31.
10 Kauer JMG, Functional anatomy of the carpometacarpal joint of the thumb, *Clin Orthop Rel Res* (1987) **220**:7–13.

28
Arthroscopic treatment of acute gamekeeper's thumb

Jaiyoung Ryu

Introduction

The treatment of choice for the collateral ligaments of human joints is generally a conservative one. An exception to this rule is with common ulnar collateral ligament (UCL) injuries of the thumb metacarpophalangeal (MP) joint, for which many open surgical treatment modalities producing better results than the conservative treatment have been advocated.

The reason for this is that the gamekeeper's thumb is often associated with a Stener lesion. In other words, should we be able to reduce the Stener lesion, a conservative treatment would be a viable option with the potential for better results than those yielded by current formal operative repairs.

With this in mind, we have treated acute gamekeeper's thumb by reducing the Stener lesions arthroscopically and then immobilizing the joint.

Technical aspects

The surgery is done under pneumatic tourniquet control. A Chinese finger trap is used on the thumb to suspend the hand vertically with the weight of the arm serving as traction. A No. 11 blade is inserted into the MP joint, just dorsal to the radial collateral ligament and radial to the extensor pollicis longus (radiodorsal portal), followed by a blunt trocar and a 1.9 mm, 15° arthroscope. Joint articular surfaces are examined, and the presence or absence of the UCL is confirmed. A second portal just volar to the radial collateral ligament (radiovolar portal) is established, and a hook is introduced. When a large amount of synovium blocks the view, a 2.0 mm full radius cutter is used for debridement through the radiovolar portal.

After the inner wall of the adductor aponeurosis is identified, a small bent probe, inserted through the radiovolar portal, is introduced along the metacarpal head, passed through the proximal edge of the aponeurosis around the anticipated origin site of the UCL and pulled toward the joint. This manoeuvre, which may be repeated if necessary, brings the distal end of the UCL inside the joint (Figure 1). The ligament's end is placed at its point of proximal phalangeal base insertion (Figure 2). In cases where no Stener lesion is present, the placement of the UCL is confirmed. A 0.045 Kirschner wire is inserted to immobilize the MP joint in a 20–30° flexed position. A thumb spica short arm cast is applied.

Postoperative care

The Kirschner wire is removed 4 weeks postoperatively, but the thumb spica cast remains for 6 weeks. Daily active and passive range of motion exercises are begun 6 weeks postoperatively under the supervision of hand therapists. Sports activity and heavy lifting are prohibited for one month after cast removal.

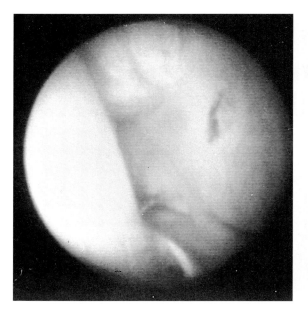

Figure 1

The ulnar collateral ligament was reduced and placed in its proper anatomical position. Note a small rent at its midsubstance. A portion of metacarpal head is shown on the left side.

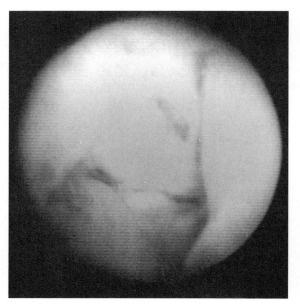

Figure 2

The ulnar collateral ligament was arthroscopically reduced and placed in its anatomical position. A portion of proximal phalangeal base is shown on the right side.

Pros and cons compared to classical techniques

The attractions of this technique are numerous:

(1) The surgical intervention is minimal with decreased surgical morbidity.
(2) The incision over the first web space is eliminated, preventing hypersensitive, insensate or contractile scarring on this highly used region.
(3) It reduces the joint stiffness with a traditional repair and tightening of the UCL and the adductor aponeurosis. Instead, it leaves the collateral ligament without any undue tension for its natural healing process, comparable to the preferred treatment of other collateral ligament ruptures where concern about the Stener's lesion does not exist.
(4) The procedure does not demand preoperative differentiation as to whether the Stener's lesion is present.

The only disadvantages of the procedure are that it requires small joint arthroscopic equipment and that a surgeon needs to go through a 'learning curve', which can be satisfactorily achieved with cadaver specimens.

Results

The initial report on the technique was based on eight cases with an average follow-up of 21.4 months (range 12–30 months).[1] The averages of tip pinch, key pinch and grip strength were measured at 13 lb, 19 lb and 97.8 lb, respectively. In most cases, these strengths were equal to or greater than non-operated sides (averages 109%, 108% and 116%, respectively). This was attributed to the dominance of that side (seven out of eight thumbs) and our aggressive hand muscle strengthening therapy after the surgery.

There was no appreciable postoperative joint laxity (greater than 10°) of the MP joints during stress examination, compared to the opposite thumbs in seven cases. One thumb could be stressed 22° more than the thumb on the opposite side. All patients could touch the fifth MP crease with the thumb tip.

The average operated thumb interphalangeal (IP) joint motion was 102°, which was 99% of the opposite thumb. The thumb's MP joint motion was 51° and 99% of that of the thumb on the opposite side. The average combined motion of IP and MP was 153° for the operated thumb and 154° for the opposite thumb. Seven out of eight patients reported no pain or functional limitation of their thumbs. One reported mild pain associated with such activities as opening jars or cutting meat.

The one complication was a pin tract infection that resulted in removal of the Kirschner wire 2 weeks early. The patient was placed on oral antibiotics and the infection was resolved with no further problems; the thumb spica splint was left in place for 6 weeks. When compared to the report by Osterman et al on primary repair of the UCL,[2] our results seem to be slightly better, with the added attraction of fewer complications.

The author continues to use the technique to date and has treated at least 12 more cases since the initial report with very similar and satisfying results.

Indications

The procedure is indicated for acute complete rupture of the thumb UCL. More importantly, it is contraindicated for chronic cases, incomplete tears or in the cases where a large intraarticular fracture is present.

References

1   Ryu J, Fagan R, Arthroscopic treatment of acute complete thumb metacarpophalangeal ulnar collateral ligament tears, *J Hand Surg* (1995) **20A**:1037–42.
2   Osterman AL, Hayken GD, Bora FW, A quantitative evaluation of thumb function after ulnar collateral repair and reconstruction, *J Trauma* (1981) **21**:854–61.

Treatment of scaphotrapeziotrapezoid arthrosis by distal scaphoid resection and capsular interposition arthroplasty

Marc Garcia-Elias, Alberto L Lluch and Angel Farreres

Introduction

Scaphotrapeziotrapezoid (STT) arthrosis is frequently found in association with degeneration of the trapeziometacarpal joint.[1-4] As an isolated condition it is quite uncommon. According to North and Eaton,[5] only 6% of 68 dissected wrists over 50 years old had an STT arthrosis in the absence of a trapeziometacarpal degeneration. Other series indicate a higher prevalence (15% according to Zemel[6]). Treatment options when an STT arthrosis becomes symptomatic, include resting splints, physiotherapy, anti-inflammatory drugs and eventually intraarticular corticoid injections. When conservative measures fail to relieve symptoms, surgery may be indicated. This usually consists of either fusion of the joint,[3,4,7] or interposition of a silicone spacer as reported by Kessler and others.[6,8] Complications of STT arthrodesis have been increasingly recognized in recent years. Painful nonunion and radioscaphoid impingement problems are the two more frequent complications reported.[9,10] Problems with silastic implants have also been found. These usually are secondary to wear or fracture of the silicone spacer, with the consequent biological response to it.[11]

In 1990, Linscheid and colleagues suggested a new approach to this problem.[2,3] They reported seven patients who sustained a fibrous arthroplasty of the STT joint, with five good results. They approached the joint palmarly, and filled the space with a slip of the flexor carpi radialis (FCR) tendon. Since 1992 we have used a modification of this technique by using a dorsal approach and a capsular flap as the interposing material.

Technical aspects

The wrist joint is approached using a zig-zag dorsolateral incision. The dorsal branches of the radial nerve are identified and carefully protected. By displacing the tendons extensor carpi radialis (longus and brevis) and extensor pollicis longus medially, and the extensor pollicis brevis and abductor pollicis longus laterally, the dorsolateral capsule is exposed. The radial artery, which crosses obliquely the distal corner of the surgical exposure, also needs to be identified, separated from the capsule and protected. A 2 cm wide, distally based, capsular flap is then fashioned with its base distal to the dorsal aspect of the STT joint. The flap is detached from the dorsal rim of both the radius and the scaphoid, and retracted distally until the whole STT joint cavity is visible (Figure 1a).

The distal articular surface of the scaphoid is then osteotomized with an oscillating saw and removed from the joint. Care must be taken not to remove too much bone so that the palmar scaphotrapezial ligaments remain attached to the waist of the scaphoid. The proximal articular surfaces of the trapezium and trapezoid are also

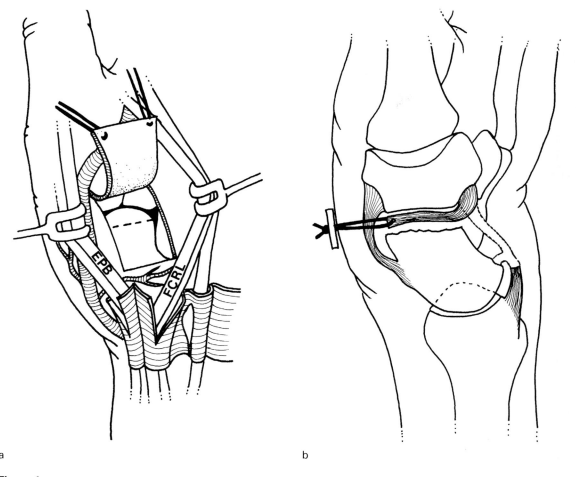

a   b

Figure 1

Schematic representation of the technique. (a) The joint capsule is approached dorsally through the interval between the first and second extensor compartments. A distal-based capsular flap is elevated and the STT joint exposed. (b) Once the distal articular surface of the scaphoid has been removed, the capsular flap is interposed within the joint using a pull-out technique. EPB, extensor pollicis brevis; FCRL, flexor carpi radialis longus.

removed with a rongeur and the joint copiously irrigated. The capsular flap is then interposed between the scaphoid and the trapezium-trapezoid bones by means of a pull-out wire technique, in a similar fashion as in the Bentzon's technique for scaphoid nonunions (Figure 1b).[12,13]

To cover the capsular defect, a portion of the extensor retinaculum can be detached medially and sutured to the capsular remnants under the extensor carpi radialis tendons. The wrist is immobilized in a below-elbow plaster slab for 2–3 weeks, followed by a controlled programme of physical rehabilitation.

Advantages and disadvantages compared to other techniques

This method uses as interposition material a biological tissue which is able to adapt histologically

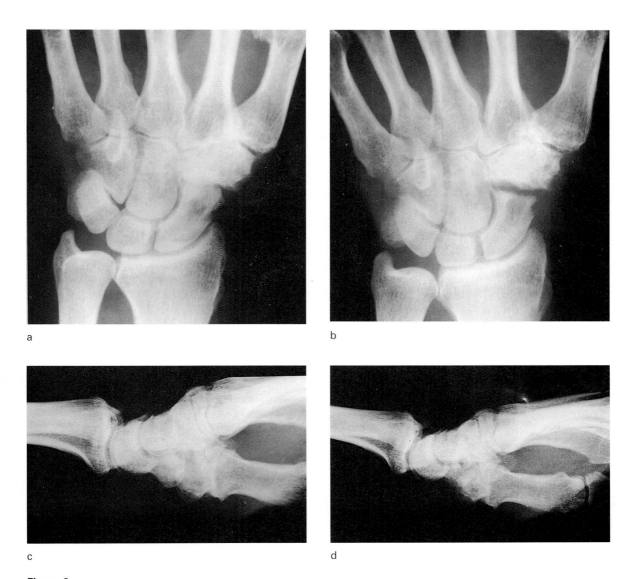

Figure 2

(a) Posteroanterior radiograph of the wrist of a 54-year-old male who complained of pain and tenderness on the lateral aspect of his dominant wrist, secondary to an isolated STT degenerative arthrosis. (b) Eighteen months after a resection-interposition arthroplasty, the patient was painfree, with full grip and pinch strength, and only a slight limitation of the flexion-extension (60–45°). Despite the patient being symptom-free, the lateral projections taken before (c) and after (d) surgery demonstrate that the nondissociative DISI pattern of carpal instability was not corrected by the procedure.

and mechanically to the newly created conditions of the joint. It does not require the use of any metal or silicone implant which may not withstand the forces transferred across the joint, and either dislocate, fracture or wear with the resulting joint dysfunction, if not a particle-induced synovitis. In other locations, such as in scaphoid nonunions, the long-term results of this type of soft-tissue arthroplasty have been found very encouraging.[13]

An alternative to this method is the fibrous interposition arthroplasty using a palmar approach as suggested by Linscheid et al.[3] This would be especially indicated in the cases where there is a tenosynovitis of the FCR, a relatively frequent association.[14] If there is not an obvious tenosynovitis, however, we prefer the dorsal approach described here for it does not violate the palmar capsule which contains the STT ligamentous complex, an important midcarpal stabilizer.[15]

Compared to an STT fusion which requires a minimum of 8 weeks of wrist immobilization, this method requires only 3 weeks, thus allowing a much faster return to the patient's activities. Furthermore, partial arthrodeses do alter significantly carpal kinematics[16] and kinetics,[17] aside from other significant complications including a high index of nonunions (from 4% to 23% according to different series[7,10]) and the frequent early development of radioscaphoid impingement problems.[9] Based on our experience, we only recommend an STT fusion when there is a substantial dorsal intercalated segment instability (DISI) pattern of carpal malalignment that needs to be corrected.[18,19] Indeed, with the method described above, this problem cannot be solved.

Results

Of the 10 patients operated on, 7 have been followed-up for more than 12 months, with an average of 19 months (range 12–37 months). Pain and functional discomfort were alleviated in all cases. Before surgery, all of them had pain rated 3 to 4 in a scale from 0 to 4. At follow-up, there was no pain in six patients, while in one moderate discomfort persisted in the extremes of motion.

Preoperatively, wrist motion was reduced relative to the contralateral side in most wrists. After surgery, the range of motion as compared to the contralateral side had slightly improved but very seldom became normal (average preoperative/postoperative: flexion 91%/93%; extension 96%/97%; radial deviation 72%/79%; ulnar deviation 83%/90%).

Wrist strength improved in all cases after surgery (average preoperative: 75% of the contralateral side; postoperative: 82%). This was especially true for the lateral pinch which increased significantly after surgery (preoperative: 67% of contralateral; postoperative: 94%; $P < 0.05$).

What surgery could not solve was carpal alignment. A nondissociative DISI pattern of instability was present in 6 of the 10 cases operated on (average preoperative radiolunate angle: 13°). At the latest follow-up a DISI pattern of malalignment was observed in 7 patients, with one having increased in comparison with the preoperative condition (average postoperative: 15°) (Figure 2). Whether or not the residual carpal malalignment will induce degenerative changes of the wrist with time is unknown. At the latest controls, however, this was perfectly tolerated.

Indications

The major indication of the resection-interposition arthroplasty described here is the symptomatic STT arthrosis with minimal carpal malalignment. It can also be an alternative in cases where the prolonged immobilization required for an STT fusion is contraindicated, or if a previous attempt of fusion has failed. When there is substantial malalignment an STT fusion would be preferable, although an arthroplasty can also be used. In this case, however, the patient should be warned about the possibility of the persisting carpal malalignment being the cause of long-term problems.

References

1   Carstam N, Eiken O, Andrew L, Osteoarthritis of the trapezio-scaphoid joint, *Acta Orthop Scand* (1968) **39**:354–8.
2   Crosby EB, Linscheid RL, Dobyns JH, Scapho-trapezial-trapezoidal arthrosis, *J Hand Surg* (1978) **3**:223–34.
3   Linscheid RL, Lirette R, Dobyns JH, L'arthrose dégénérative scapho-trapézienne. In: Saffar Ph, ed, *La Rhizarthrose* (Monographies du GEM, Expansion Scientifique Française: Paris, 1990) 185–94.
4   Watson HK, Hempton RF, Limited wrist arthrodeses. I. The triscaphoid joint, *J Hand Surg* (1980) **5**:320–7.
5   North ET, Eaton RG, Degenerative joint disease of the trapezium: a comparative radiographic and anatomic study, *J Hand Surg* (1983) **8**:160–7.
6   Zemel NP, Traitement de l'arthrose isolée de

l'articulation scapho-trapézo-trapézoïdienne. In: Saffar Ph, ed, *La Rhizarthrose* (Monographies du GEM, Expansion Scientifique Française: Paris, 1990) 194–202.

7   Rogers WD, Watson HK, Degenerative arthritis at the triscaphe joint, *J Hand Surg* (1990) **15A**:232–5.

8   Kessler I, Baruch A, Hecht O, et al, Osteoarthritis at the base of the thumb, *Acta Orthop Scand* (1976) **47**:361–9.

9   Rogers WD, Watson HK, Radial styloid impingement after triscaphe arthrodesis, *J Hand Surg* (1989) **14A**:297–301.

10 Fortin PT, Louis DS, Long-term follow-up of scaphoid-trapezium-trapezoid arthrodesis, *J Hand Surg* (1993) **18A**:675–81.

11 Khoo CTH, Silicone synovitis. The current role of silicone elastomer implants in joint reconstruction, *J Hand Surg* (1993) **18B**:679–92.

12 Bentzon PGK, Randlov-Madsen A, On fracture of the carpal scaphoid, *Acta Orthop Scand* (1945) **16**:30–9.

13 Boeckstyns MEH, Kjaër L, Busch P, et al, Soft-tissue interposition arthroplasty for scaphoid nonunions, *J Hand Surg* (1985) **10A**:109–14.

14 Irwin LR, Outhwaite J, Burge PD, Rupture of the flexor carpi radialis tendon associated with scapho-trapezial osteoarthritis, *J Hand Surg* (1992) **17B**:343–5.

15 Drewniany JJ, Palmer AK, Flatt AE, The scapho-trapezial ligament complex: an anatomic and biomechanical study, *J Hand Surg* (1985) **10A**:492–8.

16 Garcia-Elias M, Cooney WP, An KN, et al, Wrist kinematics after limited intercarpal arthrodesis, *J Hand Surg* (1989) **14A**:791–9.

17 Viegas SF, Patterson RM, Peterson PD, et al, Evaluation of the biomechanical efficacy of limited intercarpal fusions for the treatment of scapho-lunate dissociation, *J Hand Surg* (1990) **15A**:120–8.

18 Ferris BD, Dunnett W, Lavelle JR, An association between STT osteoarthritis and static dorsal inter-calated segment instability, *J Hand Surg* (1994) **19B**:338–9.

19 Oberlin C, Daunois O, Oberlin F, L'arthrose scapho-trapézo-trapézoïdienne. Son ratentissement sur le carpe, *Ann Chir Main* (1990) **9**:163–7.

Commentary

Chapter 27

Doctor Berger has shown that one can safely perform arthroscopic examination and reduction of Bennett fractures. The technique can also be used to remove loose bodies and debride early arthritis. Obviously, this is something for experienced arthroscopists only!

PCA

Chapter 28

As technical facility with the arthroscope increases, and technological advancements continue, arthroscopic treatment can be employed for more and more problems. Here we learn of a new way to manage ruptures of the ulnar collateral ligament of thumb metacarpophalangeal joint. Since the whole purpose of treatment is to get the ligament underneath the extensor aponeurosis, this would seem to be a quite effective, yet minimally invasive, method to use, provided one can get good visualization.

PCA

Chapter 29

The method proposed by Garcia-Elias et al seems a very reasonable alternative to scapho-trapeziotrapezoid (STT) fusion for cases of STT arthrosis. I have certainly been unimpressed with anchovy-type procedures in such circumstances. This seems to be a significant improvement, at least for cases without gross carpal malalignment. I agree with the authors that for care of STT arthrosis with carpal malalignment, an arthrodesis would be required.

PCA

This technique is easy to perform, provides very good results and has a high degree of patient satisfaction, even with a long follow-up (we saw a 17-year follow-up in a patient who came to be operated on the other side of the hand). During the procedure, it is easy to test the first ray stability: first ray collapse is not a problem because proximal migration is not possible. In our own practice, we have performed this procedure without interposition and without immobilization. Sufficient resection should be made to prevent scaphotrapezial impingement in any position.

PS

Treatment of Dupuytren's disease by percutaneous needle fasciotomy

Remy Bleton, Daniel Marcireau and Jean-Yves Alnot

Introduction

Since 1823, when subcutaneous fasciotomy was first suggested by Sir Astley Cooper and later by Dupuytren himself (Dupuytren 1832), the treatment of Dupuytren's contracture has remained controversial. Through the years, surgical fascial excision (SFE) appeared to be the procedure of choice, despite postoperative complications, disability and long-term recurrent deformity. Various procedures of subcutaneous fasciotomy have also been described; these usually employ a modified blade as a fasciotome (Kelly and Clifford 1959, Colville 1983). In 1979 Lermusiaux introduced the original technique of percutaneous needle fasciotomy (PNF) in the office, with promising results (Lermusiaux and Debeyre 1980). Schernberg (1994) was the first hand surgeon to try this technique. However, at four years of follow-up, he considered that the recurrence rate experienced was too high for the technique to be recommended.

Between 1992 and 1995, we have performed PNF for Dupuytren's contracture of any type and at any stage, when an operative treatment was indicated. The purpose of this chapter is to report some ways to improve the technique and make it safe. We also report our results and compare indications for this procedure in relation to surgical fascial excision.

Methods

Treatment is carried out in surgical conditions. It may be performed either in the office or in the operating theatre as an outpatient procedure. When the procedure is long (several fascio-

tomies in both hands, for example), it is better to perform the procedure in the operating theatre, for better patient comfort. The patient may receive intravenous sedative drugs if necessary and is allowed to return home immediately after the procedure.

The needle fasciotomy, as described by Lermusiaux, is performed under local analgesia (lidocaine without adrenaline or epinephrine) without a tourniquet. The cord of Dupuytren's disease is punctured by a hypodermic needle (25 gauge), for injection of 1% lidocaine without cortisone. The use of cortisone was first proposed by Lermusiaux (a rheumatologist), but in our practice it has not been shown to be of benefit.

Several punctures are made in the Dupuytren's cord to divide it. It is important to use the edge of the needle as a punch and not as a small blade. The needle must be pushed forward and backward many times to weaken the cord. It must not be mobilized transversally like a blade, to prevent damage to vascular and nervous structures. As the finger is held passively and maximally extended, the fibers of the subcutaneous cord will break at the level of the needle. Our opinion is that vascular and nervous structures are pushed backward by the needle because they are smooth and not tight, especially in the palm. Conversely, the subcutaneous cord held tightly by the forced passively extended finger cannot escape the sharp edge of the needle. The cord is weakened by several stamp punctures. Rupture of the cord is assessed by progressive gentle passive extension of the finger.

Although this procedure is performed 'blind', it is easy to avoid tendinous and vasculonervous structures in the palm. Sometimes it is difficult to feel the difference between the cord and the tendon. By asking the patient to mobilize his finger, it is possible to assess whether or not the needle is in contact with the flexor tendon. In the palm, vascular and nervous structures are usually deep and lateral to the cord. When the cord is large and adheres to the skin, the injection of anesthetic in the cord may be painful. In such cases, it is easier to inject laterally into the cord. It is also time consuming to weaken these large cords with a 25 gauge needle. An intramuscular needle (20 gauge) may be more efficient but more dangerous elsewhere and should not be used in the finger. It is important to make the puncture of the cord at the level where the cord is separated from the skin by a fat pad. If the cord is broken where it adheres to the skin, a tear of the skin will appear when the finger is extended. Distal to the distal palmar crease and in the finger, the risk of damage to digital lateral nerves is greater. Sometimes the lateral nerve is superficial to the cord and could be cut by the needle.

For the safe use of this procedure in the finger, we recommend the following. First, as already mentioned, the finger is stretched and the maximum needle size is 25 gauge. Second, it is safer to perform a local superficial skin anesthesia, without proximal injection of lidocaine. In this case, the patient is acutely aware if you contact the lateral nerve with your needle, and the patient's reported pain informs you of the position of the nerve relative to the cord. If several fasciotomies are planned during the same operating time, it is wiser to begin with the digital and distal ones. Last but not least, the neurovascular bundle is always (according to MacFarlane 1988) under the cord at the distal end of the proximal phalanx and at the level of the proximal interphalangeal joint (PIP), so the PNF must be done at this level.

No dressing is necessary unless a skin tear occurs. For most of our patients, a dynamic extension splint is applied. Patients are advised to use it at night, immediately after the procedure, for a minimum of 3 weeks. Patients are encouraged to begin active motion without restriction. Formal rehabilitation is not required.

Results

Between January 1992 and September 1994, a prospective study of 67 patients with Dupuytren's disease treated by PNF by two senior surgeons (JY Alnot and R Bleton) was undertaken. The procedure was proposed to every patient who presented with a defined fibrous cord and whose deformity would indicate a surgical treatment according to the table test: surgical treatment was proposed when the hand could not be laid down on a flat table. Patients with nodes or cords without contracture, and those with recurrent deformity after SFE, were excluded from the study. Patient age, sex, occupation, and aggressiveness or stage of the disease did not affect indications in this prospective study.

Data were collected and analysed by an independent surgeon (D Marcireau). One patient died of unrelated causes and seven were lost to follow-up. Fifty-nine patients were examined at a minimum of 6 months follow-up. There were nine women and fifty men, aged 41–86 years (mean 64 years). Bilateral involvement was usual (41 cases, 70%), and was associated with plantar fibromatosis or LaPeyronie's disease in three cases. Hereditary factors were found in 20 patients. Alcoholism, epilepsy, or diabetes were present in 20% of the patients. Half of the patients had professional occupations, 26% were manual workers. A total of 110 fingers on 67 hands were treated, because of bilateral and pluridigital involvement; 39 hands were dominant. Digital involvement is reported in Table 1.

The preoperative deformity averaged 73° of extension deficit: the mean MP joint contracture was 39°, the mean PIP contracture 32°, and the DIP contracture 2°. Over one-third were severe contractures, with overall deformity exceeding 90°, rated as grades III or IV according to Tubiana's classification (Table 2); 85% of the fingers presented a digital or digitopalmar cord, 91% were well defined, linear, string-like cords, while 9% were larger. Marked adherence of the overlying skin was noted in 24%. Nodules were

Table 1   Digital involvement: 67 hands.

Number of involved digits	n	Location	n
One digit	32	Second digit	1
Two digits	25	Third digit	16
Three digits	9	Fourth digit	39
Four digits	1	Fifth digit	54

Table 2 Rate of contracture according to Tubiana's classification.

Grade I	33 (30%)
Grade II	39 (35%)
Grade III	27 (25%)
Grade IV	11 (10%)

found in 18% of the cases. Seven patients had a needle fasciotomy after a previous surgical excision on the same hand, but the digits treated by needle fasciotomy had not been treated by this previous surgery. The time period between the two procedures was on average 2.7 years. Treatment was carried out in surgical conditions, either in the office (52 cases) or in the operating theatre as an outpatient procedure (15 cases).

We observed minor complications in 7 cases. Four skin tears healed spontaneously with paraffin dressing. A superficial infection resolved without a new operation. One patient suffered temporary paresthesia after a digital fasciotomy, without hypoalgesia. Another presented with finger numbness for some weeks after a palmar procedure, which suggested contusion or stretching of the ulnar digital nerve. At the time of the latest examination, no patient complained of paresthesia, numbness, or residual pain. Digital sensitivity measured by static two-point discrimination and compared to the opposite side was always normal (the comparative ratio of the static two-point discrimination test was 1.02 on average).

There were no major complications. Fifty-three patients (90%) returned to activities of daily living the day following the procedure. Half of the patients resumed their work immediately. One patient returned to his leisure activity 3 months after a bilateral pluridigital procedure. The satisfaction rate was 61%. If a recurrence should occur, 60% of these patients would agree to the same treatment, even if the procedure had to be repeated every 2 years, and 10% were uncertain as to whether they would prefer open surgery. Thirty-nine per cent were disappointed because of primary failure (13 cases) or recurrence (13 cases). Results are reported in Table 3, digit by digit. We used the improvement ratio (IR), defined as the gain in extension in degrees, compared to the overall preoperative deformity.

$$IR = \frac{\text{initial extension deficit} - \text{final extension deficit}}{\text{initial extension deficit}} \times 100$$

The results were classified into three groups: good results, primary failures, and recurrence. We considered 26 fingers in 13 patients (13 hands, 19%) as primary failures because of an improvement ratio of under 50% at the first postoperative examination. Every patient in this group was offered an SFE. Ten were operated upon with a good result at short term. Surgery was not more difficult due to the previous fasciotomies; PIP release was necessary in one case to obtain complete extension. Recurrence was found in another 13 patients (29 fingers from 13 hands, 24% of the initial good results). We did not include nodular recurrence without contracture, nor extension of the disease without recurrence on the initially affected fingers. In half of these patients, recurrence is still well tolerated. The most severe recurrent contractures occurred within the first 6 months after PNF. Three patients required SFE for nodular forms. A second needle fasciotomy has been performed in four patients with success.

Table 3 Results according to the improvement ratio.

	n digits (n hands)	Improvement ratio (%)	Final extension deficit (°)	Final MP deficit (°)	Final PIP deficit (°)
Good results	55 (41)	+83	13	3	10
Primary failures	26 (13)	+15	76	21	55
Recurrences	29 (13)	−2	66	38	28

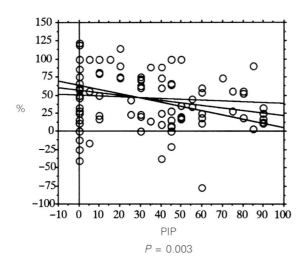

$P = 0.003$

Figure 1

There is a negative correlation between the improvement ratio and the preoperative PIP contracture ($P = 0.003$).

Table 4 Results according to location of the fasciotomies ($P = 0.23$).

	Improvement ratio
Palmar fasciotomies	29% (n = 26)
Palmar and digital fasciotomies	42% (n = 19)

Table 5 PNF results.

	Good results	Primary failures	Recur- rence	P
N+	40%	10%	50%	
N–	54%	26%	20%	0.018
Adherent cord	31%	37%	32%	
Supple cord	57%	14%	29%	0.05
Digital or digital and palmar cord	44%	29%	27%	
Palmar cord	87%	0	13%	0.05

N+, nodes; N–, no nodes.

We consider the treatment of the remaining 41 hands in 33 patients (62%) to be successful, as the IR has remained over 50% at the most recent examination. The average follow-up was 21 months. Fifty have complete extension of the MP joint, but 30 retain a mild PIP contracture (5–15°), which is well tolerated.

Age, sex, causal factors, and aggressiveness of the disease do not appear to be statistically significant predictors of results in this series. The severity of MP joint preoperative contracture also did not influence the final result. Poor results occurred after a previous surgical procedure on the same hand (average improvement rate 32%). The magnitude of the initial PIP joint contracture correlated with the prognosis; the deformity averaged 59° in failures, 25° in good results, and 29° in recurrent cases ($P = 0.0001$). Figure 1 shows a negative correlation between the improvement ratio and the preoperative PIP contracture.

In the 45 fingers with a dominant PIP contracture (always exceeding 40°), postoperative results seem better after palmar and digital fasciotomy, but the difference with isolated palmar fasciotomy is not statistically significant (Table 4). The gain in extension depends mainly on the anatomical type of the disease. The best results are obtained with the string-like palmar fibrous cords, without marked skin adherence and nodes. Knuckle pads did not have a poor prognosis. The influence of these factors in the three groups of results is reported in Table 5. The percentages indicate the proportion of treated digits for each factor. String-like palmar cords without nodes, with supple skin, and mild PIP contracture give the best and most long-lasting results. Immediate results are consistently poor in cases of skin adherence, especially in digitopalmar cords with severe PIP contracture. Nodular forms usually lead to recurrence, despite good immediate results.

Discussion

Percutaneous fasciotomy is usually presented as a blind procedure, with risks for the flexor tendons and digital nerves. Tubiana (1974) emphasized the particular risk of digital fasciotomy, nerve injuries being of greatest concern. The highest rate of nerve injury following PNF was reported by Luck (1959), with 8 cases out of 154. However, the same incidence was reported by Hoèt et al (1988), after open fasciectomy. Luck advocated removal of the nodes and transverse section of fibrous cords at levels four to six in the palm, which significantly increases the risk of nerve injury. Colville (1983), who routinely performed digital fasciotomy, just mentioned 'temporary tingling of the fingers in some patients'. Rodrigo et al (1976) reported nervous injury in 2% of their patients after palmar fasciotomy.

The needle percutaneous procedure reduces this risk. The progressive rupture of the cord by the needle is less aggressive than subcutaneous transverse section by a blade. Under pure local analgesia, the patient feels the puncture of the digital nerve, which prevents section by needle manipulation. Badois et al (1993) reported a 2% rate of temporary paresthesia and noted six digital nerve lesions and four flexor tendon ruptures in 2500 hands treated by the same procedure. Schernberg (1994) reported persistent sensory loss in one patient out of 100.

Our series (Bleton 1995) confirms that the procedure is safe, with normal sensibility at the last examination when tested by static two-point discrimination. Absence of tendon and nerves injuries could be explained by the safety of the procedure itself, and perhaps also by the fact that these procedures were done by hand surgeons who are trained in the anatomy and surgery of Dupuytren's disease.

No severe complications have been reported after percutaneous fasciotomy, nor reflex sympathetic dystrophy or postoperative stiffness, whereas this complication is frequent after SFE (10% for Rodrigo et al 1976). Minor complications, mainly superficial, may occur: skin tears, superficial infections, temporary swelling, mild haematomas. They do not impair the functional outcome. We believe our low complication rate (7% versus 18% for Badois et al 1993) is due to the fact that the procedure is performed in surgical conditions without cortisone injection, and severe or pluridigital lesions are treated in several sessions.

Except for cutaneous incidents, which require dressing and daily care, functional postoperative disability is particularly short. The use of a needle as an aponeurotome under simple local analgesia and the night splint make this a suitable outpatient procedure and facilitate an immediate return to usual activities for most patients. Luck (1959) and Schernberg (1994) stated that patients usually resume daily activities on the second day and manual work after one week. Rodrigo et al (1976) consider that the period of disability is three times shorter after fasciotomy than after SFE.

Immediate results after fasciotomy are satisfactory: the primary failure rate in our prospective study is similar to Badois et al (19%, 1993) and Schernberg (15%, 1994). These results improve in selected cases. The stage of the disease according to Tubiana seems to be a good prognostic indicator: Badois et al obtained more than 80% immediate good results for grades I to III, but only 48% for grade IV. Most authors emphasize the importance of PIP contracture, and we noted a negative relationship between the gain in extension and the initial PIP deformity. This is particularly true in severe, long standing PIP joint contractures. Nevertheless, this is also true after surgical excision.

Complete extension may be achieved by simple palmar section of a digitopalmar cord, in string-like cords with supple skin, but only modest benefit is obtained when PIP contracture is predominant. We noted no statistical difference of gain in extension between digitopalmar and isolated palmar PNF in this case, but three out of seven complications concerned the 17 hands treated by PIP PNF (20% incidence rate). However, digitopalmar cords with severe PIP contracture, considered as a contraindication, may benefit from the procedure as a preliminary to open fasciectomy. Seven patients that we have classified as failures had such initial PIP joint involvement: the gain in extension varied up to 50°, facilitating the further SFE. This indication of fasciotomy as a preliminary procedure has also been suggested by others (Rodrigo et al 1976, Colville 1983, Bryan and Ghorbal 1988). In our experience it has never complicated the further SFE. We perform the procedure in the office, in contrast to Schernberg (1994) who prefers to continue with open surgery in the operating theatre when fasciotomy fails. We were reluctant to use PIP PNF at the start of this study. However, we are now more confident with the procedure and we are currently satisfied with it, although the advantages and disadvantages of PIP PNF remain controversial and will have to be answered later.

There are very few published references to the importance of the anatomical type of the disease. Luck (1959) pointed out the role of the nodes. Colville (1983) advocated fasciotomy on string-like, bowstringing cords, with supple overlying skin. In this indication, limited to palmar predominant cords, we obtained 100% immediate good results, with 87% maintained at follow-up. Because of the different procedures, indications, and assessments of the results, it is difficult to establish whether recurrence is due to the disease or to the fasciotomy.

There are many published references to long term recurrence after SFE: most authors consider recurrence as the natural course of the disease. The recurrence rate appears to be related to the duration of follow-up rather than the type of surgical procedure: 54–63% at 5 years (Honner et al 1971, Rodrigo et al 1976, Hoèt et al 1988), 66% at 10 years (Leclercq and Tubiana 1986), 71% after 10 years (Norotte et al 1989) to 77% at 20 years (Mantero 1983).

The recurrence rate after percutaneous fasciotomy seems to be higher, although there are very few long-term published references. Bryan and Ghorbal (1988) reported 63% recurrent deformity at 5 years in patients with predominant MP involvement. Schernberg (1994) mentioned some evidence of recurrence in two-thirds of patients at 4 years follow-up. Badois et al (1993) claimed the best results with a 50% recurrence rate at 5 years. However, they included the repeated fasciotomies in the final good results, they did not consider nodular recurrence, and more than one-third of their patients were lost to follow-up.

However, it is very difficult to compare two treatments like SFE and PNF, which are so different in their principles. The aim of surgical excision is to cure definitively the disease whatever the difficulties. The cost and the difficulties of this procedure could be justified by the long-term success. The aim of the PNF is not to cure the disease, but only to improve the functional result as the contracture is decreased. It is not surprising that this procedure comes from rheumatologists who are used to treating long standing illnesses such as rheumatoid arthritis, which cannot be cured. The procedure may be repeated from time to time. Recurrence after needle fasciotomy allows simple care, while

recurrence following SFE may require difficult and uncertain treatment (Leclercq and Tubiana 1986). The needle leaves no scar; except in the case of nodular forms, we experienced recurrence as a new string-like cord without marked skin adherence. A repeated PNF gave a good immediate result in the four patients treated. Colville (1983), whose procedure differs, considers the second fasciotomy is still useful although less satisfactory. Badois et al (1993) treated recurrent deformities of grade I disease by a second needle procedure with success. We believe needle fasciotomy can be performed as many times as necessary, but have no experience of PNF as a third procedure.

Factors leading to recurrence after fasciotomy are rarely mentioned in the literature. Our findings support Luck's conviction that leaving nodes quickly leads to recurrence of the contracture, despite a good immediate result. These forms, frequently associated with strong diathesis, might deserve complete SFE. Most studies also report a higher recurrence rate after fasciotomy in young patients with aggressive disease and strong diathesis. Thus, Colville (1983) and Schernberg (1994) tend to limit indications of fasciotomy to elderly patients. We found no statistical value of sex, age, or hereditary factors in predicting the results of needle fasciotomy. We could not confirm the poor prognosis associated with strong diathesis, perhaps because of a small proportion of patients under 50 years and the short follow-up time of our study. The rate of primary failure and recurrence seems to indicate that PNF is not a miraculous solution for Dupuytren's disease with strong diathesis. In these cases, surgical procedures remain the gold standard. But we believe that young, active patients, expecting a short functional outcome, can benefit from needle fasciotomy, if they agree to a repeated procedure or a further surgical excision in case of recurrence.

Conclusion

Percutaneous needle fasciotomy is a simple and inexpensive outpatient treatment of Dupuytren's contracture. Our study demonstrates a lower complication rate than after SFE, when performed in surgical conditions. Complications, mainly superficial, resolve spontaneously and do not impair the functional outcome. Satisfactory results are obtained with a very short term disability in selected cases: a palmar predominant cord with supple overlying skin is the best indication. In the case of primary failure or recurrent severe deformity, SFE can be performed.

We believe needle fasciotomy is an interesting alternative to SFE and should take its place among the various operative procedures available. However, the technique finds its limits in patients with PIP joint predominant contracture, with digitopalmar cord, adherent skin and nodes. PNF could be tried in the first instance in a young patient with a strong diathesis, but it often leads to recurrent deformity. Such patients also have a poor prognosis with a surgical procedure, however, with a high rate of complications and stiffness.

Thus PNF can be proposed primarily as a means to improve the situation, not as a definite solution. It may also serve as a first stage procedure, so that surgical excision may be performed more easily.

References

Badois FJ, Lermusiaux JL, Massé C, et al (1993) Traitement non chirurgical de la maladie de Dupuytren par aponévrotomie à l'aiguille, Rev Rhum 60:808–13.

Bleton R (1995) Place de l'aponévrotomie percutanée à l'aiguille dans le traitement de la maladie de Dupuytren, Entretiens de Bichat. Orthopédie (Expansion Scientifique Française: Paris).

Bryan AS, Ghorbal MS (1988) The long term results of closed palmar fasciotomy in the management of Dupuytren's contracture, J Hand Surg 13B:254–6.

Colville J (1983) Dupuytren's contracture: the role of fasciotomy, The Hand 15:162–6.

Dupuytren G (1832) Leçon orale faites à l'Hôtel Dieu, Paris, Vol. In chapitre I, (Germer Baillère: Paris).

Hoët F, Boxho J, Decoster E, et al (1988) Maladie de Dupuytren: revue de 326 patients opérés, Ann Chir Main 7:251–5.

Honner R, Lamb DW, James JIP (1971) Dupuytren's contracture: long term results after fasciectomy, J Bone Joint Surg 53B:240–5.

Kelly AP, Clifford RH (1959) Subcutaneous fasciotomy in the treatment of Dupuytren's contracture, Plast Reconstr Surg 24:505–10.

Leclercq C, Tubiana R (1986) Résultat à long terme des aponévrectomies pour maladie de Dupuytren, Chirurgie 112:194–7.

Lermusiaux JL, Debeyre N (1980) Le traitement médical de la maladie de Dupuytren. In: Sèze S de, Ryckewaert A, Kahn MF, et al, eds, L'Actualité Rhumatologique 1979 Présentée aux Praticiens (Expansion Scientifique Française: Paris) 338–43.

Luck JV (1959) Dupuytren's contracture: a new concept of the pathogenesis correlated with surgical management, J Bone Joint Surg 41A:635–64.

MacFarlane RM (1988) Dupuytren's contracture. In: Green DP, ed, Operative Hand Surgery, 2nd edn (Churchill Livingstone: New York) 553–89.

Mantero R, Grandis C, Auxilia E (1983) Arteriographic findings in congenital malformations of the hand, Handchir Mikrochir Plast Chir 15:71–6.

Norotte G, Apoil A, Travers V (1989) Résultats à plus de 10 ans de la maladie Dupuytren: à propos de cinquante huit observations, Sem Hôp Paris 65:1045–8.

Rodrigo JJ, Niebauer JJ, Brown RL, et al (1976) Treatment of Dupuytren's contracture. Long term results after fasciotomy and fascial excision, J Bone Joint Surg 58A:380–7.

Schernberg F (1994) Percutaneous fasciotomy in Dupuytren's contracture. In: Kasdan M, Bowes W, Amadio P, eds, Technical Tips for Hand Surgery (Hanley and Belfus: Philadelphia): 89–90.

Tubiana R, Hueston JT (1974) Dupuytren's Disease (Churchill Livingstone).

Watson JD (1984). Fasciotomy and Z-plasty in the management of Dupuytren's contracture, Br J Plast Surg 37:27–30.

Continuous extension treatment by the TEC device for severe Dupuytren's contracture of the fingers

Antonino Messina and Jane C Messina

Introduction

The continuous elongation technique (TEC) aims to achieve extension of the retracted fingers, correction of the deformity and functional reconstruction of the hand in severe cases of Dupuytren's disease (Messina 1989). It consists of a physiologic, painless and atraumatic elongation of the very retracted aponeurotic fascia of the hands, achieved by means of a device (Figures 1 and 2). This chapter presents our experience since 1986 in the treatment of Dupuytren's disease with severe hand contractures in order to return the retracted cord to its initial appearance (Messina and Messina 1991, 1993). This advanced method always effects complete correction of the contracture, stops the evolution of the disease, improves conditions for the surgical approach and reduces the complexity of the intervention of fasciectomy.

Application of the TEC device

Under regional or block axillary anaesthesia, two self-drilling pins with continuous threads are inserted on the cubital side of the hand through the skin. The pins are inserted transversally through the fifth and the fourth metacarpal bones at the proximal and distal metaphyses (Figure 2). Clinical and radiographic control of the length and position of the inserted pins confirms that they have completely penetrated cortices of the fifth and fourth metacarpal bones. In this way we have a very stable and painless

assembly that supports the TEC device in order to achieve continuous elongation of the retracted fingers (Messina 1989; Messina and Messina 1991, 1993, 1995) (Figure 3). A Kirschner wire is then inserted transversally through the distal metaphysis of P2, through the proximal metaphysis of P3 if this is retracted, or through both metaphyses if both the proximal and the distal

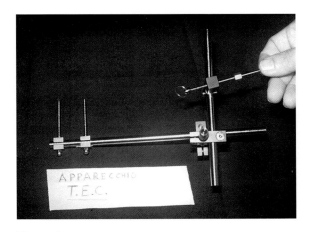

Figure 1

The continuous elongation technique (TEC) device is an advanced apparatus to perform continuous extension treatment of the fingers in severe cases of Dupuytren's contracture. The device is not cumbersome—its size can be adapted to the elongated fingers and it weighs only 190 g. The continuous extension treatment is atraumatic and painless. The height and direction of the lengthening can be calibrated according to the degree of retraction of the finger. Continuous traction can be applied simultaneously to several retracted fingers.

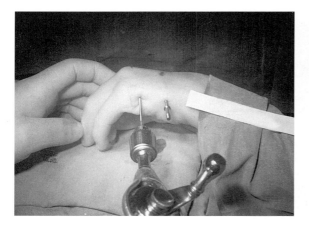

Figure 2

With locoregional anaesthesia, two self-drilling pins are inserted transversally through the proximal and distal metaphyses of the fifth and fourth metacarpal bones. In this way, a stable and painless assembly is mounted and the continuous extension device is fixed to it. The continuous lengthening is carried out by the patient at home.

interphalangeal joints are flexed together in severe contracture. The Kirschner wire is bent to form a traction loop. The TEC device is assembled on the metacarpal pins outside the operating room. The phalangeal traction loop is connected to a threaded screw allowing a 2 mm per day lengthening of the retracted finger (2 mm distributed four times a day: 8 am, 12 pm, 4 pm, 8 pm). The device is regulated with regard to adequate direction and height according to the respective extent of flexion and direction until complete elongation of the retracted finger has been achieved (Figure 4). Then the pins, the Kirschner wire and the TEC device are removed and the fasciectomy performed at the same time (Messina and Messina 1993).

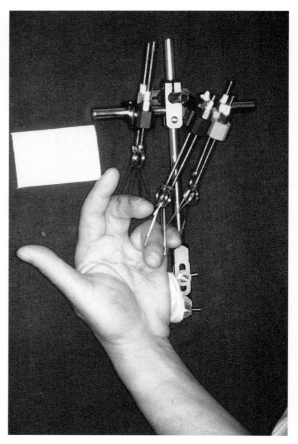

Figure 3

Patient treated by TEC device elongation of three retracted fingers in severe Dupuytren's disease in active contracture with rapid progression. The TEC procedure facilitates the intervention, reducing the complexity, length and surgical trauma. The TEC device is secured firmly to the two self-drilling pins by a rod. The continuous elongation is carried out on the retracted fingers by means of a screw, the height and direction of which are calibrated according to the degree of retraction of the finger. The screw is then progressively adjusted in relation to the elongation of the finger. It is given a half turn every 4 hours (8 am, 12 pm, 4 pm, 8 pm), which corresponds to an extension of 2 mm. In this way, the elongation is atraumatic and painless and there is no risk of vasculonervous bundle damage.

Pros and cons compared to classical techniques

The continuous elongation technique is the most advanced method for treatment of the pathologic digito-palmar fascia excision in severe and inveterate Dupuytren's contracture. This technique is a real alternative to amputation for severely retracted fingers in recurrences and in very advanced cases. At the end of the lengthening the fingers are completely extended so that the

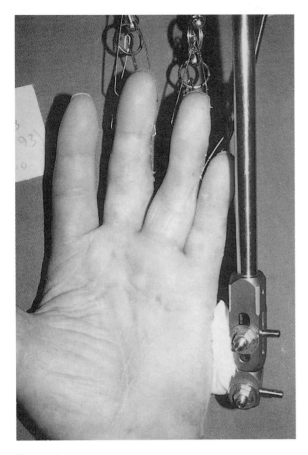

Figure 4

Middle, ring and little fingers are extended at the end of continuous elongation (2–3 weeks). The elongation is carried out by the patient at home. The patient will be monitored every week on an ambulatory basis. The fasciectomy must be performed at the same time the TEC device is removed. The surgical approach is as simple as in the first stage of Dupuytren's disease, so that every inexperienced surgeon can perform it.

and the stretching and tearing of collateral vasculonervous bundles which are the cause of devascularization and trophic difficulties in fingers retracted for many years in complete flexion. The continuous elongation technique produces an improvement of microvascularity of the retracted finger and promotes lengthening of the retracted skin (1.5 cm on average) and recovery of the skin dystrophy and of mycosis. At the end of lengthening, the 'compression test' shows that the nodule is flattened and that the pretendinous cord has disappeared (Messina and Messina 1993, 1995).

The TEC treatment is then an alternative to plastic surgery for digital or palmar skin loss, particularly when there is a need for a flap or a skin graft. It improves on the McCash 'open-palm technique' in terms of both practical application and theoretical principles and facilitates conservation and some functional reconstruction of a seriously retracted finger (this was impossible or at the limits of technical possibility with the classical operations). In the morphological field, the TEC device produces a 'stop-go-back process' of the evolution of the fascia contracture, when the patients treated represent the most severe and progressive types of contracture.

Against all these advantages, the patient must come to terms with the TEC device, which is relatively light (190 g) and of a size just adapted to the elongated fingers. The patient must wait 2–3 weeks for complete extension of the finger, when fasciectomy can be performed. The surgeon should explain the advantages of the TEC treatment, plan the technical procedure and oversee the treatment of the patient.

skin incision and surgical approach will also be easy for inexperienced hand surgeons to perform. The TEC device treatment facilitates the procedure, greatly reducing surgical trauma and the complexity, length and difficulties of operation. It avoids complementary articular interventions such as capsulotomy, arthrolysis, surgical release of check-reins, collateral ligaments and retracted lateral digital fascia; it avoids the sudden surgical extension of the retracted finger

Complications

We did not observe any trophic disturbance or vascular difficulties or any pin-tract infection in the treated fingers. Interphalangeal joint subluxation occurred in one patient. The subluxation reduced spontaneously, leaving traction at the end of the finger elongation. In three patients, after fasciectomy, we observed a swan-neck deformity of the proximal interphalangeal joint without loss of joint mobility. It is possible to prevent joint subluxation by extending the finger harmonically according to its curve. Nevertheless,

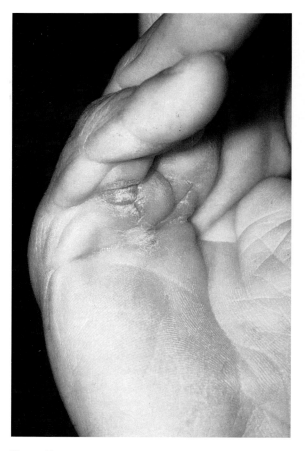

Figure 5

Another patient with a very severe recurrence of Dupuytren's disease of the fifth and fourth fingers after an operation in another hospital. Severe contracture and skin loss, trophic problems on the palmar skin and interdigital mycotic intertrigo. With the use of the TEC device the localized progression of the disease (recurrence) has so far been halted. Plastic skin surgery, including Z-plasties, skin grafts, etc, was unnecessary.

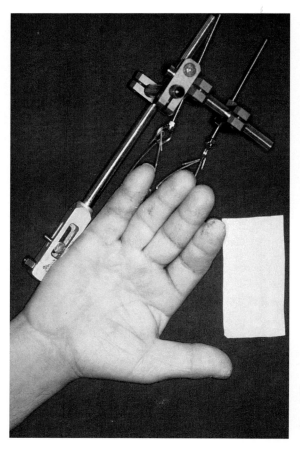

Figure 6

Ring and little fingers extended following continuous elongation treatment by a TEC device. The resulting elongation of the retracted skin was 1.5 cm, on average. A considerable improvement in elasticity, skin trophism and microvascularity of the elongated skin was observed. The skin's microbial protection also was notably improved by spontaneous healing of the interdigital mycosis affecting the skin. Fasciectomy is now very simple. The TEC device avoids complementary articular interventions and improves on the McCash 'open-palm technique' in terms of both practical application and theoretical principles.

proximal and distal interphalangeal joints must be elongated simultaneously if both are retracted in flexion. Some surgeons using the TEC technique observed oedema and algodystrophy correlated with too quickly performed elongation or intermittent traction. It is important to adhere strictly to the TEC protocol of continuous, gradual and physiological lengthening which is painless and not traumatic.

Results

The continuous elongation technique has been applied to 56 hands and 85 fingers affected by

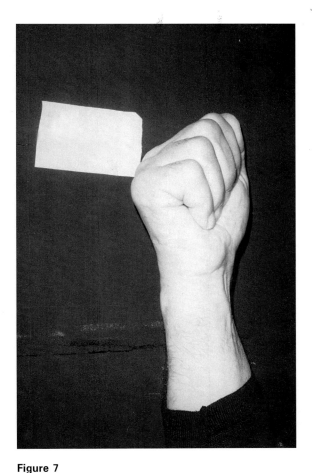

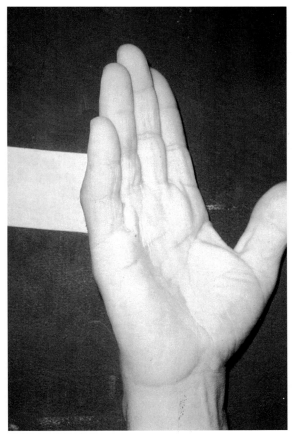

Figure 7

Functional result after continuous elongation treatment with a TEC device: active flexion of the fingers.

Figure 8

Active extension of the fingers. The TEC device is especially recommended in those cases in which the most sophisticated operating techniques prove to be inadequate in keeping the fingers rigidly retracted in flexion or in achieving satisfactory functional results.

grades III, IVa and IVb Dupuytren's contracture, according to the Tubiana classification (Tubiana 1986). The TEC device was applied to 19 previously unoperated hands and 37 hands that showed recurrence/extension after a previous operation performed in another hospital. Patients were treated from 1986 to 1991 and the features

and the functional results were 75% excellent, 15% good, 0% fair and 10% bad, according to TAM evaluation (Figures 5–8). At follow-up 6 years later, recurrence of Dupuytren's disease was observed in eight patients with the appearance of a nodule. Five patients presented with an extension of the disease on the border of the operated area, with a little nodule or cords on the radial side of the hand. No pain or painful scars were noted and skin sensitivity was found to be normal (comparable to the surrounding normal skin).

Indications

The continuous elongation technique is indicated:

(1) When maximally retracted fingers are held to be inoperable because of the impossibility of achieving secondary functional recovery;

(2) In cases of surgical indication of amputation of the retracted finger, i.e. in cases which present with long-term retracted joints, stiffness, with the evolved stage already operated on with severe recurrence and extension of disease;

(3) In loss of the finger's volar skin or of the hand's palmar surface;

(4) In severe problems of collateral vasculonervous bundles in prolonged contracted fingers (or thrombosis of the ulnar artery with vascular loss of collateral pedicles);

(5) In systemic illness (severe and unstable diabetes, immunodeficiency, serious cardiopulmonary illness);

(6) In old age.

Conclusion

The continuous elongation technique represents an alternative to finger amputation in severe cases of Dupuytren's disease, as a means of avoiding necrosis, loss of vascularity and functional impairment resulting from classical procedures. This technique is an advanced method for the excision of pathological palmar fascia in severe and inveterate Dupuytren's contracture. The TEC device always achieves lengthening of the fascia of very contracted fingers and in a very simple way enables the retracted tissues (skin, fascia, ligaments, capsu-

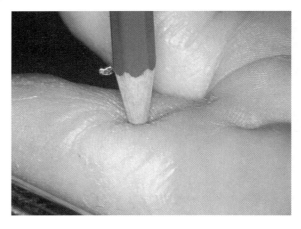

Figure 9

Compression test after treatment of Dupuytren's contracture by the continuous elongation technique.

lar tissues, etc) to revert to the first stage of onset of the disease (compression test, Figure 9).

According to a clinical and morphological view, for 165 years Dupuytren's contracture was thought to be a degenerative, progressive and irreversible disease. However, the TEC device, by bringing the contracture back to the initial stage of the disease, has shown that the histomorphological process can in fact be reversed ('stop-go-back process') (see Figures 2–8). The continuous elongation technique opens the way for new basic research into the morphological and biochemical processes of the collagen in the retracted palmar fascia (Bailey et al 1994, Brandes et al 1994). Recent research by the laboratories of cell biology and electron microscopy of the Medical School of Hanover (Brandes et al 1995) has revealed the unexpected appearance of 'stress fibres' in the endothelial cells of both arterioles and venules in the contractured fascia of Dupuytren's disease after application of a TEC device. These fibres have never been seen before in these structures. This confirms the scientific importance of the TEC method in Dupuytren's disease studies and its clinical originality. It could explain the morphological basis of the mechanism of the contracture of the fascia in Dupuytren's disease and its recurrence (Figure 10).

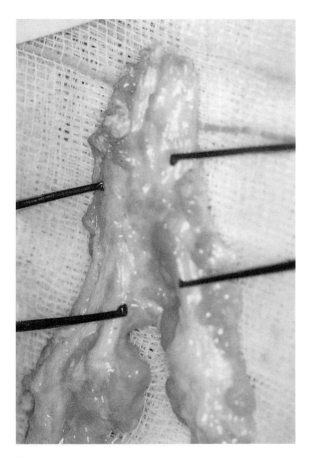

Figure 10

Lengthening of the fascia obtained after treatment with a TEC device. There is neither macroscopic nor microscopic evidence of tissue rupture or haemorrhage. The nodule is flattened. The previous firm prominent Dupuytren's bands are found to be reduced to soft fibrous ribbons which are removed by fasciectomy. The biological mechanism of the contraction process of collagen tissue is thus reversed by TEC and perhaps explained by the appearance of 'stress fibres' in the microvascular endothelium.

References

Bailey AJ, Tarlton JF, Van der Stappen J, et al (1994) The continuous elongation technique for severe Dupuytren's disease: a biochemical mechanism, *J Hand Surg* **19B**:522–7.

Brandes G, Messina A, Reale E (1994) The palmar fascia after treatment by the continuous extension technique for Dupuytren's contracture, *J Hand Surg* **19B**:528–33.

Brandes G, Reale E, Messina A (1996) Stress fibers and microvascular endothelium of the palmar fascia generated by mechanical forces applied from outside in Dupuytren's disease, *Virchows Archiv:* in preparation.

Messina A (1989) La TEC (Tecnica di Estensione Continua) nel morbo di Dupuytren grave: dall'amputazione alla ricostruzione, *Riv Chir Mano* **26**:253.

Messina A, Messina J (1991) The TEC treatment (Continuous Extension Technique) for severe Dupuytren's contracture of the fingers, *Ann Chir Main Mentr Super* **10**:247.

Messina A, Messina J (1993) The continuous elongation treatment by the TEC device for severe Dupuytren's contracture of the fingers, *Plast Reconstr Surg* **92**:84–90.

Messina A, Messina J (1995) Considerazioni sulla tecnica di estensione continua (TEC) nel trattamento dei casi gravi e le recidive del morbo di Dupuytren, *Riv Ital Chir Plast* **27**:75–81.

Tubiana R (1986) *La Maladie de Dupuytren*, 3rd edn (Expansion Scientifique Française: Paris).

Commentary

Chapter 30

This new technique certainly has some indications, particularly in elderly people or as a preoperative treatment. Its great advantage is its simplicity. However, results are considered as good by the authors (62%), 'if the gain extension is maintained over 50% at the most recent examination' after an average follow-up of 21 months. This is a modest result. Other techniques of fasciotomy have already demonstrated a high rate of recurrence. This technique, initiated by rheumatologists, has spread in France and provided some complications such as nerve and flexor tendon lacerations. Only surgeons with a good knowledge of hand anatomy and Dupuytren's surgical procedures should perform this technique, especially in the digital area. PIP contracture seems difficult to treat by this technique.

PS

Chapter 31

The concept of continuous extension for the treatment of Dupuytren's disease is certainly new and may help in cases of advanced retraction. It should not preclude fasciectomy. Recurrence is certainly less frequent after continuous extension. This technique which facilitates finger straightening without pain or severe devascularization is certainly useful in some indications.

PS

Crossed intrinsic transfers versus metacarpophalangeal joint arthroplasty in rheumatoid arthritis

William F Blair and Peter JL Jebson

Introduction

The options for surgical reconstruction of the metacarpophalangeal (MP) joint in patients with rheumatoid arthritis are varied, and depend upon the specifics of the patient's clinical problem. Two general approaches are most widely accepted: (1) soft tissue reconstruction of the MP joint[1-3] and (2) silicone implant arthroplasty.[4,5] In clinical practice, variations in each of these general approaches are exercised, resulting in a much broader range of technical practices. The more conservative option includes extensor digitorum communis (EDC) centralization in one or more fingers, with or without MP joint synovectomy, performed without a crossed intrinsic tendon transfer. A more comprehensive and formal soft tissue reconstruction includes synovectomy, EDC centralization, and crossed intrinsic transfer from the index, long, and ring fingers to the long, ring, and small fingers, respectively.[2,3] The traditional silicone implant arthroplasty includes an MP joint synovectomy, EDC centralization, and reattachment of the radial collateral ligament of the MP joint, usually to the index and long fingers.[5] Increasingly, the traditional silicone implant arthroplasty is being supplemented with crossed intrinsic transfers, usually to all three of the ulnarmost fingers.

'Hybrid' operations, in which soft tissue reconstruction alone is performed in certain fingers and implant arthroplasty in others, may also be appropriate in selected patients.

Indications

The indications for operative treatment in a specific patient with rheumatoid arthritis involving the MP joints must be carefully considered. The indications are based primarily upon pain and disability. The patient's MP joint pain must be severe enough to significantly interfere with their sense of well-being. Existing or imminent deformity of the fingers must constitute a disability. Thus, the indications for surgery, in general, are relative and must be individualized. Long finger ulnar deviation of 15° alone may be a disability in an active and employed individual whose job requires finger dexterity, even in the absence of pain. In contrast, irreducible MP joint dislocations with flexion contractures and ulnar drift in all four fingers may be a minimal disability in an individual who is retired, inactive, and has a supportive home environment. The emphasis on indications should be conservative. The appropriateness of the indication and the success of MP joint reconstruction should be judged not only on technical accomplishment, but on the patient's perception of improvement in their health status.

There are specific indications for each of the various procedures advocated for MP joint reconstruction. EDC centralization alone is indicated if ulnar deviation is present in one or two fingers (usually the long) with minimal MP joint synovitis, no pain, and no radiographic evidence of MP joint subluxation, narrowing, or erosions. More comprehensive soft tissue reconstruction is appropriate in the presence of MP joint synovitis, with or without mild pain, but with ulnar deviation that interferes with function.[1] Soft tissue reconstruction should be done when there is no more than minimal MP joint subluxation that can be corrected with passive manipulation at the time of physical examination. In addition, radiographs, including a Brewerton's view, should demonstrate an absence of significant joint space narrowing or erosions.

If the MP joint is moderately subluxed, yet reducible, a difficult dilemma presents. Formal soft tissue reconstruction can be done with temporary pinning of the MP joint in a fully extended position. However, this strategy is generally not recommended as limited MP joint motion will result. Usually, for patients with this stage of disease, no surgical treatment is recommended and the disease is allowed to progress until MP joint arthroplasty is indicated. Implant arthroplasty of the MP joint is appropriate in the patient with MP joint pain and synovitis, up to 20° of ulnar deviation, irreducible MP joint dislocations, and radiographs that demonstrate joint space narrowing and erosions.[4] Finally, MP joint implant arthroplasty combined with crossed intrinsic transfer may be appropriate if the ulnar drift is more advanced, perhaps being 30° or more.

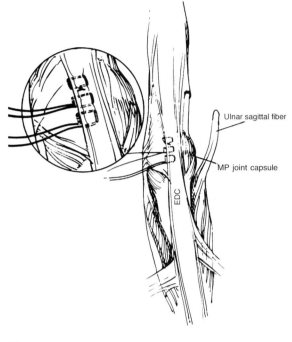

Figure 1

Imbrication of the radial aspect of the dorsal apparatus is carried out with stitches that leave the knots between the layers of tendinous tissue. EDC, extensor digitorum communis.

Technical aspects

Although the technical aspects of silicone MP joint arthroplasty are well described, the details of soft tissue reconstruction and specifically the crossed intrinsic transfer component are worth consideration. Extensor digitorum communis centralization alone requires two steps: (1) division of the radial sagittal bands to facilitate imbrication of the dorsal apparatus, and (2) release of the ulnar sagittal fibers to prevent the tendency for recurrent ulnar translation of the EDC. Precise positioning of the EDC, centrally over the metacarpal head, is critical for a successful result. The position is secured by imbrication that is best done with a nonabsorbable suture and three stitches that leave the knots between the layers of imbricated tissue (Figure 1). If the amount of MP joint synovitis justifies synovectomy, a longitudinal capsular incision is used to access the joint. The synovectomy is completed (including the recess beneath the collateral ligaments), redundant capsule is excised, and the residual capsule approximated with absorbable sutures.

A comprehensive soft tissue reconstruction includes crossed intrinsic tendon transfers. The transferred tendon is released by making an incision along the ulnar border of the EDC in the donor finger, along a distance of 2–3 cm, depending upon the size of the finger. The intrinsic tendon is then transected distally. It is then important to completely mobilize the intrinsic tendon and muscle, which are usually adherent to the ulnar side of the MP joint capsule. When adequately mobilized, gently pulling on the end of the intrinsic tendon should result in about 3 mm of excursion. The abductor digiti minimi (ADM) fibers are released along the ulnar side of the small finger MP joint. Because the ADM and flexor digiti minimi may form a conjoint tendon of insertion, only the medial most ADM fibers should be released.

A tunnel is then bluntly dissected in the deep subcutaneous tissues of the web space. The intrinsic is passed through the tunnel, and should take a free and straight-line course to the site of insertion. Our preference, in the absence of swan-neck deformity in the recipient finger, is an insertion into the radial aspect of the EDC, distal to the distalmost fibers of the radial sagittal band. The transfer is done after the EDC centralization step of the soft tissue reconstruction. Two longitudinal incisions, each 5 mm in length, are made along the radial aspect of the EDC fibers. The transfer is passed through these incisions, and then back onto itself (Figure 2). The MP joint is placed in neutral flexion and extension, and the finger is placed in neutral radial ulnar deviation. The transfer is then tightened just enough to initiate very slight radial translation of the EDC. The transfer is sewn with figure of eight stitches, using non-absorbable suture material, first to the EDC, and then back onto itself. An identical technique is used in conjunction with the MP arthroplasty, although the intrinsic tendon is mobilized at the same time the soft tissues are taken down for the MP arthroplasty. The transfer and insertion is performed only after all steps in the arthroplasty procedure are completed, including EDC centralization.

An optimum result from soft tissue reconstruction depends upon quality postoperative care. The hand is placed in plaster apposition splints with the MP joints in neutral and the fingers well aligned for approximately 7 days. When local wound conditions permit, a dynamic dorsally based MP joint extension orthotic with outriggers and rubber bands to control ulnar deviation is used. Active finger flexion exercises are initiated in the splint. The rubber bands are removed three times a day and the patient is encouraged to actively begin MP joint flexion exercises. This splint is worn until 3 weeks after surgery. At this time the dynamic splint is discontinued and limited activities of daily living are allowed. Active and passive range of motion exercises for all joints of all fingers are continued. If there is a tendency for recurrent ulnar drift, a static night splint holding the fingers in neutral is used. At 6 weeks postoperatively,

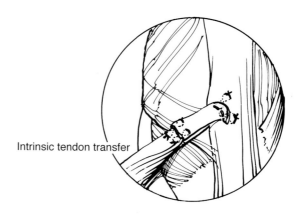

Intrinsic tendon transfer

Figure 2

The transferred intrinsic tendon is passed through longitudinal incisions along the radial aspect of the EDC fibers, and sutured to the EDC and back onto itself.

unrestricted activities of daily living are allowed, and active resisted exercises are begun.

Pros and cons

Advantages of soft tissue reconstruction of the MP joints, and specifically the crossed intrinsic transfer component, are apparent. The procedure decreases MP joint pain, corrects ulnar drift, and maintains that correction over an extended period of time.[2,6] Correction of ulnar drift of the finger improves selected motor skills, as well as the cosmetic appearance of the hand. When used in conjunction with MP arthroplasty, it protects predisposed fingers from assuming recurrent ulnar drift.

There are disadvantages to this operation. Crossed intrinsic transfers are technically difficult, implying that appropriate surgical training and experience are necessary to consistently perform the operation well. When crossed intrinsic transfers are used with MP arthroplasty, the duration of the operation is extended, increasing the utilization of both surgeon and hospital resources. In less advanced cases, the operation may correct ulnar drift, but individual fingers may be left with decreased abduction and adduction, and some loss of active MP joint motion is common. If the transfer is inserted too tightly, radial deviation of the fingers can result. Although this is seldom a functional problem, it is cosmetically nonoptimum. The transfer can be associated with adhesions about the dorsal apparatus, causing decreased PIP joint motion if rehabilitation is not instituted early.

The advantages of MP joint implant arthroplasty are similar to those of the soft tissue reconstruction procedures. MP joint arthroplasty decreases joint pain, corrects ulnar drift, and improves the functional use and cosmetic appearance of the hand.[5] Patient satisfaction is high.

A major disadvantage of MP arthroplasty is the technical expertise necessary for a successful result. Additional disadvantages associated with the implant include a fracture rate of 10–20%, infection, and dislocation.[7,8] Particular synovitis, although uncommon, may result in loss of implant stability requiring revision or resection arthroplasty.

Results

The results of EDC centralization alone are not well documented, but in our experience they are favorable when appropriately indicated. The results of soft tissue reconstruction with crossed intrinsic transfer are better defined. The operation substantially corrects ulnar drift, maintains correction over time, and results in an average of 5° of ulnar drift at 12 years follow-up.[2] The operation results in active MP joint motion of about 50°, which can represent a decrease of up to 18°.[1,2] Proximal and distal interphalangeal joint motion increase during the first few years after the operation, probably as a result of release of at least one tight intrinsic from the donor fingers.[6] The possibility of inducing or accentuating a pre-existing swan-neck deformity remains a concern. Presently, in the finger predisposed to swan-neck deformity, we transfer into the radial collateral ligament rather than the dorsal apparatus.

The results of silicone implant MP arthroplasty can be well determined from numerous resources. The most comprehensive recent publication by Kirschenbaum and co-authors is helpful in this regard.[4] The operation, on average, improves ulnar drift to a position of about 7° of residual ulnar deviation. The operation predictably increases the arc of MP joint motion to about 45°, moving it from a flexed position to a more extended and functional location. The operation also predictably decreases MP joint pain and improves the appearance of the hand. Reported implant fracture rates are approximately 10%, but have little relationship to the quality of the result.[4] The effect of supplementing MP arthroplasty with crossed intrinsic transfer is not well documented, though in our experience it increases the predictability with which ulnar drift is corrected and maintained.

References

1   Blair WF, Crossed intrinsic transfers. In: Blair WF, Steyers CM, eds, *Techniques in Hand Surgery* (Williams and Wilkins: Philadelphia, 1996) 660–6.
2   Oster LH, Blair WF, Steyers CM, et al, Crossed intrinsic transfer, *J Hand Surg* (1989) **14A**:963–71.
3   Wood VE, Ichertz DR, Yahiku H, Soft tissue metacarpophangeal reconstruction for treatment of rheumatoid hand deformity, *J Hand Surg* (1989) **14A**:163–74.
4   Kirschenbaum D, Schneider H, Adams C, et al, Arthroplasty of the metacarpophalangeal joints with use of silicone-rubber implants in patients who have rheumatoid arthritis, *J Bone Joint Surg* (1993) **75A**:3–12.
5   Nalebuff EA, Silicone arthroplasty of the metacarpophalangeal joint. In: Blair WF, Steyers CM, eds, *Techniques in Hand Surgery* (Williams and Wilkins: Philadelphia, 1996) 936–46.
6   El-Gammal TA, Blair WF, Motion after metacarpophalangeal joint reconstruction in rheumatoid disease, *J Hand Surg* (1993) **18A**:504–11.
7   Swanson AB, *Flexible Implant Resection Arthroplasty in the Hand and Extremities* (CV Mosby: St Louis, 1973).
8   Vahvanen V, Viljalkka T, Silicone rubber implant arthroplasty of the metacarpophalangeal joint in rheumatoid arthritis: a follow-up study of 32 patients, *J Hand Surg* (1986) **11A**:333–9.

Commentary

Chapter 32

Crossed intrinsic transfers were described as a part of the treatment of rheumatoid metacarpophalangeal joint deformities even before silicone implant arthroplasty, and now are experiencing something of a renaissance. Because silicone implant arthroplasty does not restore normal function, the marginal benefit which implant arthroplasty provides in patients with less severe disease is accordingly less. This is turn makes joint sparing options such as crossed intrinsic transfer/synovectomy, as described here, more appealing. This is another example of something which is not new, but which remains valuable.

PCA

33
Total wrist arthroplasty for rheumatoid arthritis

Jayasankar Menon

Introduction

Low friction arthroplasty of the hips and knees has become the standard practice to manage arthritic involvement of these joints. However, in the case of radiocarpal arthritis, fusion still remains the number one choice of a majority of surgeons. Technical difficulties associated with implantation of the prosthesis, high rate of complications,[1] and early failures were the most compelling reasons for not recommending total wrist arthroplasty. It is being increasingly accepted that preservation of wrist motion is preferable to fusion, especially when multiple joints are involved as in rheumatoid arthritis. Patients who had arthroplasty on one side and fusion on the other preferred arthroplasty to fusion. Biaxial,[2] Swanson,[3] Meuli,[4] and Volz[5] are the most frequently used prostheses in the United States. The Universal total wrist prosthesis was conceived taking into consideration the various factors that led to the failures of early wrist devices. This chapter describes the surgical technique and the design rationale of the Universal wrist prosthesis.

Preoperative evaluation

As with any major surgical procedure, a thorough history and physical examination should be carried out to assess the patient's health to withstand anesthesia. Details of medications the patient is taking should be noted. It is very important to know whether the patient is on steroids or other immunosuppres-sive drugs. Ideally the patient should not be taking more than 10 mg of prednisone per day. A combination of prednisone and methotrexate could increase the chance of postoperative infection. If the patient is planning to have joint replacements in the lower extremity, that should precede wrist arthroplasty. Evaluation of the cervical spine should be done to alert the anesthesiologist of any unforeseen problems during intubation. Examination of the wrist should include the condition of the skin, presence or absence of synovitis, any evidence of tendon ruptures, status of distal ulna, and range of motion of the wrist. Anterior–posterior and lateral radiographs of the wrist should be done to determine the quality of the bone, degree of subluxation and ulnar translocation of the carpus. It is important to know whether there is any radial deviation of the metacarpals.

Indications

Patients with chronic wrist pain unrelieved by adequate medical treatment by a qualified rheumatologist, or patients who have severe wrist deformity that interferes with function are candidates for total wrist arthroplasty. When there are combined deformities of the wrist and the fingers, wrist arthroplasty should be considered first. Wrist arthroplasty is contraindicated if there is a history of infection and in patients with systemic lupus erythematosus and wrist extensor tendon ruptures. It is also not recommended if the patient is a laborer or the hand is non-functional.

Universal total wrist prosthesis

This is a nonconstrained joint. The components are made of titanium. The articular surface of the radial component is inclined 20° similar to the articular surface of the radius. The concavity of the articular surface is sufficient to provide immediate stability when components are inserted under appropriate tension. The carpal plate is ovoid in shape and matches the cut surface of the carpal bones. It has a central peg and two peripheral holes. The central peg engages the capitate and the screws inserted through the peripheral holes capture the scaphoid and trapezoid on the radial side and triquetrum and hamate on the ulnar side. The components are fixed to the bone with methyl methacrylate. A convex high density polyethylene insert slides over the carpal plate and this articulates with the radial component.

The Universal prosthesis also has a carpal plate without the central peg. Instead of the peg, a 6.5 mm diameter and 35 mm long cancellous screw is inserted through a central hole into the capitate. Additional fixation is obtained by two peripheral screws. The radial component has a tie mesh on either side of the stem and can be inserted with or without the use of bone cement. (*Note*: the design of the carpal plate with three screws has not been released for general use in the United States.)

Surgical technique

After adequate anesthesia the hand is prepped and draped in the usual manner. The tourniquet is inflated to 250 mm of mercury. A dorsal longitudinal incision is made along the line of the third metacarpal. The skin and the subcutaneous tissue are elevated sharply from the extensor tendons and retracted medially and laterally using 3-0 silk retraction sutures. The extensor retinaculum is then opened in a step cut fashion and raised medially and laterally. One-half of the retinaculum is utilized to patch any defects in the joint capsule.

A synovectomy is then carried out, followed by inspection of the extensor tendons. The capsule over the distal ulna is then opened longitudinally and the distal 1 cm of the ulna is osteotomized

and removed. A synovectomy of the ulnar compartment is then performed. To open the radiocarpal joint the capsule is detached from the distal radius and left attached distally. The extensor retinaculum is then subperiosteally elevated radially along with brachioradialis and the tendons of the first dorsal compartment muscles from the styloid process. The branch of the posterior interosseus nerve is resected and the accompanying vessel cauterized. The wrist is now flexed and the soft tissues are protected by Hayes retractors. The radial cutting jig is aligned along the longitudinal axis of the radius. The dorsal lip and the articular surface are then removed with an oscillating saw. This exposes the carpal bones. In many instances the carpal bones have subluxed under the radius and traction on the hand is necessary to expose the proximal row. The line of osteotomy of the carpal bones goes through the proximal end of the capitate. The plane of osteotomy is perpendicular to the axis of the capitate metacarpal complex.

Osteotomy is carried out using an oscillating saw. Care is taken to positively identify the capitate prior to resection. Part of the scaphoid and the triquetrum remains after the resection (Figure 1). An intercarpal fusion is carried out by removing articular cartilage from the capitate, scaphoid, triquetrum, and hamate using a burr or curette. Any rents in the volar capsule are closed with absorbable sutures. All loose fragments of bone are removed from the joint. While the wrist is held in flexed position, a drill hole is made in the center of the capitate metacarpal complex with a 3.2 mm drill bit. A probe is introduced into this hole and the position is checked by an image intensifier in an anteroposterior and lateral plane. This is done to make sure that the tract is intraosseous. The drill has to be angled 10° dorsally to accomplish the correct alignment. Once the position is confirmed, enlarge this tract with a 3.5 mm drill bit.

The surgeon now sits at the end of the hand table in order to have an end-on view of the radius. The medullary canal of the radius is then reamed with an appropriate size broach. The broach should be inserted in valgus. Malrotation of the broach inside the medullary canal of the radius must be avoided. The second radial cutting block is aligned over the broach and the

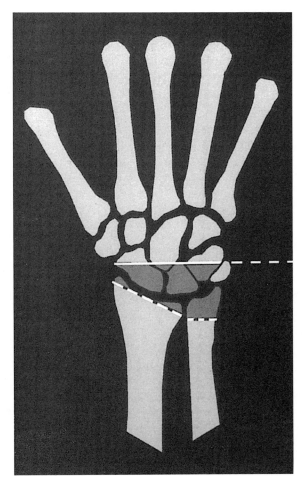 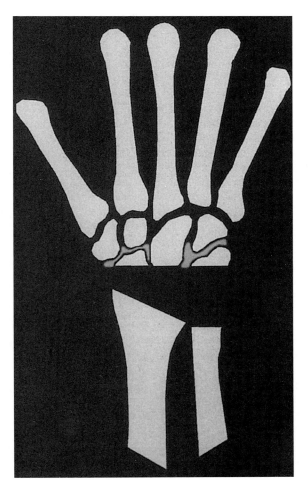

Figure 1

This shows the level of bone resection. The carpal cut goes through the proximal end of the capitate. Intercarpal fusion enhances the bony support of the carpal plate.

radius is cut to match the contour of the radial component.

Trial reduction

The stem of the trial carpal component is introduced into the opening in the capitate. A drill hole is made through the radial opening of the carpal plate, capturing the scaphoid and the trapezoid bones, using a 2.5 mm drill. A 20 mm long and 4.5 mm diameter self-tapping screw is then inserted to obtain temporary fixation. A trial radial component is then inserted into the radius. Trial plastic carpal bearing is slid over the carpal plate and the joint is reduced. If the joint is too tight, additional bone is removed until good flexion and extension, and radial and ulnar deviation are achieved. The trial components are then removed. The wound is irrigated with pulse lavage and dried.

Methyl methacrylate is introduced into the central hole in the capitate metacarpal complex.

The stem of the carpal component is then introduced into this hole and tapped all the way in. Excess cement is removed from the intercarpal area. The ulnar side of the carpal plate is drilled with a 2.5 mm bit and 4.5 mm screws are now inserted through the peripheral holes. Cancellous bone grafts are packed into the defects between the carpal bones to obtain uniform fusion. A bone plug is inserted into the medullary canal of the radius and the remaining bone cement is introduced into the medullary canal. The true radial component is then introduced into the radius. Excess cement is removed. Care is taken to place the prosthesis in valgus. The polyethylene interface is now slid over the carpal plate and the components are reduced. The joint is tested for stability. The ulnar joint capsule is tightly closed, stabilizing the distal ulna. The capsule of the radiocarpal joint is reattached to the radius. If the capsule is deficient, one-half of the retinaculum is used to cover the defects. The other half is used to reconstruct the extensor retinaculum. The skin and the subcutaneous tissue are closed in layers. A bulky hand dressing is then applied. The wrist is immobilized in neutral position for 4 weeks in a cast and then range of motion started.

Salient features of the Universal wrist prosthesis

(1) A minimal amount of bone is resected.
(2) The articular surface of the radial component is inclined 20° similar to the distal end of the radius. This feature makes the wrist easy to balance.
(3) A third generation cementing technique is used to improve bonding between the cement and the bone, thus decreasing the chance of loosening.
(4) The carpal component supports the first and the fifth ray and prevents proximal migration of these columns. Other existing designs do not support the entire carpus.
(5) If the carpal bones are deficient, the carpal height can be restored by insertion of a corticocancellous bone graft—a unique advantage of the Universal wrist prosthesis.
(6) Oblique osteotomy removes comparatively less bone from the radius. This, coupled with the configuration of the radial component, helps to transfer the load from the carpus to the radius as in vivo.
(7) Intercarpal fusion forms a solid bony support for the carpal component and reduces the chance of loosening by decreasing the toggle.
(8) Soft tissue balancing can be achieved by choosing the appropriate size polyethylene insert.
(9) Adequate bone stock is available to salvage the wrist by fusion if the prosthesis fails.

Results

Fifty-seven Universal implants were inserted in 50 patients during a period of 9 years (Figure 2). There were 13 males and 37 females; their ages ranged from 35 to 81 with a mean of 58.1 years. The majority of the patients had rheumatoid arthritis. Pain relief was obtained in 90% of patients. All patients achieved a functional range of motion of the wrist postoperatively. The most common complication was volar dislocation of the prosthesis—six patients developed this complication. The wrists were salvaged by either open or closed reduction except in one case. Due to the recurrence of dislocation, the wrist was fused in one patient. Loosening of the radial component occurred in two cases. In these two cases the radial component was uncemented. Both cases were revised with a cemented radial component.

There has not been any loosening of the carpal component with three screw fixation. One patient developed staphylococcus infection a year and a half postoperatively. This patient was on high doses of steroids and methotrexate and had multiple sites of infection. The prosthesis had to be removed in this case. Another patient developed systemic candidiasis along with involvement of the wrist joint. This patient survived the infection and the wrist was salvaged. In two cases the carpal bones were deficient and a corticocancellous iliac bone graft was used to restore the carpal height. In both cases the bone graft incorporated well with the remaining carpal bones. Two patients had spontaneous fusion of the radiocarpal joint in malposition preoperatively. Following insertion

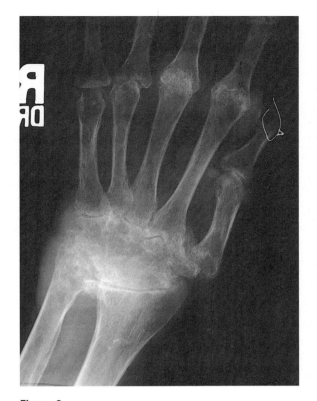 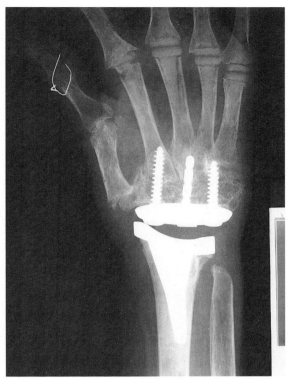

Figure 2

(a) Preoperative radiograph of the wrist of a patient with rheumatoid arthritis. (b) Radiographic appearance after insertion of a Universal wrist prosthesis.

of the Universal prosthesis these patients obtained good correction of their deformity and gained adequate range of motion. The Universal prosthesis also allows the patient to balance the wrist (i.e. bring the wrist to the neutral position by volition) relatively easily, as this design does not disturb the lever arms of the muscles acting across the wrist joint to any significant extent. (The most common postoperative ulnar deviation deformity results from the increased pull of the flexor carpi ulnaris tendon due to the change of length of the lever arm i.e. the distance from the center of rotation of the wrist to the axis of the FCU tendon.)

Overall, long-term results with this device have been very good. With improvements in instrumentation and the future availability of prostheses of varying sizes, the outcome of total wrist arthroplasty can be further improved to match that of hips and knees.

References

1   Cooney WP, Beckenbaugh RD, Linscheid RL, Total wrist arthroplasty. Problems with implant failures, *Clin Orthop* (1984) **187**:121–8.

2   Rettig ME, Beckenbaugh RD, Revision total wrist arthroplasty, *J Hand Surg* (1993) **18A**:798–804.

3   Davis RF, Weiland AJ, Dowling SV, Swanson implant arthroplasty of the wrist in rheumatoid patients, *Clin Orthop* (1982) **166**:132–7.

4   Meuli HC, Fernandez DL, Uncemented total wrist arthroplasty, *J Hand Surg* (1995) **20A**:115–22.

5   Menon J, Total wrist arthroplasty using the modified Volz prosthesis, *J Bone Joint Surg* (1987) **69A**:998–1006.

34
Uncemented total wrist arthroplasty for rheumatoid arthritis

Hans Christoph Meuli

Introduction

Our first total wrist prosthesis was designed in 1970, and a first publication of the clinical outcome followed in 1973.[1] In the course of time the prosthesis has been continuously improved. Improvements in the surgical technique, careful selection of patients and better observation of the indications have also helped to avoid failures and to significantly reduce the revision rate. However, some problems still had to be solved, such as centering of the prosthesis, fixation of the prosthesis in the carpus, the use of cement, and polyethylene wear. Therefore the prosthesis design and the surgical technique were modified in 1986.

Technical aspects

The prosthesis MWP III (Meuli wrist prosthesis, third revised implant) is composed of titanium 6-aluminum 7-niobium wrought alloy Protasul 100. The surface is corundum rough blasted. The ball head is coated with titanium nitride. The cup inset is made of UHMW-polyethylene chirulen. The special design of the carpal component in the right and left hand versions helps to center and balance it. The radius part can be used for both the right and left hand prosthesis, the head being offset to the ulnar side. The prosthesis is designed for use without cement. The prongs can be contoured to adapt to the position of the metacarpals and to the intramedullary canal of the radius. The prosthesis functions as an unconstrained ball and socket joint (Figure 1).

The details of surgical technique, which must be strictly observed, have been described in a

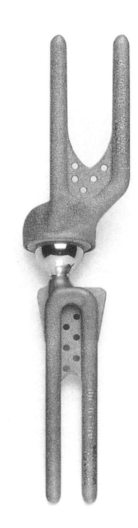

Figure 1

The MWP III (Meuli wrist prosthesis, third revised implant) total wrist prosthesis.

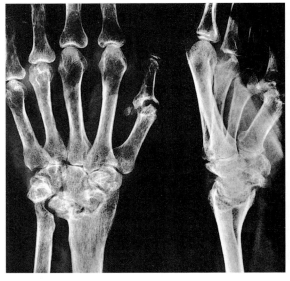
a

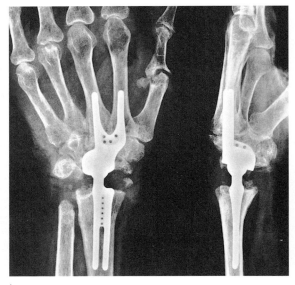
b

Figure 2

Correctly implanted wrist prosthesis in a 72-year-old female patient with rheumatoid arthritis. (a) X-ray film before surgery and (b) X-ray film after surgery. The prosthesis is centered with axial alignment and restores carpal height. The prosthesis is firmly fixed in the carpal bone stock, with no palmar protrusion.

previous report.[2] The most important step is correct placement of the prosthesis. Bone resection must be minimal. It is absolutely necessary to preserve bone support at the palmar side of the carpus to guarantee a solid anchorage of the carpal component of the prosthesis. Intra-operative fluoroscopic X-ray control is routinely performed before and after reduction of the prosthetic parts (Figure 2).

Active exercises are started 1 week after the operation. The wrist is maintained in a neutral position for up to 2 weeks while the wound heals. Then the flexion–extension exercises are gradually increased, but a resting splint should be worn for 6 weeks and at night. Excessive range of motion exercises should be avoided in favor of maximum stability. When the position is incorrect, or there is a tendency to contract, a dynamic splint is used.

Pros and cons compared to classical techniques

During the past 25 years numerous wrist prostheses have been designed and used in patients.[2-4] It is remarkable that, in all current wrist implants, cementing is an important prerequisite. However, the use of methyl-methacrylate in the carpus is difficult because, instead of one solid bone, an assemblage of several small bones with joint spaces between them is present. Cementing is therefore often insufficient. In cases of instability the wear products of cement lead to granulomatous soft tissue reactions, resulting in local osteolysis with severe subsequent reduction of the bone stock.

Indeed, loosening and migration of the carpal component appears to be the most common complication associated with total wrist replacement, and has repeatedly been emphasized by several authors.[2-5] This is particularly true for voluminous carpal implants that are not solidly fixed within the carpus and in which ultimate stability depends entirely on the metacarpal anchorage with bone cement. Even the use of longer prongs may result in late loosening due to the absence of bony support of the prosthesis proximally. Functional loading in these instances may be responsible for bending and torsional stresses of the implant, micromotion, and progressive loosening of the metacarpal bone–cement interface.

Since long-lasting fixation of a noncemented prosthesis is solely dependent on bony ingrowth on the implant surface (osseointegration), maximal coverage of the prosthetic parts during implantation is imperative. Whenever the local bone stock is insufficient, bone grafting (autologous iliac bone) is strongly recommended. In addition, the carpometacarpal joints II and III have to be stabilized with bone grafts.

Obviously it is more difficult to balance a nonconstrained ball and socket joint than a semiconstrained prosthesis or a prosthesis with an ellipsoid head. The ball joint, however, allows motion in all planes without impingement as well as a slight distraction. Thus, any unfavorable stresses on the anchorage of the parts in bone are greatly reduced. The prosthetic parts require precise placement, the center of motion being within the head of the capitate bone.

Polyethylene wear continues to be a certain problem also in this new prosthesis, as it is in all current wrist implants. Perhaps metal-to-metal pairing will be the solution of the future.

Results

The preliminary results of a series of 50 prostheses have been carefully analyzed.[2] It could be clearly demonstrated that a solid fixation of the wrist prosthesis is possible without the need for bone cement.

Between 1986 and 1991 50 prostheses were implanted in 45 patients, 33 with rheumatoid arthritis, 12 with traumatic arthrosis. Evaluation included questioning of the patient on pain, satisfaction, and ability to perform daily activities, motion and grip strength measurements and radiographic findings. The final result was rated as excellent in 24 wrists, good in 12, fair in 5 and poor in 8 wrists. Initially the problems associated with malalignment and poor bone quality were not recognized and accounted for the complications observed in the early period of this study. Thereafter the results were highly satisfactory.

Indications

Total wrist replacement may be indicated when there is severe painful destruction and instability of the wrist due to rheumatoid arthritis or posttraumatic arthrosis. However, it should be undertaken only if a reconstructive, motion preserving procedure is no longer feasible and wrist arthrodesis is being considered. In contrast to wrist fusion, total wrist arthroplasty is a motion preserving operation designed to prolong wrist function in time, which is most appreciated by patients with rheumatoid arthritis. Loosening of the implant can always be salvaged with arthrodesis at a later date.

Wrist arthrodesis is still the preferred procedure if there are definite contraindications for a total wrist replacement, for example in workers engaged in heavy manual labor and in patients who must rely on walking aids. In the presence of insufficient bone stock, severe extensor tendon deficiencies, or malposition of the metacarpophalangeal joints with hyperflexion a total wrist prosthesis is also contraindicated.

References

1   Meuli HC, Arthroplastie du poignet, *Ann Chir* (1973) **27**:527–30.
2   Meuli HC, Fernandez DL, Uncemented total wrist arthroplasty, *J Hand Surg* (1995) **20A**:115–22.
3   Beckenbaugh RD, Linscheid RL, Arthroplasty in the hand and wrist. In: Green DP, ed, *Operative Hand Surgery* (Churchill Livingstone: New York, 1982) 167–214.
4   Beckenbaugh RD, Arthroplasty of the wrist. In: Morrey BF, ed, *Joint Replacement Arthroplasty* (Churchill Livingstone: New York, 1991) 195–215.
5   Cooney WP III, Beckenbaugh RD, Linscheid RL, Total wrist arthroplasty. Problems with implant failures, *Clin Orthop* (1984) **187**:121–8.

Surface replacement arthroplasty for the proximal interphalangeal joint and trapeziometacarpal joint

Ronald L Linscheid

A number of innovative approaches has been made to prosthetic replacement arthroplasty of the small joints of the hand in the last several decades. The design of such implants must take into account the anatomy of the joint, the kinematics of joint movement, the material properties of prosthetic components, the feasible mechanical equivalent of the joint, the biologic compatibility of the material, the method of fixation to bone, and the surgical approach that guarantees the best postoperative response. This section will briefly review our design concepts and experience with surface replacement prostheses of the proximal interphalangeal (PIP) and trapeziometacarpal (TMC) joints.[1]

The proximal interphalangeal joint

Introduction

When we first designed a two component surface replacement prosthesis for the PIP, our assumptions were:

(1) An unconstrained surface replacement (SR) prosthesis would give a more physiologic articulation.
(2) Minimal bony excision with optimal preservation of the collateral ligaments would provide a more stable joint particularly to lateral forces.

(3) A properly centered anatomical configuration would restore balanced tendon moments to the joint.
(4) Diversion of some of the transverse forces and axial torques to the collateral ligaments and lateral cortices would diminish the stresses on the prosthesis–endosteal interface and decrease the mechanical contribution to osteolysis and subsidence.
(5) The most suitable fixation was polymethylmethacrylate (PMMA) for the following reasons: (a) irregular intramedullary cavities make design of a congruent contoured stem difficult; (b) the finger bones are of differing shapes and sizes; (c) there is inadequate joint space to allow a sintered metal backing for the distal component; (d) proper centering and alignment are enhanced by the ability to position the components within the cement.[1,2]

The PIP joint is a diarthrodial hinge joint that normally has 115° arc range of motion. Joint stability is attributable to the bicondylar configuration and the collateral ligaments with secondary help from the lateral bands of the extensor apparatus and the retinacular structures.

Technical aspects

A proximal component of CoCr alloy simulates the normal contour of the proximal phalanx. The distal component of ultra high molecular weight

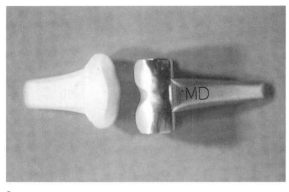

a

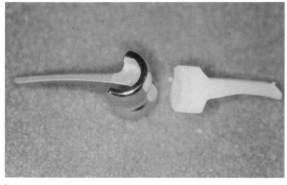

b

Figure 1

(a,b) Surface replacement prostheses for the PIP joint.

the alignment of the trial components under the image intensifier. Full extension and flexion to at least 80° was sought. PMMA was injected from a syringe and both components inserted. The joint was held in extension under firm compression until the cement set. Any loose or extruded cement was then removed. The extensor apparatus was repaired by midline closure.

Progressive flexion exercises followed by a return to full extension were practised under the supervision of a hand therapist beginning at 10–12 days. A daytime dynamic extension assist splint and a nighttime static splint were used up to 6 weeks. More recently exposure has been achieved through a dorsal approach by reflection of a distally based central slip. This permits some adjustment of the tension on the central slip and earlier mobilization of the joint.

Pros and cons compared to classical techniques

We were dissatisfied with our results in PIP arthroplasties in the late 1970s. A custom metallo-plastic hinged prosthesis required extensive bony excision and developed loosening problems.[1] One piece silicone flexible implants[3,4] lost motion progressively and were often unstable in our hands. The SR prosthesis requires exacting alignment and soft tissue preservation and repair for optimal function.[5]

Clinical material

A surface replacement PIP arthroplasty was performed on 66 joints over a 16-year period. The average age was 58 years. Thirty-seven joints were replaced for degenerative joint disease, 16 for traumatic arthritis and 13 for inflammatory arthritis.

Preoperative motion varied widely. Static deformities included swan neck in eight, boutonnière in four and lateral deviations from 10 to 35° in 21 fingers. Three were radially deviated. Partial bone loss from trauma was present in five. Three had an unsatisfactory previous silicone rubber arthroplasty. Grip and pinch strength varied widely, and were primarily dependent on the

polyethylene (UHMWPE) has a bifaceted biconcave surface that fits flush against the cortical rim of the midphalangeal base. Both have intramedullary stems that extend beyond the respective midpoints of the phalanx (Figure 1).

Exposure: an ulnar approach which attempted to preserve the central slip insertion was used in the initial 13 cases. Alignment and positioning difficulties led to the adoption of a palmar approach in 10 subsequent cases. A dorsal approach was used in the remainder of the cases. The central slip was split and either side with its lateral band was swept laterally to expose the joint. Collateral ligaments were protected while the joint surfaces were removed. The intramedullary cavities were broached. It was found to be desirable to repeatedly check

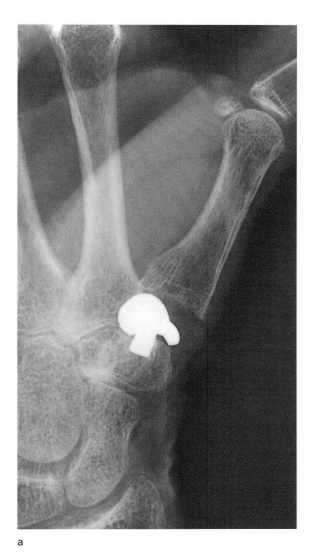
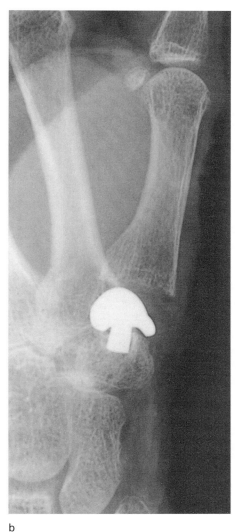

a   b

Figure 2

Radiographs of a surface replacement TMC joint in place, showing range of motion in flexion/extension.

overall involvement of the hand and proximity of the involved digit to the thumb.

Results

An average follow-up of 54 months was available on 63 of the 66 original joints from 1 to 14 years.

Postoperatively, 56 joints were pain free, six had mild aching, and four had discomfort with activity. Preoperatively the average range of motion was 11–46° (arc 35°). Postoperatively the average was 14–61° (arc 47°), a gain of 12°. Postoperative motion reflected the type of motion arc present preoperatively. All but three patients returned to their original work or life style. Preoperatively 18 joints had ulnar deviation (UD) of 10° or more

Table 1   Results of surface replacement PIP arthroplasty on 66 joints.

Diagnosis	good	fair	poor
DJD	22	11	4
TA	5	5	6
RA	5	3	5
Totals	32	19	15

DJD, degenerative joint disease; TA, traumatic arthritis; RA, rheumatoid arthritis.

(10–35°) as opposed to three postoperatively. Radial deviation (RD) of 10° was present in three joints preoperatively and one postoperatively.

The results (Table 1) were graded as good, fair or poor based on motion, stance, function and radiographic appearance.

Complications

There were a significant number of complications, sometimes more than one in each joint in this series. These tended to reflect the preoperative status. Instability noted preoperatively persisted in five joints. Recurrent ulnar deviation of 15° or greater occurred in three of these joints and one redeveloped a 25° radial deformity.

Recurrent swan neck deformity occurred in five joints. Three joints were rated poor for having only a few degrees of active flexion. Persistent or recurrent flexion deformity was noted in two joints which were also unstable preoperatively. Extension lags of 45° occurred in eight otherwise stable joints with satisfactory additional motion. These occurred primarily in fingers which had the lateral or palmar approaches early in the series.

Seven joints with less than 15° of active motion had previous extensive trauma. Twelve secondary surgeries were carried out on 11 fingers. This included two extensor plications for a flexion lag, three tendolyses of the extensor apparatus for flexion deficit, one realignment of the proximal component, and radial collateral ligament reconstruction for ulnar deviation. Two late amputations were done, and two skin grafts were inserted on palmar incisional scars for flexion contractures.

The alignment of seven components was 10° or more offline from the longitudinal axis of the phalanx on postoperative radiographs. This occurred primarily in fingers approached laterally or in traumatically deformed or rheumatoid fingers. Radiographic evidence of loosening has been remarkably absent in this series.

Indications

Pain, deformity, and limited motion were indications for surgery. Excessive bone or soft tissue loss or scarring are contraindications.

The trapeziometacarpal joint

Introduction

The trapeziometacarpal (TMC) joint is a frequent site of degenerative arthritis. A variety of surgical procedures has been suggested for advanced degenerative disease. The very number of proposed procedures attests to the difficulty in finding a consensus on the most efficacious treatment.

Technical aspects

Joint kinematics and pathomechanics

The TMC joint lies in a complex kinematic chain of the thumb axis. The double saddle configuration has been compared to a universal joint that allows only 2° of freedom. Flexion/extension occurs about an instant center of rotation in the trapezium in a plane set at approximately 80° to the plane of the adjacent metacarpals. Abduction/adduction occurs about a center of rotation in the base of the first metacarpal which is roughly perpendicular to the flexion plane. Opposition is a combination of the two motions. The trapezial surface is wider radially than ulnarly. This facilitates the circular arc described in the oppositional movement. A modest incongruence of the surfaces permits a small axial rotation.[6] Zancolli[7] describes an area of increased joint congruence radially which increases joint contact area during oppositional pinch.

The axial compression force at this joint has been shown to be an order of magnitude higher than the output force at the thumb tip. The shear stress produced on the joint during pinch appears to be the result of a posteroradially directed composite force vector.[8,9] This force is normally held in dynamic equilibrium by the joint contact force with little reliance on ligamentous tension.[6] There is general agreement that the pathomechanics of degenerative arthritis results from progressive dorsal and radial displacement of the base of the first metacarpal base on the trapezium.[10] This is associated with erosive narrowing of the articular cartilage from the ulnavolar facet of the metacarpal base and the corresponding anterior facet of the trapezium. The flatness of the joint surfaces has been shown to be more pronounced in women as had long been suspected.[11] Pelligrini has suggested attritional attenuation of the 'beak ligament' is a contributing factor in instability of the joint.[10]

An additional factor in the pathogenesis of the disease may be cantilever bending of the trapezium from its support on the base of the second metacarpal and trapezoid even though it is partially supported by the scaphoid proximally. This may be especially relevant in rheumatoid disease. This is resisted by ligaments arising from the second and third metacarpal bases and the trapezoid.[12] Radial angulation of the trapezium increases the tendency for the metacarpal to displace dorsoradially. Erosion of the joint surfaces radially and enchondral new bone formation ulnarly further increase the trapezial cant and aggravate the displacement of the metacarpal base.

Prosthetic design

A two component surface replacement device with matching symmetrical hyperbolic paraboloid sections may closely mimic the kinematics of the normal joint by integrating joint movement to the distribution of muscular forces disposed around the joint. The under surface of the proximal component provides for a wide contact area on the trapezium for maximum dispersion of joint contact forces. A central 6 mm long peg on the under surface provides additional fixation. The use of PMMA cement aids fixation on the prepared trapezial surface.

The enchondral changes ulnarly and erosive changes radially are most easily recognized and measured on a Robert's view. To correct this increased slope of the trapezial surface it is necessary to sculpt away more bone ulnarly than radially.

The distal component stem extends past the midpoint of the first metacarpal shaft. This reduces side forces on the metaphyseal flare. The stem is offset dorsally to conform to the anatomic alignment of the metacarpal. The flat dorsal surface makes alignment with the dorsal surface of the thumb easier. The flare at the base of the prosthesis allows contact with the cortices of the metacarpal for three point stabilization. A slight incongruence allows for modest axial rotation as part of a conjunct circumduction motion (Figures 2 and 3).

Surgical exposure

A posterior approach allows the dorsal superficial sensory nerves and the radial artery to be gently mobilized. The posterior capsule is reflected proximally. The proximal 3 mm of the base are removed. The intramedullary cavity is prepared with a custom broach.

The trapezium is inspected and the anterior recess cleared of redundant synovium and debris. Most of the cortical surface is leveled with a sagittal saw angled to correct the radial slant of the surface. A dumbbell shaped cutting burr is applied to the trapezial surface in a to and fro motion. This contours the remaining surface to the shape of the undersurface of the proximal component. A drill template for the peg hole is positioned ulnarly on the trapezial surface and checked under the image intensifier in the Robert's position. Trial components are fitted sequentially and such further revisions as necessary to ensure fit and alignment are made. The joint is reduced and a range of motion carried out passively. When satisfactory the components are cemented. A thin covering of cement is placed on the raw surface of the trapezium. The metacarpal component is inserted first and any excess cement removed. The thumb is distracted and the

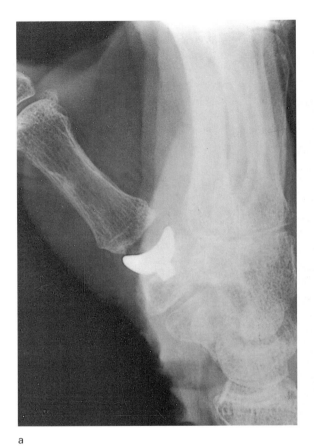

a

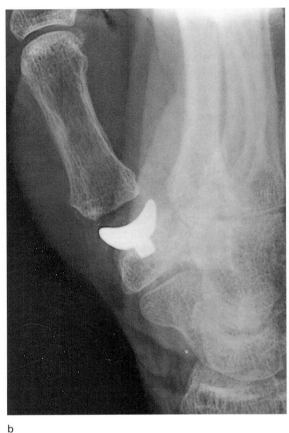

b

Figure 3

Radiographs of a surface replacement TMC joint in place, showing range of motion in abduction/adduction.

proximal component seated. The anterior recess is cleared of any residual cement and the joint reduced and compressed until the cement is set. The posterior capsule is resutured to the posterior lip of the metacarpal base and the skin is closed with subcuticular absorbable sutures.

A splint dressing which allows movement of the distal phalanx is applied with the thumb in opposition. A removable splint is applied when metacarpophalangeal motion is started at 3–5 days and progressive metacarpaltrapezial motion is added at 10 days with supervision during the 6 week rehabilitation period. Radiographs and progress are reviewed at 2 week periods.

Pros and cons compared to classical techniques

Most total joint arthroplasties use a ball and socket configuration that places the pivot point within the trapezium and places the joint compressive load on a small trabecular area. This may lead to subsidence and loosening. Interposition arthroplasties of polymeric substances are subject to degradation. Suspension arthroplasties often show progressive proximal migration of the metacarpal and occasional metacarpotrapezoidal or scaphotrapezoidal impingement. We recognized that the attenuated ligament system would be further compromised by resection of the metacarpal base. Therefore the curvature of the surfaces was slightly increased to provide more inherent stability.

Results

The initial response of a small group of 10 patients with over a 2-year follow-up who have undergone this procedure has been encouraging both from the standpoint of patient satisfaction and functional result, but a suitable number of patients studied in a prospective manner and compared to a matched series treated by a comparable technique is necessary to confirm the appropriateness of this surface replacement approach (Figure 3).

Indications

The trapeziotrapezoidal joint should be stable. Its involvement in rheumatoid arthritis is a contraindication. Suspension arthroplasty would be the most likely salvage operation for a failed surface replacement arthroplasty.

References

1 Linscheid RL, Dobyns JH, Total joint arthroplasty. The hand, *Mayo Clin Proc* (1979) **54**:516–26.

2 Beckenbaugh RD, Linscheid RL, Arthroplasty in the hand and wrist. In: Green DP, ed, *Operative Hand Surgery,* 3rd edn, Vol 1 (Churchill Livingstone: New York 1993) 146–84.

3 Swanson AB, Maupin BK, Gajjar NV, et al, Flexible implant arthroplasty in the proximal interphalangeal joint of the hand, *J Hand Surg* (1985) **10A**:796–805.

4 Lin HH, Wyrick JD, Stern PJ, Proximal interphalangeal joint silicone replacement arthroplasty: clinical results using an anterior approach, *J Hand Surg* (1995) **20A**:123–32.

5 Uchiyama S, Linscheid RL, Cooney WP, et al, Kinematics of the proximal interphalangeal joint of the finger after surface replacement, *J Hand Surg* (1996) in press.

6 Imaeda T, Niebur G, Cooney WP, et al, Kinematics of the normal trapeziometacarpal joint, *J Orthop Res* (1995) **12**:197–204.

7 Zancolli EA, Zaidenberg C, Zancolli E Jnr, Biomechanics of the trapeziometacarpal joint, *Clin Orthop* (1987) **220**:14–26.

8 Cooney WP, Chao EYS, Biomechanical analysis of static forces in the thumb during hand function, *J Bone Joint Surg* (1977) **59A**:27–36.

9 Lbath F, Rumelhart C, Comtet JJ, Étude biomécanique in vivo de l'articulatio trapézo-métacarpienne à l'aide de l'IRM. Détermination de l'effort résultant et modélisation articulaire, *La Main* (1996) **1**:13–21.

10 Pelligrini VD, Osteoarthritis of the trapeziometacarpal joint: the pathophysiology of articular cartilage degeneration. II Articular wear patterns in the osteoarthritic joint, *J Hand Surg* (1991) **16A**:975–82.

11 Ateshian GA, Rosenwasser MP, Van Mow VC, Anatomic forms of male and female carpometacarpal joints. In: Schuind F et al, eds, *Advances in Biomechanics of the Hand and Wrist* (Plenum Press: New York, 1994).

12 Bettinger PC, Linscheid RL, Berger RA, et al, Anatomic study of the stabilizing ligaments of the trapezium and trapeziometacarpal joint, *J Hand Surg* (1996) (submitted).

Commentary

Chapters 33 and 34

There are a number of ways to manage severe wrist involvement in patients with rheumatoid arthritis. Currently, my own practice is to involve many more arthrodeses than arthroplasties. Often a radiolunate arthrodesis will suffice but occasionally in more advanced cases a complete wrist arthrodesis may be necessary. I find the results of wrist arthrodesis, whether or not complete, to be more predictable than the results of wrist arthroplasty but clearly there are many patients for whom a complete loss of motion is unacceptable and for these, arthroplasty is certainly an option. The silicone implant arthroplasty option seems to be less popular currently. The cemented metal and plastic options including the Biaxial, Meuli, and Universal implants,

appear to have some role. Here Jay Menon describes one currently used wrist arthroplasty technique, using the Universal implant. Results seem similar to those which have been reported by Beckenbaugh for the biaxial wrist. Professor Meuli has taken an approach of modifying his well known implant to be used without cement. His early results seem worthwhile.

PCA

Chapter 35

These new cemented metal–plastic surface replacement implants represent a potential advance in our ability to treat hand arthritis.

PCA

External fixation for distal radius fractures

Andrew Ellowitz, Matthew D Putnam and Melissa Cohen

Introduction

Controversy continues to exist pertaining to several aspects of external fixation as a treatment for distal radial fractures. In this chapter, it is our goal to use the latest available information in order to clarify some of these issues.

Indications

As with any fracture, treatment options must be individualized to each patient and depend upon the goals of treatment. An elderly nursing home patient with multiple medical problems who sustains an isolated fracture of the distal radius may do well with a less than anatomic result, while someone with higher demands and longer life expectancy may require more aggressive treatment to restore desired function.

Knirk and Jupiter found that the most critical factor in achieving a satisfactory result in the treatment of distal radius fractures was restoration of the articular surface when an intraarticular fracture component was greater than 2 mm.[1] Critical evaluation of patient outcomes has made it clear that clinical results correlate highly with the restoration of the normal preinjury anatomy. Closed reduction and plaster immobilization is an acceptable method to gain an anatomic result when fractures are primarily extraarticular and not associated with a significant degree of dorsal or volar comminution. When these components are present it has been observed that fracture reduction is unlikely to be maintained in the anatomic configuration by plaster alone.[2,3] This can often be predicted on the basis of the original injury film and the first closed reduction radiograph.[2,4] Current indications in the literature for surgical intervention include the following:

(1) A fracture pattern with significant dorsal or volar comminution with or without articular involvement;
(2) A fracture with a displaced intraarticular component—the radiocarpal or distal radio-ulnar joint;[1]
(3) Open fractures;[5]
(4) Multiple trauma;
(5) Loss of reduction with cast treatment;
(6) The presence of die punch fragment;[3]
(7) Bilateral distal radial fractures.[6,7]

Figures 1–3 show three examples of distal radius fractures treated with external fixation.

Several classifications of distal radius fractures exist. Fracture classifications are useful as long as they include important components of the injury which are predictive of treatment or prognosis. Eponyms are not descriptive and are often misused.

External fixation has been shown to be an effective treatment modality to maintain reduction of distal radius fractures.[4,5,8,9] It is most commonly employed in displaced intraarticular fractures, but it is also used in extraarticular fractures with comminution and open fractures where soft tissue wound care and the prevention of infection are important issues.[6,7] Other potential advantages of external fixation include its versatility, as it may be adjusted to correct deformities in several planes. It also facilitates early motion of adjacent joints while maintaining skeletal stability in the appropriately applied frame.[7]

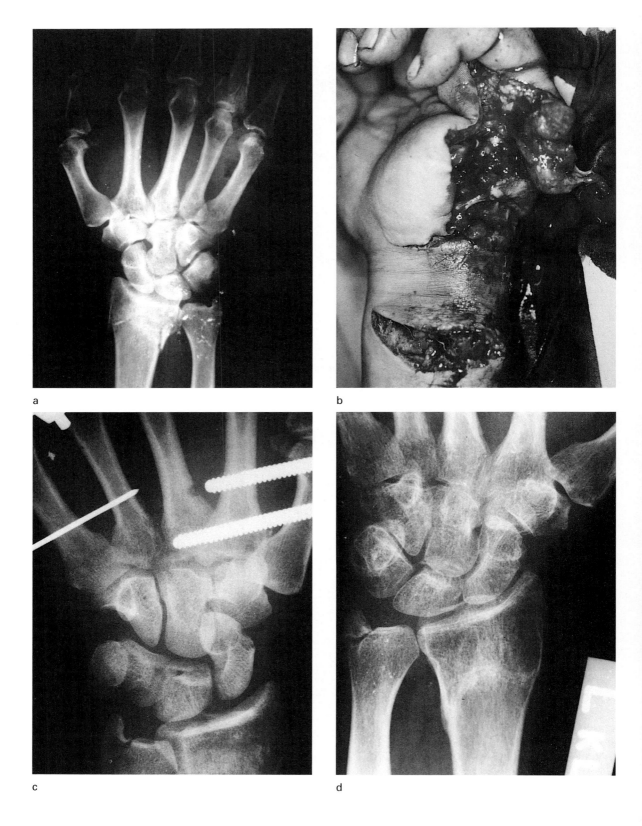

a

b

c

d

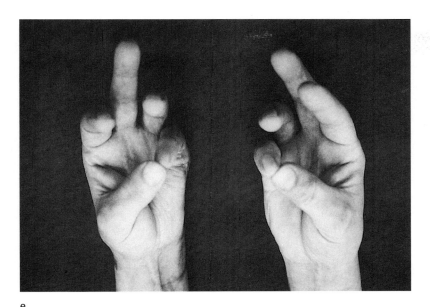

Figure 1

(a) Anteroposterior radiographg of an open distal radius fracture with an associated fifth metacarpal fracture. (b) Photographic representation of the soft tissue injury. The patient had no disruption of nerve function. (c) External fixation and reduction of the fracture. (d) Postoperative radiograph demonstrating a healed fracture at 6 months. (e) Soft tissue healing at the forearm, wrist and hand.

e

Table 1   Physical comparison data. (Reproduced with permission from Frykman et al.[12])

Fixator	Stiffness index	Weight (g)	Cost	Dynamic	Controlled adjustment
Hoffman C Series Unilateral	5.2	174	840	No	Yes
Hoffman Dynamic	5.8	389	1926	Yes	Yes
Agee Wrist Jack	7.1	212	1200	Yes	Yes
Lima	8.2	136	1358	Yes	Yes
Clyburn	8.4	88	948	Yes	Yes
Ace Colles'	10.3	123	985	No	Yes
Pennig	10.7	135	1810	Yes	Yes
Small AO	13.7	88	1188	No	No
Roger Anderson	14.8	126	340	No	No
Richard Colles's	17.5	96	722	Yes	No
Hoffman C Series Bilateral	18.8	247	1142	No	Yes
Methyl Methacrylate	22.1	107	250	No	No
Orthofix	42.3	264	1520	No	Yes

Principles and types of external fixation for distal radial fractures

Ligamentotaxis is the continued distraction across the fracture site which allows an intact soft tissue sleeve to reduce and maintain otherwise unstable fragments into an acceptable alignment. External fixation utilizes this concept in the management of distal radius fractures. In order to accomplish this goal, the construct must anchor bony fragments across the fracture site and provide longitudinal support. Stability of the construct depends upon several factors such as material stiffness, number and diameter of pins, pin to bone purchase[10] (Figure 4), pin to pin distance, limb to bar distance, and intrinsic geometric stability at the fracture site.[11]

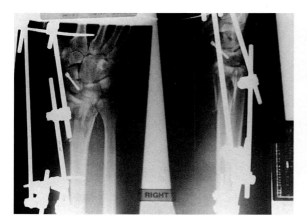

a

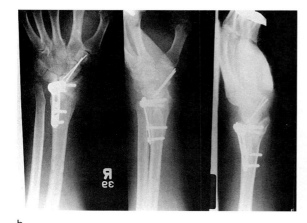

b   c

Figure 2

(a) Case demonstrating inability of ligamentotaxis to obtain intraarticular reduction. (b,c) Reconstruction of the early radial malunion where external fixation was used for interoperative distraction in the application of a plate, in addition a corrective osteotomy was performed.

While it is not known exactly what the optimal rigidity is for a given external fixation system to facilitate union of distal radius fractures, it is believed that the greater the stiffness, the better the construct. Frykman et al tested the rigidity of 13 commercially available external fixator devices for fractures of the distal radius and found that the OrthoFix (EBI Inc, Parsippany, NJ, USA) device was by far the most rigid.[12] Rigidity, however, is but one factor in the decision of which device to use. This must be weighed against the ease of application, weight and cost of each device (Table 1). In fact, Frykman et al did not recommend any one fixator based on their study, and stressed the point that no particular device is optimal in all distal radial fractures. Recent reports have demonstrated good results with the use of the Hoffman external fixator at an average of about 3 years follow-up,[4] and the small AO fixator at 12 years follow-up.[8]

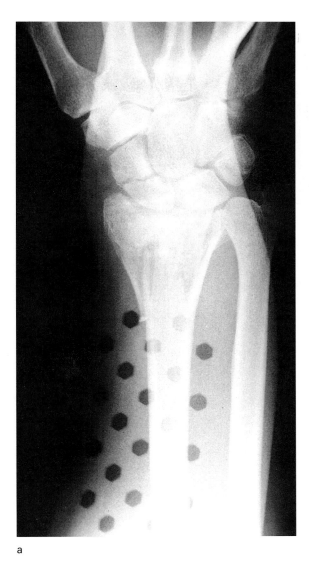

a

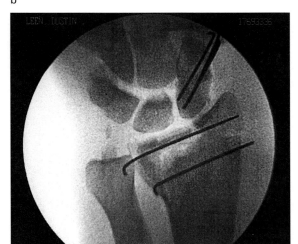

b

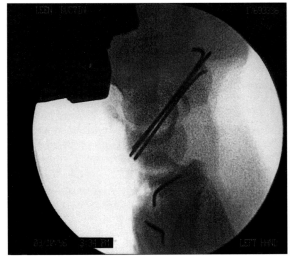

c

d

Figure 3

(a) Prefixation radiograph of comminuted extra- and intra-articular radius fracture with an associated unstable scaphoid fracture. (b) Intraoperative distraction using the Wagner limb lengthener to assist in the assembly of the displaced joint fragments through an incision separating dorsal compartments 3 and 4. The distraction was left in place as a fixator. (c,d) Postoperative reduction anteroposterior and lateral radiographs. The articular surface was reduced with Kirschner wires. Distraction of the carpal elements did not exceed the patient's extrinsic glide.

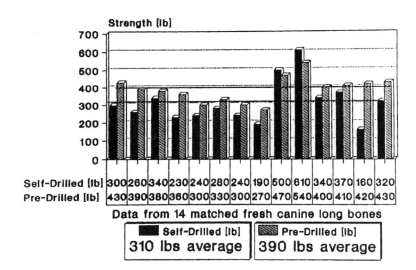

Figure 4

Bar graph demonstrating individual pull out test results in 14 identically matched pairs of canine femora. (Reproduced with permission from Seitz et al.[10])

| Self-Drilled [lb] | 300 | 260 | 340 | 230 | 240 | 280 | 240 | 190 | 500 | 610 | 340 | 370 | 160 | 320 |
| Pre-Drilled [lb] | 430 | 390 | 380 | 360 | 300 | 330 | 300 | 270 | 470 | 540 | 400 | 410 | 420 | 430 |

Data from 14 matched fresh canine long bones

■ Self-Drilled [lb]	▨ Pre-Drilled [lb]
310 lbs average	390 lbs average

Theory and techniques of application

The technique of application of external fixators plays a large role in the avoidance of complications associated with this fracture fixation method.[5] Behrens characterized limb segments into corridors based upon anatomical structures contained therein.[13] Safe corridors are defined as those which contain no musculotendinous units or neurovascular bundles such as the subcutaneous metacarpals and anteromedial tibia. Hazardous corridors are those in which musculotendinous units exist but no neurovascular bundles are present. Unsafe corridors contain both neurovascular structures and musculocutaneous units. In the case of the radius, no safe zone exists as this bone is surrounded by muscle tendon units, nerves and blood vessels. It has therefore been recommended that a mini open technique of application for the proximal radial pins be employed.[5] This has been shown to decrease the incidence of eccentric pin placement which can lead to loosening and fixation failure. Also, damage to the superficial branch of the radial nerve and extensor tendons is less likely since they are directly visualized.

Mini open technique

Many complications such as pin loosening, pin tract infection, fracture through drill holes, and soft tissue damage may be avoided by the use of surgical techniques which allow direct visualization of the bony target.

The technique proposed may be used with any fixation device of half-frame design; however, we have employed and recommend a device that allows primary insertion of the pins followed by application of the device itself and then reduction of the fracture (Figure 5).

Following the preparation of the entire upper extremity, the first step is to insert the proximal pin. A point between 10 and 12 cm proximal to the radial styloid is marked over the radial aspect of the forearm with the arm held in a neutral position of pronation and supination. A 2.5 cm incision is centered over this point. Directly under the incision is the musculotendinous junction of the brachioradialis, the extensor carpi radialis longus tendon, and between these two tendons, the radial sensory nerve. The nerve is dissected from its soft tissue surroundings, retracted, and the interval between the two tendons is incised to the periosteum. Frequently,

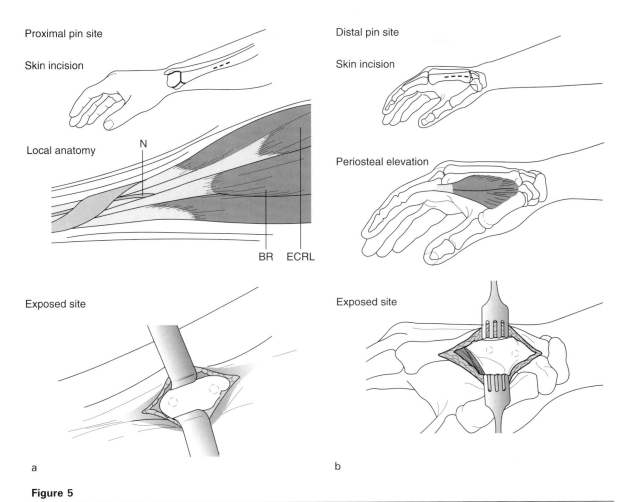

Proximal pin site

Skin incision

Local anatomy

N

BR   ECRL

Exposed site

a

Distal pin site

Skin incision

Periosteal elevation

Exposed site

b

Figure 5

(a) The top drawing depicts the incision over the radial aspect of the forearm centered approximately 10–12 cm proximal to the radial styloid. The middle drawing demonstrates the local anatomy with the radial sensory nerve (N) emerging from under the brachioradialis (BR) at its myotendinous junction and lying between it and the extensor carpi radialis longus (ECRL) tendon. The bottom drawing demonstrates the exposure of the radius for central drilling and in insertion with the soft tissues protected. (b) The top drawing demonstrates the dorsal skin incision over the base of the index metacarpus. In the middle drawing the anatomy can be seen. The first dorsal interosseous muscle must be carefully elevated from its attachment to the shaft of the index metacarpal. The bottom drawing shows the soft tissues protected by retractors with the base of the index metacarpal exposed for central drilling and pin insertion. Note: the most proximal pin should be placed at the tubercular flair of the metacarpal base. This allows insertion across bases of both index and long metacarpals without violation of the interosseous muscle compartment. The more distal pin should be placed only through the shaft of the index metacarpal.

the pronator teres is seen. These should not be detached but can be partially elevated. While the soft tissues are protected with Bennett retractors, a drill guide is used to predrill and two 3.2 mm drill bits are left in place. These are then sequentially replaced with 4 mm self-tapping threaded half pins through both the inner and outer cortices. The soft tissues are closed loosely.

The distal pin placement is prepared by palpation of the dorsoradial aspect of the index metacarpal to locate the tubercle of its most proximal flair. A 2.5 cm incision is centered over this proximal pole along its dorsal radial aspect. Terminal branches of the radial sensory nerve can be identified and protected during dissection. Retraction of the first dorsal interosseous then permits excellent visualization of the entire radial portion of the index metacarpal base. Under direct vision and with appropriate soft tissue protection, two 3.2 mm drill bits are placed into the second and third metacarpals. The first drill bit is placed with the use of image intensification control through the bases of the second and third metacarpals. A second drill bit is then inserted through both the radial and ulnar cortices of the second metacarpal shaft but not into the third metacarpal to avoid violation of the second interosseous compartment. The drill bits are again replaced with 4 mm self-tapping half pins. The soft tissues are loosely closed.

Device application and reduction: the loosened device is then placed on the fixator pins in the hand and forearm. The loosened device is malleable enough to allow free motion in three planes. The fracture fragments are manipulated into their reduced position, and the assembled device is secured in place by tightening of the four appropriate square nuts. A fifth square nut is tightened after final reduction has been achieved. Evaluation of fracture fragment alignment is usually completed with an image intensifier. If additional ligamentotaxis or reduction is necessary, the device is lengthened or loosened as appropriate. The procedure is finished when reduction is satisfactory. However, if articular depression and/or substantial bone loss exists, additional internal fixation and bone grafting may be necessary and should be completed at this time.

Adjuvant techniques

Percutaneous Kirschner wire fixation is a useful adjunct in the treatment of distal radial fractures. Ligamentotaxis alone is often not sufficient to reduce displaced intraarticular fragments or restore volar inclination.[14]

Arthroscopically assisted reduction of impacted, intraarticular fragments greater than 2 mm has been reported by Geissler.[15] The advantages include direct articular visualization, the ability to irrigate away joint debris secondary to the fracture, and access for primary repair of the radiocarpal and triangular fibrocartilage ligament structures.

Bone grafting is another useful adjunct which can be used with external fixation. Although indications for bone grafting may vary, it is often necessary in order to fill the void after reduction of an impacted lunate fossa articular fragment.[16,17]

Lastly, external fixation itself can be used as an adjunctive technique when intraoperative distraction is required to reduce a difficult distal radius fracture. This may be a helpful technique in the application of a plate during open reduction and internal fixation.

Postoperative care

The immediate postoperative care consists of next day referral to the hand therapy department for active and active-assisted range of motion of the fingers, forearm, elbow and shoulder (Figure 6). Postoperative dressings are removed in 5–7 days by the therapist and patient education and pin care are begun. The patient is allowed to shower without dressings at day 10.

Timing of external fixator removal

From the moment an external fixator is placed across the wrist for the treatment of a distal radius fracture the race is on between the ability of the fracture to heal and the onset of deleterious effects of immobilization, but there are few scientific data on which to base recommendations of duration of fixator treatment. Kaempffe et al found increased pain and decreased wrist motion, grip strength, and overall function were associated with an increased amount and duration of distraction.[18] Given these data it follows that one would prefer to leave the joint distracted no longer than necessary, but since collapse has been reported as a complication following early removal of the external fixator, the experience of the surgeon, geometry of the fracture, and patient factors will play a significant role in the decision of when to remove the external fixator.

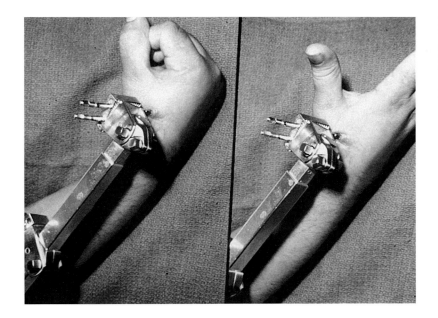

Figure 6

Demonstration of extrinsic extensor glide which should be obtained with the external fixator in place. (Note full motion of metacarpophalangeal joints.)

Complications of external fixation

Complications reported in the literature secondary to external fixation include pin tract infections, pin loosening, pin tract osteomyelitis, loss of reduction, iatrogenic fracture, tendon and nerve injury, arthrofibrosis, carpal tunnel syndrome, and reflex sympathetic dystrophy.[2,8,19–22]

Many of these problems can be addressed with careful surgical technique. The mini open technique previously described for insertion of the proximal threaded half-pins has been utilized in order to avoid soft tissue complications which include nerve and tendon entrapment.[5,23] The mini open technique not only helps to avoid soft tissue damage, but it also increases the surgeon's ability to place the threaded half-pins into the center of the bone. This provides a stronger bond at the all important pin–bone interface and is relevant because eccentric pin placement may lead to pin loosening, infection, loss of fixation, and fracture.

Expected results

Gartland and Werley[24] defined satisfactory results in the treatment of distal radius fractures as follows:

Wrist range of motion:	45° of extension, 30° of flexion, 50° pronation, 50° supination, 15° radial deviation, 15° ulnar deviation
Pain:	occasional discomfort with heavy use
Disability:	none
Cosmetic deformity:	minimal

Table 2 Guidelines for distal radius fracture reduction.

	Acceptable	Normal
Radial inclination	12°	23°
Radial length	5 mm	12 mm
Palmar tilt	−10°	11°
Ulnar variance	2 mm	—
Articular congruity	<2 mm	—

Modern technical advances in surgical technique, external fixation devices, and techniques of augmentation should make it easier for the surgeon to obtain the above criteria. Although differences in opinion still exist as to what acceptable indices of reduction are, general guidelines which may be useful are shown in Table 2.

Conclusion

External fixation has been historically associated with extremely high rates of complications beyond the annoying problem of pin site drainage. Studies have demonstrated that the mini open technique is beneficial in reducing the number of soft tissue and bony complications. With adherence to meticulous surgical technique and the use of the mini open approach, good results can be obtained and complications minimized but not eliminated.

Several methods of enhancing external fixation of distal radius fractures can be used. Internal fixation with Kirschner wires, bone grafting, and arthroscopy are all used with reportedly good results. Although external fixation is an excellent method of fracture management, adjuvant techniques are sometimes required for the most optimal outcome. This is especially true when ligamentotaxis alone is unable to reduce an intraarticular fragment.

References

1   Knirk JL, Jupiter JB, Intra-articular fractures of the distal end of the radius in young adults, *J Bone Joint Surg* (1986) **68A**:647.

2   Weber SC, Szabo RM, Severely comminuted distal radial fractures as an unsolved problem: complications associated with external fixation and pins and plaster techniques, *J Hand Surgery* (1986) **11A**:157.

3   Seitz WH, Fromison Al, Leb R, et al, Augmented external fixation of unstable distal radius fractures, *J Hand Surg* (1991) **16A**:1010–16.

4   Suso S, Combalia A, Segur J, et al, Comminuted intra-articular fractures of the distal end of the radius treated with a Hoffman fixator, *J Trauma* (1993) **35**:61–6.

5   Seitz WH, Putnam MD, Dick HM, Limited open surgical approach for external fixation of distal radius fractures, *J Hand Surg* (1990) **15A**:288–93.

6   Seitz WH, External fixation of distal radius fractures: indications and technical principles, *Orthop Clin N Am* (1993) **24**:255–64.

7   Putnam MD, Walsh TM, External fixation for open fractures of the upper extremity, *Hand Clin* (1993) **9**:613–23.

8   Steffen Th, Eugester Th, Jakob RP, Twelve years follow-up of fractures of the distal radius treated with an external fixator, *Injury* (1994) **25**:S-D44–S-D54.

9   Raskin KB, Melone CP, Unstable articular fractures of the distal radius, *Orthop Clin N Am* (1993) **24**:275–86.

10 Seitz WH, Fromison Al, Brooks DB, et al, External fixator pin insertion techniques: biomechanical analysis and clinical relevance, *J Hand Surg* (1991) **16A**:560–3.

11 Behrens F, A primer of fixator devices and configurations, *Clin Orthop Rel Res* (1989) **241**:5–14.

12 Frykman GK, Peckham RH, Willard K, et al, External fixators for treatment of unstable wrist fractures: a biomechanical, design feature, and cost comparison, *Hand Clin* (1993) **9**:555–65.

13 Behrens F, General theory and principles of external fixation, *Clin Orthop Rel Res* (1989) **241**:15–23.

14 Braun RM, Gellman H, Dorsal pin placement and external fixation for correction of dorsal tilt in fractures of the distal radius, *J Hand Surg* (1994) **19A**:653–5.

15 Geissler WB, Arthroscopically assisted reduction of intra-articular fractures of the distal radius, *Hand Clin* (1995) **11**:19–29.

16 Putnam MD, Seitz WH, Advances in fracture management in the hand and distal radius, *Hand Clin* (1989) **5**:455–69.

17 McBirnie J, Court-Brown CM, McQueen MM, Early open reduction and bone grafting for unstable fractures of the distal radius, *J Bone Joint Surg* (1995) **77B**:571–5.

18 Kaempffe FA, Wheeler DR, Peimer CA, et al, Severe fractures of the distal radius: effect of amount and duration of external fixator distraction on outcome, *J Hand Surg* (1993) **18A**:33–41.

19 McQueen MM, Michie M, Court-Brown CM, Hand and wrist function after external fixation of unstable distal radial fractures, *Clin Orthop Rel Res* (1992) **285**:200–4.

20 Hove LM, Nerve entrapment and reflex sympathetic dystrophy after fractures of the distal radius, *Scand J Plast Reconstr Hand Surg* (1995) **29**:53–8.

21 Kozin SH, Wood MB, Early soft-tissue complications after fractures of the distal part of the radius, *J Bone Joint Surg* (1993) **75A**:144–53.

22 Sanders RA, Keppel FL, Waldrop JI, External fixation of distal radial fractures: results and complications, *J Hand Surg* (1991) **16A**:385–91.

23 Eglseder AW, Open half-pin insertion for distal radial fractures, *Mil Med* (1993) **158**:708–11.

24 Gartland JJ, Werley CW, Evaluation of healed Colles' fracture, *J Bone Joint Surg* (1951) **33A**:895–907.

Limited open reduction of the distal radius

William H Seitz Jr and Rick F Papandrea

Introduction

The treatment of distal radius fractures has evolved significantly since Colles' description of the dorsally displaced, extraarticular metaphyseal fracture. Improvements in treatment technique have parallelled a better understanding of the variety and complexity of fracture patterns. Of paramount importance is the reduction of any intraarticular extension involving both the radiocarpal and the distal radioulnar joints. Articular congruity has a direct impact on the outcome of the treatment of the distal radius fracture.[1] As always, the most anatomic result with the least amount of intervention is desired. Recent advances in the management of distal radius fractures include multiple approaches, with several different types of fixation, for limited open reduction.

Technical aspects

A limited open approach is useful for reduction of articular incongruencies. In a classic study of the effects of intraarticular distal radius fracture, Knirk and Jupiter studied 40 young adults with intraarticular fractures of the distal radius:[1] 91% of the 24 wrists with any degree of articular stepoff, and 100% of the 8 wrists with stepoff of more than 2 mm, developed arthritis; late arthritis was seen in only 11% of the 19 wrists that healed with a congruous joint surface.

Many subsequent studies have supported the surgical treatment of radiocarpal joint incongruity of 2 mm or more. Stepoff greater than 1 mm should be reduced if possible. A limited open approach can be useful to assist in anatomic reduction of intraarticular extension of the distal radius fracture. It is particularly useful for the reduction of a 'die punch' or lunate fossa fragment.[2,3]

Limited open approaches for management of unstable distal radius fractures can be carried out in five principal ways:

(1) Reduction of unstable or irreducible dorsal, volar lunate facet or radial styloid fragments;
(2) Insertion of internal fixation devices;
(3) Insertion of subchondral supportive bone graft;
(4) Application of external fixation; or
(5) Fixation or excision of distal ulnar fracture fragments with ligamentous repair.

The approach depends on the fracture pattern and location of the articular incongruity.

The dorsal approach is made through a 2.5 cm longitudinal skin incision usually centered over Lister's tubercle. Dissection proceeds between either the third and fourth or the fourth and fifth dorsal wrist compartments, opening the septum and mobilizing the extensor pollicis longus (EPL) tendon to avoid later rupture. Soft tissue dissection is minimized to avoid capsular violation and secondary stiffness. Fluoroscopy should be used to guide the dissection, as well as the reduction. The radial styloid is fixed to the shaft with one or two oblique 0.062 Kirschner wires. Using the Kirschner wire as a joystick in the displaced fragments the 'die punch' fragment can then be elevated using a Kirschner wire, awl, or periosteal elevator, manipulating the fragment into anatomic position using fluoroscopy guidance. As the reduction is held, one or two

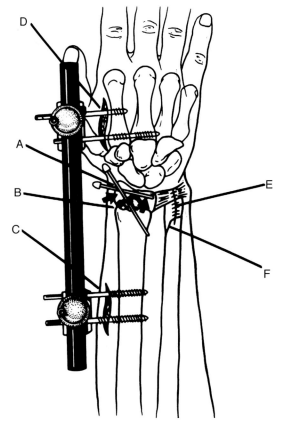

Figure 1

(A) Placement of Kirschner wires for holding a reduced distal radius fracture with 'die punch' fragment. The radial styloid pin is placed first, followed by the second pin from radial to ulnar taking care to stay subchondral and avoid the distal radioulnar joint. (B) Bone graft, either allograft with autogenous marrow or autogenous cancellous bone, should be packed into the void left after reduction. (C) Placement of proximal half-pins for external fixator through a limited open approach. (D) Placement of distal half-pins of external fixator through a limited open approach. Note that the proximal pin obtains purchase in four cortices while the distal pin above obtains purchase in two cortices, for a total of six cortices. (E) A longitudinal incision for subperiosteal resection of distal ulna. (F) Resection of distal ulna at sigmoid notch. This should be beveled to avoid radioulnar impingement. The soft tissue reconstruction described in the text prevents subluxation.

transverse Kirschner wires are placed from the prefixed radial styloid in an ulnarward direction, avoiding violation of the distal radioulnar joint. These Kirschner wires should be placed just

beneath the subchondral bone of the articular surface to maintain reduction and prevent early collapse (A on Figure 1). If a sagittal gap exists between the fracture fragment and the radius itself, a bone reduction forcep can be placed through the skin incision onto the displaced fracture fragment and on the skin overlying the radial styloid. This is then used to close the sagittal displacement while the fracture is pinned with a transverse Kirschner wire.

After reduction of the fragment, any subchondral metaphyseal void left by the impaction of cancellous bone should be grafted. This provides support for the articular fragment, facilitates healing, and helps prevent late collapse (B on Figure 1). While the autogenous bone graft is the 'gold standard', we have had excellent results using irradiated freeze dried cancellous banked allograft and autogenous marrow percutaneously aspirated from the posterior iliac crest. This limits the complications of autogenous cancellous bone harvest while still providing autogenous osteogenic graft material. The preoperative plan for surgical treatment of the distal radius fracture should include an estimation of the amount of initial shortening; more than 5 mm of shortening is an indication for primary bone grafting.[4]

Before a limited dorsal approach is undertaken, an attempt to reduce a die punch-type fragment can be made with a Kirschner wire in a joystick fashion percutaneously. If reduction is obtained, this can be pinned as described above without an open approach, limited or otherwise, and a small 1 cm incision can again be made over Lister's tubercle for purposes of graft insertion, remembering to decompress the EPL tendon.

A limited dorsal approach is also useful in aiding in the reduction of irreducible extraarticular fractures that may have soft tissue interposition.

External fixation should be used in conjunction with a limited open approach for fractures with metaphyseal and/or diaphyseal comminution or bone loss. Placement of an external fixator is performed by pin insertion through a limited open approach at both the proximal index metacarpal and the radius.[5]

Proximal pin insertion is centered at a point approximately one hand's breadth proximal to the radial styloid (10–12 cm) (C on Figure 1). The arm should be held in a neutral position of pronation and supination and a 2.5 cm longitudinal incision is centered over the radius with dissection proceeding down between the brachioradialis and the extensor carpi radialis longus. Initially care is taken to protect any terminal branches of the lateral antebrachial cutaneous nerve in the subcutaneous tissue. Subfascial dissection proceeds between the two tendons. The radial sensory nerve is identified as it emerges from between them at their myotendinous junction. If encountered, the pronator teres should be partially elevated, but not detached. After the periosteum is incised, two Bennett retractors should be placed around the radius for protection, followed by directly visualized predrilling and insertion of self-tapping half-pins in a radioulnar direction through a drill guide.

Distal pin placement is performed through a 2.5 cm incision centered over the proximal dorsoradial aspect of the index metacarpal (D on Figure 1). Superficial dissection is done with care to identify and protect terminal branches of the radial sensory nerve. Sharp elevation and retraction of the first dorsal interosseous allows the radial portion of the index metacarpal to be visualized. The proximal hole is drilled across the base of the index and long finger metacarpals, obtaining purchase through all four cortices. The second drill is placed through both cortices of the index metacarpal only. After pin insertion and closure of the limited incisions, the fixator is applied and used to provide ligamentotaxis and aid in the reduction of the articular fragments.

Four part fractures with displaced volar fragments frequently require open reduction. Formal open reduction and internal fixation can be undertaken with these fractures. Geissler and Fernandez have described a limited open approach to these fractures.[6] The volar surgical approach is more extensive than that on the dorsal surface because of the need to enter and proceed through the carpal canal. An extended incision for carpal tunnel release is used. The wrist is flexed to release tension on the flexor tendons and allow better visualization. A small dorsal arthrotomy can be made or an arthroscope used to identify the volar fragment, but care is taken not to violate soft tissue attachments. Fixation of this volar fragment, if small, can be undertaken with a single Kirschner wire placed from the volar surface through the surgi-

cal exposure, out through the dorsal surface. The dorsal aspect of the pin should penetrate proximal to the fracture, and is then withdrawn so that the distal aspect of the wire no longer protrudes through the volar fragment. Larger fragments can be fixed with screw fixation or an AO small or mini fragment (L or T) plate used as a buttress. Only the proximal holes of the buttress plate are filled, as distal holes obtain poor purchase in the small fragment, and may block reduction of the dorsal fragments. The dorsal fragment can then be reduced via ligamentotaxis or a limited open dorsal approach and stabilized with Kirschner wires.

Radial styloid fractures may be reduced and fixed percutaneously with Kirschner wires. Because of the importance of articular reduction, and the neutralization of forces at the radio-scaphoid articulation, a limited open reduction and internal fixation can be beneficial in the treatment of these fractures. Dissection is through a radial approach over the first dorsal wrist compartment. Care is taken to protect the dorsal radial sensory nerve as the subcutaneous dissection is undertaken. The first dorsal wrist compartment is entered and the abductor pollicis longus and and the extensor pollicis brevis tendons are released and retracted. Subperiosteal dissection is then undertaken over the radial aspect of the radial styloid itself. Stable internal screw fixation can then be obtained. Use of two buried headless fixation screws (Herbert™, Zimmer Inc, Warsaw, Indiana or Acutrak™, Accumed, Beaverton, OR, USA) can avoid the need for subsequent removal of irritating prominent screw heads (Figure 2). The use of two screws prevents rotation and the headless design prevents irritation of the tendons. The tendons are then placed back into the first dorsal wrist compartment and the retinaculum is closed, with care to prevent any overtightening. Usually this is accomplished by a relaxed Z-plasty reconstruction of the retinaculum to prevent an iatrogenic de Quervain's tenosynovitis. This type of stable fixation of a radial styloid fracture can allow early range of motion which may not be afforded with simple Kirschner wire fixation.

Concomitant fractures to the ulnar neck or head, while not common, present a challenging problem in the management of distal radius fractures. While some authors advocate delayed treatment of this type of injury, we have had excellent results with primary management at

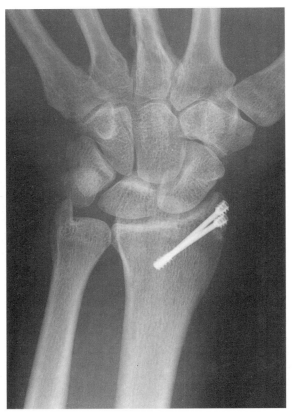

Figure 2

An anteroposterior radiograph demonstrating anatomic reduction of a radial styloid fracture after limited open approach and internal fixation with two Herbert screws.

periosteum of the distal ulna through the distal radioulnar joint capsule (E on Figure 1). Careful subperiosteal dissection is performed to preserve a continuous periosteal-capsular sheath. When comminution precludes fixation, excision of the distal ulna just proximal to the sigmoid notch is performed (F on Figure 1). Avoiding violation of the extensor carpi ulnaris tendon sheath and a tight closure of the periosteal sleeve prevent postoperative subluxation of the distal ulnar stump. Beveling of the distal ulna helps prevent radioulnar impingement, and preservation of the pronator quadratus insertion promotes anatomic positioning of the distal ulna. Through this same incision, access to a defect in the distal radial metaphysis is easily obtained and the excised fragments of bone from the head of the distal ulna can be inserted to provide the necessary subchondral supportive bone graft.

Pros and cons

Fracture care continues to evolve. Current techniques in fracture management emphasize the importance of the preservation of the soft tissues surrounding the fracture itself. Limited open reduction and internal fixation can afford access with minimal violation of soft tissue attachments, allowing accelerated bony healing, while preventing disastrous outcomes from stripping the fracture site of its vascularity. This technique is technically demanding.

The reconstruction of an intraarticular distal radius fracture is as much an art as it is a science. The limited open approach provides access to anatomically reduce these fragments, but careful imaging must be used in conjunction, as the entire joint surface cannot be adequately visualized through the surgical approach. Recent reports have suggested improved visualization by the use of arthroscopy. This however requires skill, experience and has a steep learning curve, and has yet to be proven efficacious and safe in larger series.

An articular stepoff of more than 1 mm has been shown to result in poor outcomes in these fractures.[1] Limited open reduction provides the benefit of decreased dissection and therefore reduced capsular and ligamentous fibrosis, while restoring articular congruity. This minimal soft

the time of distal radius fixation. Occasionally fixation of single large fragments by a lag screw or tension band is possible. More often, excision with repair of the triangular fibrocartilage complex in continuity with the ulnar collateral ligament distally and ulnar periosteal sleeve proximally, decompresses and stabilizes the all important distal radioulnar joint and ulnocarpal relationship.

A 2.5 cm oblique skin incision is made from proximal-ulnar to distal-radial after the radius fracture is fixed. The extensor retinaculum is step cut and a longitudinal incision made in the tissue dissection, combined with optimally placed implants, prevents irritation of the surrounding tendons and soft tissues, allowing earlier return of normal tissue compliance to these structures.

Results

The results of the limited open surgical approach for placement of an external fixator have reduced the associated complications. In a study of 66 patients with unstable distal radius fractures treated by external fixation through a limited open approach, complications were seen in only three (4.5%): this was limited to five loose pins secondary to pin tract infection. There were no eccentric placements of pins, no open section defects from eccentric placement of pins, no tendon damage and no damage to the radial sensory nerve.[5]

Geissler and Fernandez published the results of 40 patients with intraarticular fractures of the distal radius treated with percutaneous limited open reduction of the articular surface.[6] The percutaneous reduction was undertaken in 21 patients through a small limited open approach with minimal soft tissue dissection. The limited open approach was done through a 2 cm long dorsal incision between the fourth and fifth dorsal compartments. All 40 patients' radiographs were reviewed at an average of 4 years postoperatively: 15 patients exhibited articular stepoff of 1–3 mm while 20 patients showed no articular stepoff; 37 patients (92.5%) had an articular depression of less than 1 mm at this long-term follow-up. All 31 patients retrieved for clinical follow-up had good functional results of the hand and wrist.

Indications

Using the Universal Classification of distal radius fractures,[7] the following fractures may benefit from treatment with limited open approach and internal fixation:

Nonarticular displaced fractures that are irreducible may have soft tissue interposition that can be removed through a limited open approach. The nonarticular displaced fracture that is reducible, and the fracture that was initially irreducible and then became reducible once the soft tissue fragments were removed, may be unstable. If the instability from the extra-articular fragment is due to metaphyseal bone loss, the limited open dorsal approach should be undertaken to primarily bone graft the void (with autogenous graft or allograft mixed with autogenous marrow as described above).

The primary indication for limited open approach is the displaced intraarticular fracture. If the fracture is reducible closed, an open approach would not need to be undertaken. If a closed reduction is obtained but is unstable and the articular fragments need support, a limited dorsal approach should be undertaken to provide bone graft and Kirschner wires. An irreducible, articular, displaced fracture is an excellent indication for a limited open approach. This should be done through either the dorsal, or less commonly the volar or combined approach, to reduce the displaced articular fragment as described above. Bone grafting should be used whenever a void is left from the impaction of the cancellous bone. With comminution of the distal metaphysis and/or diaphysis, support of an external fixator is frequently needed to prevent malunion.

The complex articular displaced fracture may possibly benefit from a limited open approach. Extensive comminution and multiple fragments may prevent adequate reduction with this limited type of approach however, and may require a more extensile exposure.

Other indications for limited open reduction of distal radius fractures are for radial styloid fractures and concomitant distal ulna fractures.

Conclusion

The limited open approach for distal radius fractures has evolved to become an integral part of the treatment of displaced distal radius fractures, especially the intraarticular variant. This technique affords anatomic articular reduction while respecting soft tissue around the fracture and ligamentous attachments to the fracture fragments.

References

1   Knirk JL, Jupiter JB, Intra-articular fractures of the distal end of the radius in young adults, *J Bone Joint Surg* (1986) **68A**:647–59.

2   Axelrod T, Paley D, Green J, et al, Limited open reduction of the lunate facet in comminuted intra-articular fractures of the distal radius, *J Hand Surg* (1988) **13A**:372–7.

3   Seitz WH Jr, Froimson AI, Leb R, et al, Augmented external fixation of unstable distal radius fractures, *J Hand Surg* (1991) **16A**:1010–16.

4   Seitz WH Jr, Froimson AI, Leb RB, Autogenous bone marrow and allograft replacement of bone defects in the hand and upper extremities, *J Orthop Trauma* (1992) **6**:36–42.

5   Seitz WH Jr, Putnam MD, Dick HM, Limited open surgical approach for external fixation of distal radius fractures, *J Hand Surg* (1990) **15A**:288–93.

6   Geissler WB, Fernandez DL, Percutaneous and limited open reduction of the articular surface of the distal radius, *J Orthop Trauma* (1991) **5**:255–64.

7   Cooney WP, Agee JM, Hasting H II, et al, Symposium: Management of intra-articular fractures of the distal radius, *Contemp Orthop* (1990) **21**:71.

Dynamic external fixation for unstable distal radius fractures

T Greg Sommerkamp

Introduction

Unstable fractures of the distal part of the radius have repeatedly demonstrated an inherent tendency toward loss of reduction after nonoperative treatment. In 1929, Bohler lamented that

'reduction of this type of fracture—dislocation is obtained relatively easily ... however, in the most severe cases, the fragments cannot usually be maintained in good position by an unpadded plaster cast'.[1]

Since the maintenance of reduction of an unstable distal radius fracture with cast immobilization alone has proved difficult, a number of alternative types of treatment have evolved over the last several decades. These have included percutaneous pinning, pins and plaster, external fixation, ORIF, and external fixation followed by open reduction internal fixation (ORIF) and iliac crest bone grafting.

The duration of immobilization and the distraction across the radiocarpal and midcarpal joints associated with external fixation has been said by some to result in residual loss of mobility of the wrist. This, in part, stimulated the concept of so-called 'flexible' external fixation in 1977, when Jones modified a Roger Anderson fixator with a flexible linkage at the wrist to provide continuous distraction while allowing early motion.[2] In 1987 Clyburn introduced a so-called 'dynamic' external fixator with a hinged (ball-joint) design to allow for early motion of the wrist.[3] Early mobilization of the wrist in such a dynamic external fixation frame was intended not only to allow for an earlier and more complete return of mobility of the wrist, but also to stimulate articular

cartilage repair, to assist the so-called molding of articular fragments, and to diminish the development of periarticular osteopenia. In order to investigate these potential benefits, we designed a prospective, randomized study comparing dynamic external fixation with static external fixation in the treatment of unstable fractures of the distal radius.

Technical aspects

From 1986 to 1990 we conducted a prospective randomized comparison of a dynamic external fixator (Clyburn/Zimmer) and a static external fixator (AO/Synthes) in the treatment of 75 high energy comminuted unstable distal radius fractures (Figure 1). A distal radius fracture was considered to be unstable if it met one or more clinical or prereduction radiographic criteria: dorsal angulation of more than 20°, loss of radial length of more than 10 mm, intraarticular extension, severe dorsal metaphyseal comminution, open fracture, bilateral fractures, or polytrauma.

The dynamic fixator group consisted of thirteen Frykman type VIII, five type VII, three type VI, one type III, two type II, and one type I injury. Prereduction radiographs revealed an average dorsal angulation of 28°, radial length 4 mm, and radial deviation 7°. The static fixator group consisted of ten type VIII, five type VII, one type VI, one type V, six type IV, one type III, and one type II injury. Prereduction radiographs revealed an average dorsal angulation of 21°, radial length 4 mm, and radial deviation 13°. The technique for application of the Clyburn fixator followed that described in Clyburn's monograph,[3] and that for application of the AO/ Synthes

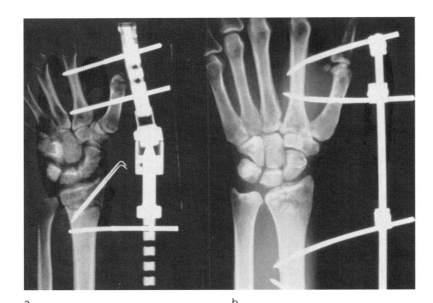

a   b

Figure 1

Radiographs showing (a) the Clyburn dynamic fixator and (b) the AO/ASIF static fixator.

external fixator followed the original description by Jakob and Fernandez.[4] When a reduction had not been successfully obtained by closed means, adjunctive percutaneous pinning or ORIF with Kirschner wires and iliac crest bone graft through a limited dorsal approach was performed.

The postoperative protocol for the static fixator group naturally consisted of no wrist motion for an average of 9–10 weeks. The dynamic fixator group was allowed flexion from 0 to 30° at 2 weeks, and 30° extension at approximately 4 weeks. This continued until the time of fixator removal at an average of 10 weeks. For patients with severe metaphyseal comminution or die punch lesions, mobilization was delayed until 4 weeks or longer as dictated by the individual fracture anatomy.

Pros and cons compared to classical techniques

The advantages of dynamic external fixation include the aforementioned theoretical benefits:

earlier and more complete return of range of motion of the wrist, stimulation of articular cartilage repair, and a decrease in periarticular osteopenia. The disadvantages would naturally include any potential complication associated with early motion: loss of reduction, fixator instability, hardware fatigue failure, and increased pin drainage/infection rates.

Results

In the dynamic group, radiographic assessment revealed an average radial length of 5 mm pre-reduction, 15 mm postapplication of external fixator, and 11 mm at the time of fixator removal.[5] In the static fixator group, the corresponding values were 4, 13 and 12 mm. The loss of 4 mm of radial length in the dynamic fixator group over the 10-week course of treatment was significantly greater than the 1 mm loss in the static fixator group (two-way repeated measures analysis of variance with interaction, $P < 0.001$).[5] Assessment of the restoration/maintenance of volar tilt and radial deviation revealed no significant difference between the two treatment groups.

Lidstrom radiographic grades were determined on radiographs made after application of the fixator and at the time of fixator removal. The dynamic group, on average, lost one Lidstrom grade or more over the 10-week course of treatment. This was significantly different from the static fixator group (McNemar test for effect of time on paired readings, $P < 0.05$).[5]

The range of motion of the wrist was measured at the time of removal of the fixator and at 1, 6, and 12 months afterward. Early mobilization of the wrist in the dynamic fixator group provided little gain in the mean motion of the wrist at the time of fixator removal or at the 1, 6, or 12 month evaluation. The static fixator group had greater flexion at 6 months (static 60°, dynamic 50°) and at 12 months (static 59°, dynamic 52°) which were statistically significant (two-sample t test, $P < 0.05$). The static fixator group had greater radial deviation at 1 month (static 9°, dynamic 3°) which was also statistically significant (two-sample t test, $P < 0.05$). The dynamic fixator group fared better only in ulnar deviation at 1 month (static 21°, dynamic 28°) which was statistically significant (two-sample t test, $P < 0.05$).

Grip and pinch strengths were measured at all intervals and although the mean values were consistently greater for the static fixator group, only the difference in the 6 month grip strength (static 70%, dynamic 50%) approached statistical significance ($P < 0.08$). Gartland and Werley[6] demerit point scores were assessed at the 6 and 12 month evaluations, and at 1 year the static group had 92% excellent/good results versus 76% in the dynamic group. Articular incongruity and subsequent posttraumatic osteoarthrosis was evaluated by the method of Knirk and Jupiter.[7] There was no association between early motion of the wrist and an increased rate of articular incongruity at the time of fixator removal. In addition, there was no difference in the prevalence of posttraumatic osteoarthritis or osteopenia between the two groups at the 1 year evaluation.

Complications, overall, were more frequent in the dynamic fixator group. Notably, pin drainage rates were slightly higher in the dynamic group (52% versus static group 40%). Transient neuritis of the superficial radial nerve was somewhat higher in the dynamic group. Two dynamic fixators experienced fatigue failure at the ball-joint, and three became unstable after spontaneous hex nut loosening. In one patient, the fixator instability resulted in a loss of reduction that required a repeat reduction under anesthesia. No static fixators broke or became unstable, however two Schanz pins broke at the time of fixator removal.

Indications

Dynamic external fixation, as introduced by Clyburn in 1987,[3] was proposed to reduce the disability associated with an unstable fracture of the distal part of the radius by facilitating the return of motion of the wrist. The results of our research fail to support the contention that mobilization with a dynamic fixator decreases the morbidity associated with this injury. Moreover, the dynamic group experienced a significant loss of reduction over the 10-week course of treatment; the difference with regard to the loss of radial length (4 mm dynamic group versus 1 mm static group) was the most striking and significant ($P < 0.001$). Clyburn himself noted the loss of reduction in both radial length and volar tilt until he delayed wrist extension to week 4.[3] Even after wrist extension was delayed, loss of radial length was still a significant problem. Lennox et al reported a prospective study of 20 patients treated with a Clyburn fixator with excellent to good results in 18.[8] However, only 4 of 20 wrists were mobilized, and the earliest was at week 4, with few details given regarding the maintenance of reduction in these four patients.

In our own cadaveric studies,[9] as well as those of Cooney,[10] Frykman,[11] and others, visible motion was evident at the fracture site, both grossly and fluoroscopically, as the dynamic fixator was mobilized. The motion was more evident in the extension arc than in the flexion arc. It also appeared that decreased tension or ligamentotaxis was generated by the fixator in the terminal arc of extension, with resultant motion of the dorsal comminuted fragments. Although the motion was slight, cyclical repetitive loading could have resulted in a gradual loss of reduction. Clinically, in our study, a marked loss of reduction was clearly related to early radiocarpal motion adjacent to these comminuted fracture fragments.

An additional argument for dynamic external fixation might be that a so-called 'slight' loss of reduction,[3] and hence a 'slight deformity', is a small price to pay for a shortened course of disability and increased final range of motion. However, in nearly all of the parameters studied, including range of motion, grip and pinch strengths, Gartland and Werley scores, etc, the static group consistently fared better than the dynamic group.

The rate of complications was slightly higher in the dynamic fixator group, especially with regard to pin erythema/drainage and hardware failure. Early mobilization in a dynamic fixator may cause increased shear stresses at the pin–bone interface and could plausibly increase pin related problems, according to Perren.[12] The high prevalence of material failure of the dynamic fixators raises the question of whether or not the ball-joint design and metallurgy can withstand the repetitive cyclical loading in the flexion–extension arc. Lennox et al also reported breakage of the fixator at the ball-joint, in one patient (of 20), after a fall;[8] however, neither of the two fixators that broke in our study did so after a fall or accident. In clear contrast, none of the AO/ASIF fixator bars broke and none of the 4.0/2.5 mm clamps loosened.

Since the late 1980s, more and more dynamic hinged external fixators have been introduced to the orthopaedic marketplace: Clyburn–Zimmer (1986), Colles' Fracture Frame—Richard's (1987), Mini-Hammer—Biomet (1987), Orthofix-Pennig (1990), Cheveigne–Judet (1991), Colles' Gold Wrist Fixator—Smith and Nephew (1995), and Dynafix–EBI (1995). Not only has biomechanical stability been a matter of concern,[11,13,14] but it has also been worrisome that no statistical evidence of the safety and efficacy of these new devices has been presented.

Hollister[14] and others have raised significant questions about the biomechanical rationale of the various dynamic external fixators. Many of these fixators attempt to 'center' their hinge or ball-joint apparatus over the instant center of rotation of the carpus—the head of the capitate.[15] It is extremely difficult, if not impossible, to replicate the true axis of rotation of the carpus with an external fixator whose articulating segment is offset some 5–6 cm from the head of the capitate. To compound the problem, even if the carpal instant center of rotation could be repli-

cated, one must realize that the normal kinematics of the carpus with respect to combined flexion/extension, radial/ulnar deviation, and circumduction will be significantly altered by longitudinal distraction and ligamentotaxis.

The AO group is currently attempting to address some of these deficiencies with a modification of the small AO external fixator, incorporating a kinematic pair consisting of a spherical shell and two discs linked together in a sliding mechanism.[16] Theoretically, with a spherical radius of 50 mm, the center of rotation is not in the device itself but rather in the wrist itself—the head of the capitate. Limited multicenter clinical trials are currently underway in Europe.

Conclusion

One must be concerned about such a wave of enthusiasm for devices that have yet to be scientifically proven superior to the traditional static external fixator. Further detailed biomechanical bench studies must be performed on experimentally reproduced distal radius fractures in cadaver prosections to demonstrate (1) replication of the carpal instant center of rotation in a kinematic model altered by ligamentotaxis, and (2) maintenance of reduction after 'dynamization'. Until this is proven scientifically, then dynamic fixators should not be mobilized until week 6 or beyond, if at all. It was interesting to note in our series a small group of patients in the dynamic group, lost to follow-up until week 6 or so and thus excluded from the study, who when mobilized experienced no loss of reduction whatsoever. At least for the final 4 weeks, these patients were allowed to experience some of the theoretical benefits of early motion.

The main goal of treatment of any severe intraarticular or juxtaarticular fracture is the restoration of anatomic alignment and position of the fragments with stable fixation so as to allow early motion of the adjacent joints. This concept should be no different for the unstable distal radius fracture. However, the whole concept of early motion is based on the premise that one truly has stable fixation to guard against a loss of reduction. To advocate early motion without such stability is to risk a loss of reduction.

References

1   Bohler L, *The Treatment of Fractures*, 5th edn, vol 1 (Grune and Stratton: New York, 1956), 796–811.

2   Jones KG, A modification of the use of extraskeletal immobilization for comminuted fractures of the distal radius, *Clin Orthop* (1977) **123**:83–6.

3   Clyburn TA, Dynamic external fixation for comminuted intra-articular fractures of the distal end of the radius, *J Bone Joint Surg* (1987) **69**:248–54.

4   Jakob RP, Fernandez D, The treatment of wrist fractures with the small AO fixation device. In: *Current Concepts of External Fixation of Fractures* (Springer-Verlag: Berlin–Heidelberg, 1982).

5   Sommerkamp TG, Seeman M, Silliman J, et al, Dynamic external fixation of unstable fractures of the distal part of the radius, *J Bone Joint Surg* (1994) **76A**:1149–61.

6   Gartland JJ Jnr, Werley CW, Evaluation of heated Colles' fracture, *J Bone Joint Surg* (1951) **33A**:895–907.

7   Knirk JL, Jupiter JB, Intraarticular fractures of the distal end of the radius in young adults, *J Bone Joint Surg* (1986) **68A**:647–59.

8   Lennox JD, Page BJ, Mandell RM, Use of the Clyburn external fixator in fractures of the distal radius, *J Trauma* (1989) **29**:326–31.

9   Sommerkamp TG, Dynamic external fixation of unstable distal radius fractures, presented at Distal Radius Trauma Symposium, American Society for Surgery of the Hand Specialty Day, American Academy of Orthopedic Surgeons 57th Annual Meeting, Orlando, Florida, 19 February 1995.

10   Cooney WP III, Distal radius fractures. Instructional course at the Annual Meeting of the American Society for Surgery of the Hand, San Antonio, Texas, 12 September 1987.

11   Frykman GK, Biomechanical comparison of external fixators, presented at Distal Radius Trauma Symposium, American Society for Surgery of the Hand Specialty Day, American Academy of Orthopedic Surgeons 57th Annual Meeting, Orlando, Florida, 19 February 1995.

12   Perren SM, Biomechanical aspects of the prevention of pin loosening in the fixateur externe, *AO/ASIF Dialogue* (1988) **1**:11–13.

13   Frykman GK, Tooma GS, Boyko K, et al, Comparison of eleven external fixators for treatment of unstable wrist fractures, *J Hand Surg* (1989) **14A**:247.

14   Hollister AM, Biomechanics of the wrist—is there a rationale for dynamic external fixators? Presented at Distal Radius Trauma Symposium, American Society for Surgery of the Hand Specialty Day, American Academy of Orthopedic Surgeons 57th Annual Meeting, Orlando, Florida, 19 February 1995.

15   Youm Y, McMurtry RY, Flatt AE, et al, Kinematics of the wrist I. An experimental study of radial–ulnar deviation and flexion–extension, *J Bone Joint Surg* (1978) **60A**:423–31.

16   Goslings JC, Tepic S, Brockhuizen AH, et al, Three dimensional dynamic AO external fixation of distal radial fractures—a preliminary report, *Injury* (1994) **25**:85–9.

Arthroscopic reduction of intraarticular fractures

Terry L Whipple

Introduction

Proper management of intraarticular fractures about the wrist poses many challenges not necessarily associated with extraarticular fractures. To function through a stable, pain free range of movement the carpus requires smooth, perfectly matched articular surfaces. There are 27 articular surfaces in the normal wrist. In addition to the distal end of the radius, many of the carpal bones are almost completely covered with articular hyaline cartilage. Any fracture of a carpal bone, therefore, will most likely involve at least one articular surface.

Intraarticular fractures of the distal radius

Fractures of the distal radius are commonly sustained by violent, axial loading forces. Impact of the proximal carpal row on to the articular facets of the radius frequently explodes or depresses segments of the joint surface. Additionally, angular forces that would typically disrupt ligaments about the wrist may also cause avulsion fractures from the ligament attachments on the radius, carpals or metacarpals. Avulsion fractures may extend onto the joint surface.

One of the primary tenets for the management of any articular fracture is accurate restoration of the articular surface. The movement of one bone on another under compression should occur across well lubricated, friction free surfaces. Fracture gaps or step-offs in the articular surface increase abrasive wear on the opposing surface. Without the capacity to regenerate, hyaline cartilage wear spells ultimate doom for a joint surface.

Traditional efforts to manipulate fracture fragments about the wrist by nonoperative means have involved gross and crude attempts by the treating physician to push bone fragments together accurately either blindly or under fluoroscopic control, or to pull them into position by traction applied through ligaments attached to the margins of the fragments. So-called 'ligamentotaxis' depends on periosteal attachments to the fragment to limit distraction of the fracture and to hinge the fragments together. Control or correction of the angulation of fragments using these techniques is limited. Moreover, it is not likely that impacted, depressed or displaced articular fragments which have little or no capsule attachment can be reduced by ligamentotaxis or external pressure manipulation.

Traditional operative reduction of articular fractures typically requires detachment or incision of critical ligaments about the wrist to visualize the articular surface, and monitor the reduction of fragments. Extrinsic wrist ligaments are vitally important to the normal mechanical function of the joint, and maintenance of the integrity of carpal alignment after healing. Scarred ligaments restrict motion. It is therefore desirable to minimize ligament disruption in the treatment of articular fractures. Moreover, the wrist is highly visible in typical wearing apparel, and extensive surgical scars pose a cosmetic concern, especially for younger, female patients.

Many attempts have been made to reduce articular fractures of the wrist under fluoroscopic control with percutaneous manipulation of the fragments using sterile pins. Fluoroscopy provides a limited, two-dimensional image of bony structures, and poor representation of most articular surfaces which lie in a parallel plane to the roentgen beam.

With these many limitations of traditional means of fracture reduction, inaccurate articular restoration has been rationalized as 'adequate' or 'satisfactory' in spite of certain consequence of accelerated articular wear following the malunion. For the best possible functional results in terms of durability, comfort, range of motion, stability and mechanical advantage, the treating physician must make every reasonable attempt to restore smooth articular surfaces to the wrist, even though it is, by comparison, less critical than in articular fractures of weight-bearing joints in the lower extremity.

Arthroscopically assisted reduction of intraarticular fractures in the wrist has evolved with the development of predictable, minimally invasive techniques for intraarticular visualization,[1] and the development of small, sturdy instruments to facilitate fracture reduction. The treatment of articular fractures of the distal radius under arthroscopic control followed favorable experience with arthroscopic management of tibial plateau fractures.[2] Arthroscopy provides a three-dimensional view of articular surfaces with adequate illumination and magnification to facilitate accurate fracture reduction. By arthroscopy, visual access is obtained with far less surgical trauma to ligaments and capsule tissues, nerves, vessels and tendons compared with traditional open approaches.

There is always more fracture debris in a joint than is evident by radiography or CT scan. Small fragments or slivers of bone, chips of articular cartilage, synovial fragments and fibrin precipitated from the associated hemarthrosis are abundant in comminuted fracture patterns, and are not uncommon even in simple articular fractures (Figure 1). Most of this debris can be cleansed from the joint by athroscopic lavage or with the assistance of small motorized shavers or grasping forceps. If the joint is purged of such fractured debris this further reduces the abrasive grit between articulating surfaces and secondarily reduces the inflammatory reaction this debris might evoke.

With adequate stabilization of accurately reduced fracture fragments, earlier mobilization of the wrist becomes plausible. Closed reduction without stabilization, or open reduction with incised or released ligaments require longer initial periods of immobilization. Early movement of a traumatized joint improves lubrication and nutrition of the articular hyaline cartilage, im-

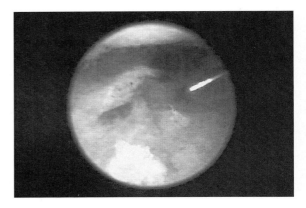

Figure 1

Arthroscopic view of the radiocarpal space of an intraarticular distal radius fracture. Notice the fibrin clot and small chips of articular cartilage and cancellous bone. The field of view in acute fractures is typically hazy as bleeding continues from the fracture line even under tourniquet control.

proves the flexibility of ligaments and capsule, permits earlier gliding of tendons crossing the joint,[3,4] and increases the sense of progress toward recuperation for patients psychologically. These advantages together are compelling justification for using minimally invasive arthroscopic techniques to facilitate reduction and stabilization of fracture fragments.

If that were not enough, considerations for the timely treatment of associated intraarticular soft tissue injuries are worthy of comment. A recent multicenter study of intraarticular fractures of the distal radius treated arthroscopically revealed a 72% incidence of associated significant soft tissue injuries.[5] The structure most commonly involved was the triangular fibrocartilage complex, followed by injuries to the scapholunate ligament, the lunotriquetral ligament, articular cartilage surfaces of the proximal carpal row and volar extrinsic ligaments in successive order. The advantage of recognizing these injuries and treating them acutely, or immobilizing the wrist in positions most advantageous for concurrent ligament healing, can abbreviate the total time under treatment. It also potentially improves the ultimate functional outcome by addressing occult lesions associated with the obvious fracture that might otherwise go unnoticed.

Technique

Reduction of fractures about the wrist under arthroscopic control is tedious but straightforward in most cases. Timing is important. The optimum opportunity for fractures of the distal radius is 2–4 days postinjury. Attempts earlier than 2 days may encounter persistent bleeding from fracture planes which obscures visualization; after 4 days fibrin clot from the hemarthrosis may become so dense and tenacious that excessive time must be spent with the shaver cleansing the joint of fracture debris and blood products.

Good quality radiographs are essential. Efforts should be made to fully understand the number, size and orientation of all fracture planes. This also defines the number and orientation of fracture fragments. The size of articular fragments, the degree of separation and whether or not they may be impacted should be anticipated preoperatively.

Initially, the best possible closed reduction should be obtained by the use of appropriate anesthesia with conventional manipulation techniques and ligamentotaxis.[6] If the reduction is imperfect, a CT scan is indicated. Particular attention should be paid to the anterior, posterior and radioulnar dimensions of the distal radius compared, if necessary, with the opposite side. Look closely for evidence of depressed fragments by obtaining radiographic views parallel with the articular surface.

When computerized tomography is performed, the extremity should be placed in the gantry so as to obtain cuts perfectly parallel with the articular surface of the radius. The plane of these cuts may be slightly different than the usual palmar tilt because of fragment displacement. Routine cuts made perpendicular to the long axis of the radius, however, will not show realistic orientation of articular fragments, nor their depression.

CT cuts should also be made in coronal and sagittal planes to confirm the degree of fragment separation and depression.

Surgical technique

Arthroscopic reduction and internal fixation should be considered if fracture lines are non-uniform, if the fragments are angulated or remain depressed, or if the AP or lateral dimen-sions are increased more than 1 or 2 mm[7,8] (Figure 2). In the surgical setting, the extremity is placed in a traction tower (Linvatec Inc, Largo, FL) that permits simultaneous traction and angular positions of the wrist. Finger trap traction should be applied to the index and long fingers (Figure 3). In elderly or rheumatoid patients, or others with fragile skin, ring finger traction is added to distribute skin pressure over a larger surface area. Fifteen to twenty pounds of traction are applied. The wrist is placed in flexion, extension, radial or ulnar deviation depending on the direction of angular displacement.

Typically, an inflow line is established in the 6-U portal. A 2.7 mm arthroscope can then be inserted in the 3-4 or the 1-2 portal. The 1-2 portal allows visualization of dorsal rim fractures of the distal radius which cannot be seen easily from the 3-4 portal.[1]

Hemarthrosis is washed from the joint. A small shaver inserted in the 4-5 or 6-R portal can be used to remove clots, small bone crumbs and cartilage debris. Fracture lines on the articular surface are surveyed, and their displacement and depression are noted. If necessary, impacted fragments can be pried loose by the insertion of a small arthroscopic dissector through an accessory portal, into the fracture plane, and the impacted fragment is gently lifted under the subchondral plate. Alternatively, a 3 mm Steinmann pin can be drilled percutaneously through the dorsal cortex 5 mm or so proximal to the depressed fragment, and the fragment levered upwards.

Once all displaced fragments have been disimpacted and mobilized with a dissector or Steinmann pin, individual 0.045 inch (1.2 mm) Kirschner wires are drilled into the largest fragments, aimed toward an adjacent fragment to cross the fracture plane at an angle that would minimize the risk of redisplacement. It is helpful to insert a hypodermic needle across the joint in the anticipated direction of the Kirschner wire. If the needle is positioned across the fracture plane obliquely, the Kirschner wire can be drilled parallel with the needle.

Fracture fragments are reduced by manipulation of the Kirschner wires in each fragment, and by external pressure applied by the surgeon. When the fracture lines are observed to close arthroscopically, the Kirschner wires are

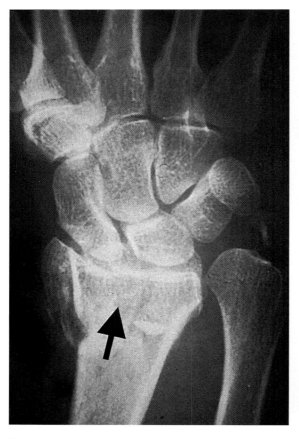

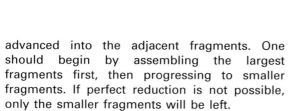

Figure 2

Radiograph of right wrist with comminuted intraarticular fracture of the distal radius and avulsion of the ulnar styloid. Notice the coronal dimension of the radius is increased. There is a depressed articular fragment below the proximal pole of the scaphoid adjacent to the sagittal ridge of the radius. Depressed fragments in this location should raise suspicion of an associated occult fracture of the proximal pole of the scaphoid. This fracture requires CT scan of the distal radius before arthroscopic reduction of the depressed fragment.

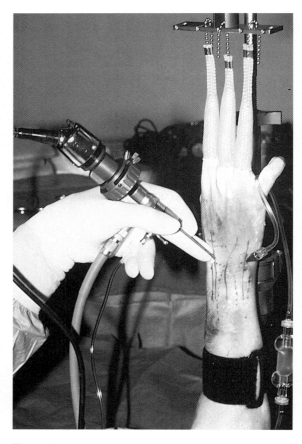

Figure 3

Right wrist suspended in traction tower (Linvatec Inc, Largo, Florida). Soft nylon finger traps are applied to the index, long and ring fingers in elderly and rheumatoid patients with fragile skin. The arthroscope is inserted in the 3-4 portal for fracture reduction.

advanced into the adjacent fragments. One should begin by assembling the largest fragments first, then progressing to smaller fragments. If perfect reduction is not possible, only the smaller fragments will be left.

A 0.045 inch (1.2 mm) Kirschner wire will fit through the bore of a 14 gauge hypodermic needle. Use of such a needle as a cannula for the Kirschner

wire helps prevent injury to subcutaneous sensory nerve branches and allows the surgeon to direct the orientation of the wire while applying additional pressure to the cortex of the fracture fragment.

Attempts should be made to place the Kirschner wire immediately beneath the subchondral bone plate. The wires will then

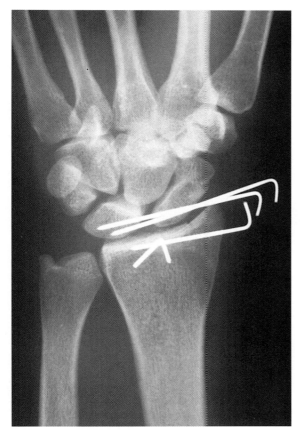

Figure 4

Postreduction radiograph of intraarticular fracture of right distal radius with an associated tear of the scapholunate ligament. Notice the articular surface of the radius has been restored to normal contour with no depression. The coronal dimension of the radius is normal and the epiphyseal cortices have been aligned normally. The three Kirschner wires stabilizing the radius fracture are placed immediately beneath the subchondral bone which provides support as well as fixation. Bone grafting defects beneath elevated fragments is rarely necessary if the Kirschner wires support the subchondral bone plate.

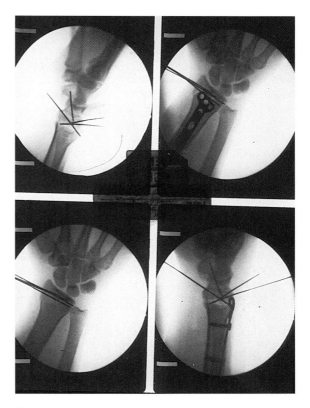

Figure 5

Interoperative radiographs of an unstable intraarticular right distal radius fracture. Top and bottom left: views of arthroscopically reduced articular surface with Kirschner wire fixation. Top and bottom right: stabilization of epiphysis to diaphysis with a supplementary dorsal buttress plate.

provide a subflooring for the articular surface which will help maintain reduction during early mobilization of the wrist.

One need pay little attention to the reduction of nonarticular cortical contours during the arthroscopic portion of the procedure. The first priority is re-establishment of normal contours to the articular surface. If the articular fragments are normally aligned, the nonarticular cortices will be as well (Figure 4). Fluoroscopy is unnecessary during pin placement. However, efforts should be made to avoid injury to extensor tendons as well as major nerves and arteries.

After radiographic confirmation of satisfactory articular surface reduction, the second consideration is to reduce and stabilize the epiphysis to the diaphysis. In many cases no additional fixation is necessary. In others, oblique Kirschner wires from the radial styloid to the opposite diaphyseal cortex will be sufficient once appropriate length and palmar tilt of the radius is restored.

Many intraarticular fractures of the radius will have extensive comminution of the metaphyseal cortex. These fractures are inherently unstable. In these cases a volar or dorsal plate may be necessary to reduce and secure the epiphysis to the diaphysis (Figure 5). The plate can be applied with the extremity suspended in the traction tower without concern for the position of the epiphyseal pins. If bone grafting is deemed necessary, it can be performed at this stage.

Occasionally, loss of metaphyseal bone may be so extensive that an external fixator is the only feasible means of maintaining appropriate length of the radius. Left in place more than 3 or 4 weeks, external fixators risk chronic stretch injuries to the joint capsule with subsequent stiffness that may be very difficult to overcome.[9] The author prefers plates with bone grafting to external fixators, as early motion can still be permitted and wrist stiffness is minimized.

Postoperative management of arthroscopically reduced fractures involves a relatively aggressive program of hand therapy. The Kirschner wires are bent and cut short. They may be wrapped with an antibiotic impregnated gauze and buried beneath a cast or splint initially. The splint should be removed as early as possible for supervised daily, gentle, passive range of motion by a hand therapist. This may be as early as the second or third week postoperatively, depending on the bone density, and the security of pin fixation in the bone cortices. Gentle traction should be applied to the index and long fingers during passive motion exercises. Generally, patients are not able to supervise their own initial mobilization exercise routines.

The Kirschner wires can be removed without anesthesia 3–5 weeks postoperatively. Again, the degree of bone density, fracture, comminution and metaphyseal support should govern this judgement. After 2 or 3 weeks, a functional range splint can be applied if the fracture fragments are stable, but beware of the potential for early fracture settlement if there is any comminution of the metaphyseal cortex.

Carpal bone fractures

Articular fractures of carpal bones other than the scaphoid usually involve avulsion of bone margins or tubercles where dense ligaments attach. Occasionally, articular compression fractures occur, usually on the proximal pole of the lunate associated with die punch fractures of the radius. Compression fractures are almost impossible to reduce, and may be evident only by the unusually soft texture of articular cartilage overlying the fracture. One should be particularly suspicious is the cartilage appears cracked as well as soft.

Avulsion fractures can usually be reduced anatomically and cross-pinned using the same principles as described for the radius. The fracture is observed arthroscopically and a 0.045 or 0.035 inch (1.2 or 0.9 mm) Kirschner wire is drilled into the fracture fragment with a hypodermic needle used for a cannula. The fracture is manipulated into a reduced position, and cross-pinned to the fracture bed.

Postoperatively, a brief period of immobilization is followed by gentle range of motion exercises. The pins typically can be removed 4 weeks postoperatively.

Scaphoid fractures

Fractures of the scaphoid present a unique challenge. Early anatomic reduction and internal stabilization of scaphoid fractures offers the distinct advantage of early mobilization of the carpus before fracture healing. Tenuous blood supply to the proximal pole of the scaphoid risks a 10% incidence of scaphoid fracture nonunion. Prolonged periods of immobilization, sometimes up to 6 months' duration, lead to poor nutrition of articular cartilage throughout the carpus, stiff ligaments and osteopenia.[10]

Intramedullary fixation of waist fractures of the scaphoid achieves greater fracture stability than can be accomplished with cast immobilization alone, and may reduce the incidence of nonunion. Once the fracture fragments are secure, many patients can resume productive use of the extremity even before fracture healing occurs. This earlier return to function may ultimately reduce the overall cost of these unfortunate injuries.

The arthroscopic portion of the procedure for minimally invasive internal fixation of acute scaphoid fractures involves only the assurance of fracture reduction and the accurate placement of the target hook of the guide barrel through which the intramedullary screw is introduced.[11] In a sense, this procedure is not strictly an arthroscopic one; it is an arthroscopically assisted procedure. The principle advantage is that the proximal pole of the scaphoid need not be exposed surgically, as is typically for open reduction and internal fixation of the scaphoid. A volar approach to the scaphoid as described by Russe[12] or Herbert[13] requires transection of the important volar radioscaphocapitate ligament. This ligament provides the primary volar support for the scaphoid, maintains its normal flexion mechanics and contributes to the proper orientation of the scaphoid to the lunate in the proximal carpal row. Arthroscopic placement of the target hook of the fixation jig obviates exposure of the proximal scaphoid pole and allows one to preserve the integrity of this important ligament.

There are many devices available for stabilization of scaphoid fractures including Kirschner wires as the simplest, several screw designs, hook plates and cortical struts of bone graft. I have tried all of these over a 21-year period, and ultimately designed a modification of the Herbert™ screw (Zimmer Inc, Warsaw, Indiana) that is stronger and cannulated for easier, more accurate insertion over a preliminary guidewire. The Herbert–Whipple screw is made of titanium and has self-tapping, variably pitched threads of the same diameter as the noncannulated stainless steel Herbert screw. Titanium provokes less bone reabsorption than stainless steel, and the larger diameter of the central, nonthreaded shaft of the screw provides over three times the bending strength (Newport ML, unpublished work).

A compression jig facilitates accurate placement of the preliminary guidewire, measurement of screw length and fracture stabilization whether the procedure is performed with arthroscopic assistance or by conventional open surgical approach.

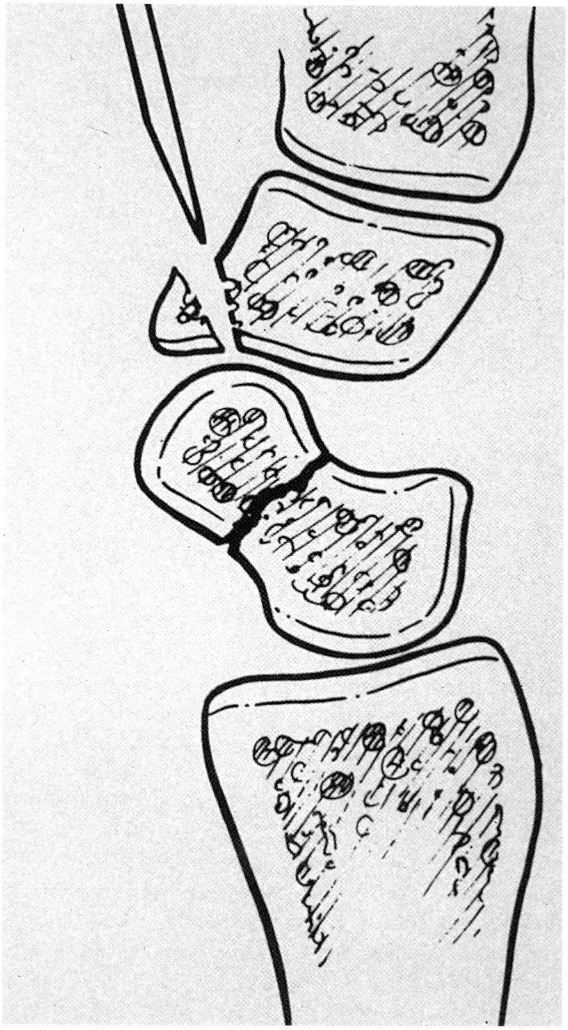

Figure 6

Illustration of excision of the volar tubercle of the trapezium, lateral view. One must see the margin of articular cartilage on the distal pole of the scaphoid to obtain axial placement of the guidewires and Herbert–Whipple Screw.

Technique

Scaphoid fractures appropriate for early arthroscopically assisted internal fixation include those waist fractures that are nondisplaced, minimally displaced or displaced and reducible. Major humpback deformities, comminuted fractures and fractures of the proximal pole represent contraindications. Proximal pole fractures can sometimes be successfully reduced and stabilized by techniques described for fractures of carpal bones other than the scaphoid.

Scaphoid waist fractures are best operated on within 2–3 weeks of injury. A radially curved incision about 15 mm long is centered over the scaphotrapeziotrapezoid joint just radial to the

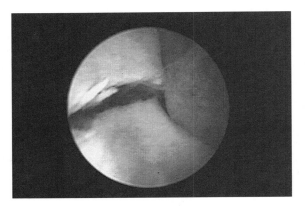

Figure 7

Arthroscopic view of a scaphoid waist fracture, right wrist, seen in the midcarpal space. Simple smooth fractures are easiest to reduce but are most unstable as they lack interdigitating contours on the fracture surface.

flexor carpi radialis tendon.[14] The scaphotrapezial joint is opened by subperiosteal dissection over the trapezium. A generous portion of the tubercle of the trapezium is excised sufficient to expose the articular margin of the distal pole of the scaphoid (Figure 6). One should then identify and mark the midportion of the distal pole in its radial to ulnar dimension. It is vitally important to avoid insertion of the fixation device through the volar radial scaphoid prominence. Such placement will risk cutting through the volar cortex with the device. The best axial placement of an intramedullary screw is gained by entering the bone just radial to the midpoint of the radioulnar dimension.

After exposure of the distal pole of the scaphoid, confirm that the fracture can be anatomically reduced and apply the fixation jig. Place the wrist in the traction tower with 5–10 lb (2.5–4.5 kg) axial traction applied through fingertraps on the index and long fingers. Insert a 2.7 mm or 1.9 mm arthroscope in the radial midcarpal portal. This portal lies midway between the base of the second metacarpal and the dorsal, distal edge of the radius on the line extended proximally from the radial border of the third metacarpal.[1] The radial midcarpal portal enters the midcarpal space between the proximal pole of the scaphoid and the head of the capitate.

Irrigation inflow is supplied through the arthroscope sheath.

Follow the concave contour of the scaphoid distally until the fracture is encountered (Figure 7). Lavage the joint to provide a clear field of view. Usually an acute fracture of the wrist can be reduced by decreasing traction, by pressing the dorsal aspect of the scaphoid, or by inserting a Kirschner wire into the proximal or distal poles percutaneously for manipulation. If the fracture cannot be satisfactorily reduced by these methods, one should proceed to conventional open reduction and internal fixation. Anatomic reduction and complete closure of the fracture line is of paramount importance.

The telescope is then transferred to the 4-5 portal which is located just distal to the dorsal rim of the radius between the fourth and fifth extensor compartments. The extensor digitorum communis tendon to the little finger is usually palpable. Looking in a radial direction, establish a 1-2 portal in the dorsal aspect of the anatomic snuffbox, near the intersection of the extensor carpi radialis longus and the extensor pollicis longus tendons. The radial artery emerges from beneath the first extensor compartment to course distally in the volar aspect of the anatomic snuffbox. Positioning the 1-2 portal in the dorsal aspect provides a margin of safety from vascular injury.

Through the 1-2 portal, introduce the target hook of the fixation jig. Seat the hook 1 or 2 mm radial to the scapholunate ligament on the horizon of the scaphoid proximal pole as visualized from the 4-5 portal. While maintaining the target hook position, assemble the guide barrel of the jig. Hyperextend the thumb to pull the trapezium dorsally on the proximal pole, and seat the teeth of the guide barrel against the scaphoid at the point previously marked midway along the articular cartilage margin of the distal pole.

The jig should not be overly compressed. Tighten it sufficiently to maintain its position and to close the fracture gap. Fracture compression however is the function of the Herbert–Whipple screw with variably pitched threads. If the fracture is overly compressed by the jig before the screw is inserted, the leading threads of the screw are unable to compress the fracture further and will lose their purchase in the proximal fragment.

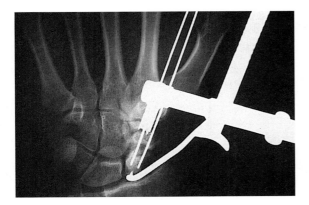

Figure 8

Interoperative radiograph of a reduced left scaphoid fracture. The fracture reduction jig is properly placed with the target hook on the proximal pole of the scaphoid adjacent to the scapholunate interval, and the guide barrel on the distal pole of the scaphoid midway between its radial and ulnar margins. The primary guide wire is centrally located in the scaphoid. The accessory guide wire is more peripheral, and stabilizes the fracture fragments while the scaphoid is drilled and the screw is inserted.

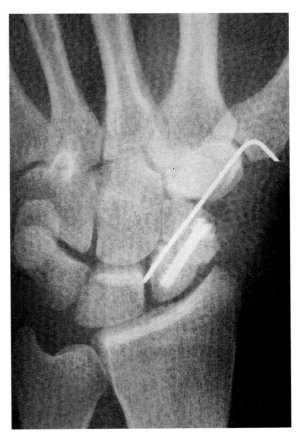

Figure 9

Postoperative radiograph of left scaphoid fracture internally fixed with Herbert–Whipple screw. The accessory guide wire can be left in place for two to three weeks for additional rotational control of the fracture if necessary.

Insert a Z-wire (diameter 0.040 inch) (Zimmer Inc, Watson, Indiana) through the guide barrel to the indicated depth. Insert a second Z-wire through the jig parallel to the first to control rotation of the fracture fragments when the first wire is over-reamed. Do not substitute K-wires, which are of a different diameter.

At this point the position of the central wire should be confirmed radiographically (Figure 8). Intraoperative fluoroscopy is especially helpful. There should be at least 2 mm of bone around all sides of the central wire to assure that the fixation device does not cut out of the scaphoid. Reposition the jig and the guide wires if they are not ideally located. Then advance the primary guide wire 2 mm to be sure it is well fixed in the proximal pole and will not be removed with the cannulated drill.

A special step drill is available for preparing the route for the screw. When the proper length Herbert–Whipple screw is installed over the guidewire, the variably pitched threads compress the fracture 1 mm. Another radiographic examination of the the wrist is necessary to confirm fracture reduction and screw placement. Proper placement of the screw and its inherent compression mechanism provide rigid stabilization of the scaphoid (Figure 9).

Postoperatively, the wrist can be immobilized in a splint or cast for 10–14 days to allow the incision to heal. Then mobilization and gentle use of the wrist are encouraged to avoid the stiffness, chondromalacia and osteopenia associated with prolonged immobilization. Patients are advised to avoid impact and torque on the wrist until there is conclusive radiographic evidence of fracture healing. Nevertheless, the hand and wrist can be used for most tasks prior to fracture union, analogous to the ambulation capability provided by modern intramedullary femoral and tibial nails.

This technique has won excellent patient acceptance with a high union rate. In a multi-center study, 15 of 16 acute fractures healed per primum.[15] One delayed union ultimately healed following an application of an electrical stimulator coil. By restoring earlier functional capabilities and allowing patients to return to work earlier than is usually possible with cast immobilization alone, primary intramedullary fixation of the scaphoid may be less costly than nonoperative treatment.

References

1   Whipple TL, Marotta J, Powell J, Techniques of wrist arthroscopy, *Arthroscopy* (1986) **2**:244–52.

2   Caspari RB, Hutton PJ, Whipple TL, et al, The role of arthroscopy in the management of tibial plateau fractures, *Arthroscopy* (1985) **1**:76–9.

3   Culver JE, Andersen TE, Fractures of the hand and wrist in the athlete, *Clin Sports Med* (1992) **11**:101–28.

4   Whipple TL, The role of arthroscopy in the treatment of wrist injuries in the athlete, *Clin Sports Med* (1992) **11**:227–38.

5   Whipple TL, Fracture management in the wrist—intra-articular fractures and associated soft tissue injuries. Presented at the 50th Anniversary Meeting of the American Society for Surgery of the Hand, San Francisco, CA, 14 September 1995.

6   Palmer AK, Fractures of the distal radius. In: Green DP, ed, *Operative Hand Surgery, 2nd edn* (Churchill Livingstone: New York, 1988) 1003–5.

7   Geissler WB, Arthroscopically assisted reduction of intraarticular fractures of the distal radius, *Hand Clin* (1995) **11**:19–29.

8   Whipple TL, *Arthroscopic Surgery: The Wrist* (JB Lippincott: Philadelphia, 1992) 143–8.

9   Weber SC, Szabo RM, Severely comminuted distal radial fracture as an unsolved problem. Complications associated with external fixation and pins and plaster techniques, *J Hand Surg* (1986) **11A**: 157–65.

10 Ruby LK, Stinson J, Belsky MR, The natural history of scaphoid nonunion. A review of 55 cases, *J Bone Joint Surg* (1985) **67A**:428–32.

11 Whipple TL, Stabilization of the fractured scaphoid under arthroscopic control, *Orthop Clin North Am* (1995) **26**:49–54.

12 Russe O, Fracture of the carpal mevicular. Diagnosis, nonoperative treatment, and operative treatment, *J Bone Joint Surg* (1960) **42A**:759–68.

13 Herbert TJ, *The Fractured Scaphoid* (Quality Medical Publishing: St Louis, 1990) 84–7.

14 Whipple TL, *Arthroscopic Surgery: The Wrist* (JB Lippincott: Philadelphia, 1992) 148–56.

15 Pereles DJ, Whipple TL, Athroscopic reduction and internal fixation of scaphoid fractures using the Herbert–Whipple screw—preliminary experience in three centers. Presented at the Arthroscopy Association of North America Annual Meeting, Orlando, FL, 30 April 1994.

Commentary

Chapter 36

External fixation of distal radius fractures is often necessary. This chapters nicely reviews the science behind the technique. I have found that careful attention to the details of pin placement and insertion is essential if one wishes to avoid complications. The advice here is sound. I believe that the particular brand of fixator chosen is not nearly as important as the principles one uses in its application.

PCA

Chapter 37

We have come a long way from Colles' attitude that fractures of the distal radius function acceptably even after poor reductions. It seems quite clear that, particularly for intraarticular fractures, accurate reduction of the joint surface is necessary. Furthermore, for young active persons something close to an anatomical reduction seems an appropriate goal, as less accurate results are often associated with poor function. In some cases closed reduction and external or percutaneous fixation may be all that is necessary. In some cases, however, an open reduction will be necessary either to restore impacted fragments or to add bone graft, or both. This chapter nicely reviews the surgical approach in such cases.

PCA

Chapter 38

Here is an example of a new technique which has not proved worthwhile. Dynamic external fixation for unstable distal radius fractures was introduced a decade or so ago with the idea of permitting early wrist motion. The goal was to improve the final motion of the wrist by permitting early mobilization while maintaining distraction. Although this has been fine in theory, in practice it has not worked out and Doctor Sommerkamp's work has been extremely valuable in this regard.

One might question why dynamic external fixation has not worked for the wrist. It may well have to do with the complex center of motion of the wrist joint, which cannot be mimicked by an external hinge the way, for example, elbow or knee motion can be. It seems unlikely that transarticular distraction of the wrist will be compatible with early wrist mobilization. Other options, which limit fixation to the radius, would seem to hold more promise if the clinician wishes to begin early wrist motion. Such options would include external fixation limited to the radius, or newer sorts of internal fixation devices which may be usable in more comminuted fractures.

PCA

Chapter 39

This method is an interesting way to reduce fragments of an intraarticular distal radius fracture, especially impacted central fragments. Even with the great experience of the author, it is a difficult technique which should be balanced against open treatment, reduction and grafting. Fractures with small comminuted fragments are a limitation to this technique. For scaphoid fractures, arthroscopic reduction appears to be rarely needed. This technique may be used for nondisplaced, minimally displaced or displaced and reducible fractures and it is essentially a method of control rather than reduction; this control may be achieved by the use of fluoroscopy.

PS

Ulnar styloid impaction syndrome

Steven M Topper*, Michael B Wood and Leonard K Ruby

Abstract

We present a previously undescribed etiology of ulnar sided wrist pain in a series of eight patients. Each patient had an excessively long ulnar styloid that was impacting the triquetrum and causing chondromalacia, synovitis, and pain. Four patients developed symptoms as a result of a definable injury and four secondary to chronic repetitive strain. The average age at the time of surgery was 34 years. There were three males and five females. The average follow-up was 34 months. All patients were treated by open partial ulnar styloidectomy. Outcome was evaluated clinically and by means of patient questionnaire and radiographs. Pain reliably improved from a preoperative average of 3.5 to a postoperative average of 1.25 which equates to mild pain requiring no medication. All but one patient returned to their previous employment unrestricted. The average preoperative ulnar styloid length was 7.38 mm and the average ulnar styloid process index was 0.41, which is almost twice normal. There were no complications. We found that an excessively long ulnar styloid has important implications on the kinematics of the lunatotriquetral interval. Details of the diagnosis of this condition, including a new provocative test, and operative management are discussed.

Introduction

Ulnar wrist pain remains a diagnostic and therapeutic challenge to the hand surgeon. This is an area of high anatomic complexity where multiple structures are frequently involved in the pathologic processes that produce symptoms. As with other wrist pain syndromes the complexity of the pathology is further compounded by the psychodynamics of work related injury. The literature has been replete with articles which discuss ulnar sided wrist pain over the last 15 years. This heightened interest has resulted in clinical and biomechanical data which have improved our understanding and management of these conditions which affect the distal radioulnar and ulnocarpal joints. Specifically the manifestation of ulnocarpal impaction syndrome has been well described.[1] This condition, which results from excessive positive ulnar variance, responds well to decompression of the ulnocarpal articulation by recessing the ulna.[2,3]

The authors report a series of patients who presented with symptoms of ulnocarpal impaction syndrome but who had neutral or negative ulnar variation. Furthermore, these patients are distinctly different from the better known form of ulnocarpal impaction in that the radiographic evidence of chondromalacia did not involve the proximal pole of the lunate and ulnar head, but rather the proximal pole of the triquetrum and the ulnar styloid. All patients in this report had an excessively long ulnar styloid.

This chapter reports on an etiology of ulnar sided wrist pain caused by an impingement between an excessively long ulnar styloid and the triquetrum. Diagnosis and clinical results

*The opinions expressed are those of the authors and do not necessarily reflect those of the US Air Force, or the Department of Defense.

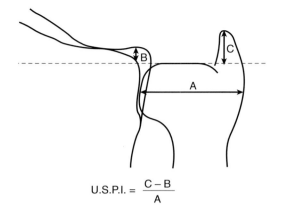

$$U.S.P.I. = \frac{C - B}{A}$$

Figure 1

The ulnar styloid process index (USPI) is calculated by subtracting the ulnar variance (B) from the length of the ulnar styloid process (C) and dividing that by the transverse diameter of the ulnar head (A).

Table 1 The scoring system for pain.

Pain scale	
0	No pain
1	Mild pain, no use of pain medication
2	Modest or intermittent pain, occasional use of nonprescription pain medication
3	Modest or intermittent pain, frequent use of nonprescription pain medication
4	Moderate pain that is not continuous but is disabling when present; occasional use of prescription pain medication
5	Severe, continuous, disabling pain; continuous use of prescription pain medication

achieved with partial ulnar styloidectomy are discussed.

Materials and methods

The study group consisted of eight patients from three institutions who were diagnosed with impingement between the ulnar styloid and the triquetrum and were treated with partial ulnar styloidectomy. There were three male patients and five females. The average age at the time of operation was 34 years (range 15–53 years). Four had a history of injury and four had a history of overuse. The average follow-up was 34 months (range 12–74 months).

In order to compare ulnar styloid lengths between patients we utilized a method originally described by Garcia-Elias.[4] This method controls for radiographic magnification variations, individual bone size, and ulnar variance by creating a ratio of styloid length minus ulnar variance divided by the width of the ulnar head (Figure 1); it is called the ulnar styloid process index (USPI). Standard styloid lengths and ulnar variance were also recorded for each patient. These measurements were compared to published norms in

order to assess relative styloid lengths of the patients in our series. Garcia-Elias compared the USPI of 76 patients who had sustained a dorsal triquetrum fracture to 100 asymptomatic controls who had not.[4] The average USPI of the 100 controls was 0.21 ± 0.07. Biyani and colleagues studied radiographic ulnar styloid morphology in 400 asymptomatic volunteers and found that an average ulnar styloid length is between 3 and 6 mm.[5]

Outcome was assessed with a questionnaire. Pain was rated by a scoring system both pre- and postoperatively (Table 1). Additional questions were asked regarding return to work and satisfaction with the procedure.

Provocative test

A provocative test to help distinguish ulnar styloid impaction syndrome from ulnocarpal impaction syndrome was developed by one of the authors (LKR). It is performed with the patient's elbow resting on the examining table. The forearm is initially positioned in neutral rotation. The examiner then maximally dorsiflexes the wrist, and then rolls the forearm into maximum supination (Figure 2). If this maneuver reproduces the patient's pain it is considered positive.

Dorsiflexion of the wrist brings the triquetrum into a dorsal position relative to the forearm. The wrist starts in neutral rotation so the ulnar styloid is positioned directly ulnar. As the forearm is

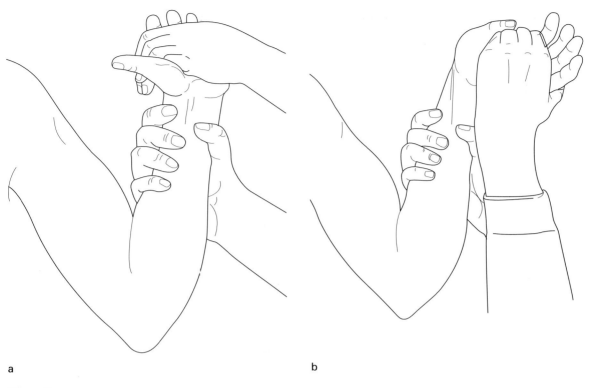

a   b

Figure 2

The ulnar styloid impaction test is performed by starting with the forearm in neutral rotation and the wrist dorsiflexed (a). The examiner then rolls the forearm into a position of maximum supination (b).

rotated into supination the ulnar styloid is brought into a dorsal position relative to the carpus. It is in this position that the impingement between the ulnar styloid and the triquetrum occurs. Forearm supination causes a recession of the ulnar head relative to the distal radius, so this maneuver would not be expected to reproduce pain caused by ulnocarpal impaction syndrome, although in the face of a torn triangular fibrocartilage complex it can.

All of the patients in this series had a positive ulnar styloid impaction test preoperatively.

Surgical procedure

The procedure is done with the elbow flexed and the forearm in neutral rotation. Either a curvi-

linear incision centered over the ulnar styloid or a straight incision over the sixth dorsal compartment is used and the dorsal sensory branch of the ulnar nerve is identified, retracted volarly, and protected. The ulnar collateral ligament and the ulnar wrist capsule are divided sharply in a longitudinal fashion directly over the ulnar styloid. A 1.2 mm Kirschner wire is then placed in the approximate location of the base of the styloid (Figure 3b). A posterior anterior radiograph is then taken so that the level of the osteotomy can be judged from the location of the Kirschner wire. In most patients the osteotomy was made flush with the distal aspect of the ulnar head (Figure 3c). In patients with particularly long styloids only the distal two-thirds of the process was resected. Osteotomy at either level will allow for adequate decompression without detachment of important ligaments

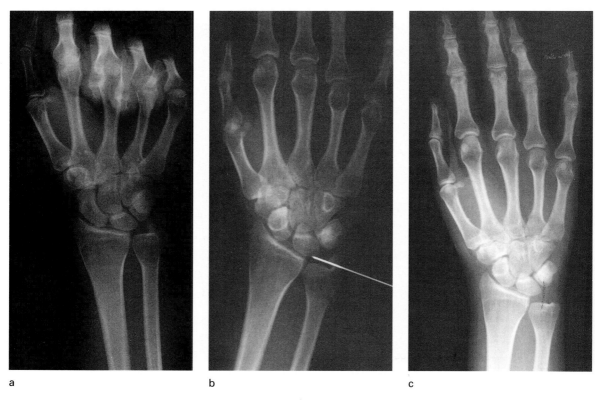

a   b   c

Figure 3

Preoperative posteroanterior radiograph which demonstrates the excessively long ulnar styloid (a). Intraoperative radiograph which demonstrates placement of the Kirschner wire used to judge the level of the osteotomy (b). Postoperative radiograph which demonstrates partial ulnar styloidectomy at the appropriate level (c).

at the base of the ulnar styloid.[6,7] We have found a small sharp osteotome to be the safest and most effective tool for the osteotomy. After completion of the osteotomy the Kirschner wire is removed and the styloid fragment is grasped and displaced ulnarly as all remaining capsular attachments are cut sharply. The ulnar collateral ligament and ulnar wrist capsule are then reapproximated followed by skin closure.

Postoperative care

The wrist is supported in a Munster splint for 2 weeks after which time motion is begun. Aggravating or stressful activities are avoided for 6 weeks. None of our patients were high performance athletes however, the authors would advise competition should be avoided for 6 weeks after this operation.

Results

Radiograph review

None of the patients in this series had a positive ulnar variance (Table 2). The average ulnar variance was negative 1.38 mm (range 0 to −2).

Table 2   Results.

Patient	Mechanism	Ulnar styloid length (mm)	USPI	Ulnar variance (mm)	Preop pain score	Postop pain score	Patient satisfaction	Return to prior employment	Associated factors
1	RS	7	0.39	0	5	2	Excellent	No	Rheumatoid arthritis
2	RS	10	0.53	0	1	0	Excellent	Yes	
3	Injury	9	0.39	−2	3	0	Excellent	Yes	
4	RS	7	0.29	−2	3	0	Excellent	Yes	
5	RS	7	0.43	−1	3	0	Excellent	Yes	
6	Injury	7	0.39	−2	5	3	Excellent	Yes	2 previous wrist surgeries (LT fusion)
7	Injury	7	0.44	−2	3	3	Good	No	3 previous wrist surgeries (SLC fusion)
8	Injury	5	0.44	−2	4	2	Excellent	No	PO wrist injury

RS, repetitive stress; USPI, ulnar styloid process index; LT, lunatotriquetral; SLC, scapholunocapitate; PO, postoperative.

All patients except one demonstrated an excessive ulnar styloid length when compared to the previously stated published norm of 3–6 mm.[5] The average ulnar styloid length was 7.38 mm (range 5–10 mm). All patients had an elevated USPI when compared to the previously stated published norm of 0.21 ± 0.07.[4] The average USPI was 0.41.

Pain relief

The average preoperative pain level was 3.5 (Table 2) which equates to modest to moderate pain, which is disabling when present and requires frequent use of pain medication. The average postoperative pain level was 1.25 which equates to mild pain requiring no medication (Table 2). All of the patients in the series except one (patient 7) improved. Four of the eight patients were pain free. Of the patients who reported persistent pain, all of them had extenuating circumstances. One of them (patient 1) had a rheumatoid flare postoperatively which diminished her pain relief assessment from an early postoperative level of 0 to 2. Two of the patients had multiple previous wrist surgeries (patients 6 and 7) including limited intercarpal arthrodesis. The last patient (patient 8) injured the wrist postoperatively which diminished the pain relief from the procedure from a level of 1 to 2. Two of the patients were receiving workman's compensation benefits at the time of follow-up (patients 7 and 8).

Employment status

Five of the eight patients returned to their previous employment without physical restrictions. One patient (patient 7) with a history of multiple previous wrist surgery changed his job to a position not requiring heavy manual activities. Two of the patients (patients 1 and 8) stopped working because of persistent wrist symptoms thought not to be directly related to their surgery (Table 2).

Satisfaction

Seven out of the eight patients described themselves as enthusiastic about the procedure and stated that they would recommend it to others in similar circumstances. One of the patients described himself as satisfied though incompletely relieved of pain. None of the patients were dissatisfied (Table 2).

Complications

No postoperative wound problems or nerve injuries occurred. On follow-up examination the stability of the distal radioulnar joint (DRUJ) was assessed by manual stress in each patient and all were judged stable to an equal degree as the opposite upper limb.

Discussion

Although the authors do not believe that ulnar styloid impaction syndrome has been previously described, an excessively long ulnar styloid has been implicated as a cause of ulnar sided wrist pathology. Fikry and associates identified what they called 'ulnar styloid overshooting' as a risk factor for the development of isolated lunatotriquetral instability in 13 patients.[8] Levy et al[9] and Garcia-Elias[4] in independent studies noted that the majority of dorsal triquetrum fractures are due to compressive forces rather than tensile forces and tend to occur in patients with long ulnar styloid processes. In our series half of the patients developed symptoms as a result of a single injury and half as a result of presumed repetitive stress injury (Table 2). None of the patients at the time of surgery had an associated lunatotriquetral ligament tear or a dorsal triquetral fracture. All of the patients were found to have chondromalacia involving the ulnar styloid tip and the proximal triquetrum. This observation suggests a pathologic sequence of events in patients with an excessively long ulnar styloid. Singular or repetitive impaction between the ulnar styloid tip and the triquetrum results in contusion which leads to chondromalacia of the opposing articular surfaces, synovitis, and pain.

One of the patients in our series (patient 6) developed symptoms and radiographic findings which suggested ulnar styloid impaction only after a lunatotriquetral fusion for isolated lunatotriquetral instability (Figure 4). This is understandable when normal lunatotriquetral rotation is considered. There is some degree of triquetrum rotation relative to the lunate with wrist motion in all directions (Table 3). Of particular interest is the rotation that occurs in ulnar deviation. Flexion of the triquetrum allows it to avoid impaction with the ulnar styloid on wrist

Table 3   Normal lunatotriquetral rotation with wrist motion.

Wrist motion	Triquetrum rotation relative to the lunate
Neutral–60° extension	Extends 9.8°
Neutral–60° flexion	Flexes 8.2°
Neutral–15° radial deviation	Radially deviates 3.6°
	Extends 2.9°
Neutral–30° ulnar deviation	Ulnarly deviates 3.4°
	Flexes 4.3°

An A, personal communication, 1995.

motion in this direction. If this normal rotational motion is prevented by a lunatotriquetral fusion an ulnar styloid impaction syndrome may be induced. We agree with Fikry and associates[8] that an excessively long ulnar styloid should be considered a potential risk factor for injury to the lunatotriquetral ligament leading to lunatotriquetral instability. These authors suggested that decompression of the ulnocarpal articulation with a diaphyseal ulnar shortening was an important adjunct to stabilization of the lunatotriquetral interval. We suggest that a simple ulnar styloidectomy, performed concomitantly with lunatotriquetral stabilization, accomplishes the same goal with less operative morbidity. This approach is of course reserved for patients with ulnar styloid impaction syndrome rather than patients with ulnocarpal impaction syndrome. In the latter the impaction area will require ulnar head recession in order to be effective.

The importance of maintaining the integrity of the ligamentous attachments to the ulnar styloid has been emphasized. The question then arises as to how much of the ulnar styloid can safely be resected. We chose to make the osteotomy flush with the distal aspect of the ulnar head. In most patients there is a recessed notch between the ulnar styloid and the ulnar head in the area where the ligamentum subcruatum inserts. With this method this typically preserves 1–2 mm of styloid process. Palmer and associates have demonstrated that the fibers which anchor the triangular fibrocartilage complex (TFCC) to the ulnar styloid attach at the base.[6,7] Preservation of the integrity of these fibers contributes to DRUJ stability; however, there are also fibers which anchor the TFCC to the ulnar head. Kauer observed that the entire styloid process is invested in an extensive fibrous mass which

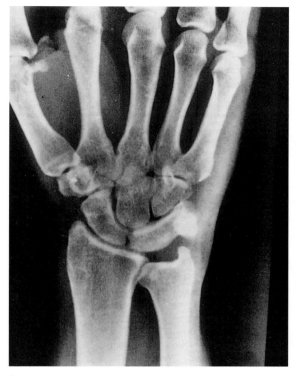

a

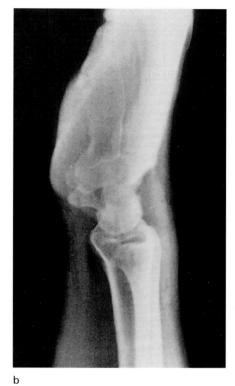

b

Figure 4

(a) Preoperative posteroanterior and (b) lateral radiographs which demonstrate the previous lunatotriquetral arthrodesis. (c) Postoperative radiograph after ulnar styloidectomy.

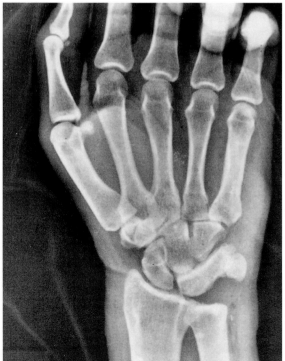

c

extends from the dorsal ulnar edge of the distal radius to the base of the fifth metacarpal.[10] This fibrous tissue which wraps and spirals around the ulnar aspect of the wrist also has connections to the head of the ulna, the triquetrum, the pisiform, and the base of the fifth metacarpal. Exposure of the ulnar styloid from an ulnar approach requires a longitudinal incision through a portion of this fibrous mass. We suggest that the integrity of this structure is not adversely affected after removal of a portion of the ulnar styloid followed by direct repair because of its extensive connections to multiple bony sites. No patient in our series developed an unstable DRUJ postoperatively.

Three of the patients in this series underwent diagnostic arthroscopy just prior to ulnar styloidectomy during the same operative procedure. This approach affords the surgeon the opportunity to confirm the diagnosis based on the presence of chondromalacia between the opposing articular surfaces of the ulnar styloid and triquetrum. It also allows for careful evaluation of the stability of the lunatotriquetral interval. Arthroscopic ulnar styloidectomy is not recommended due to the difficulty in visualizing the styloid secondary to the overlying synovium and the danger of injuring the precariously close ulnotriquetral and ulnolunate ligaments.

The diagnosis of this condition is made by radiographic evidence of an excessively long ulnar styloid in combination with a positive ulnar styloid impaction test. An excessively long ulnar styloid has a USPI greater than 0.21 ± 0.07 and/or an overall styloid length greater than 6 mm. One of the patients in this series (patient 8) had an ulnar styloid process length which was within the normal range (5 mm) but an excessive USPI. This observation underscores the importance of assessing the radiographic measurement relative to the individual patient by the USPI technique. We have also found that an injection of 1 ml of lidocaine placed directly over the tip of the

ulnar styloid helpful to establish the diagnosis.

In conclusion we present a previously undescribed etiology of ulnar sided wrist pain as well as a new provocative test for this condition. An excessively long ulnar styloid should be considered as a possible etiology for ulnar styloid impaction syndrome as well as isolated lunatotriquetral instability. Conversely, a lunatotriquetral arthrodesis may induce ulnar styloid impaction syndrome in patients with an elevated USPI. Ulnar styloid impaction syndrome reliably responds to the relatively simple procedure of partial ulnar styloidectomy.

References

1   Friedman SL, Palmer AK, The ulnar impaction syndrome, *Hand Clin* (1991) **7**:295–310.
2   Chun S, Palmer AK, The ulnar impaction syndrome: follow-up of ulnar shortening osteotomy, *J Hand Surg* (1993) **18A**:46–53.
3   Linscheid RL, Ulnar lengthening and shortening, *Hand Clin* (1987) **3**:69–79.
4   Garcia-Elias M, Dorsal fractures of the triquetrum—avulsion or compression fractures, *J Hand Surg* (1987) **12A**:266–8.
5   Biyani A, Mehara A, Bhan S, Morphological variations of the ulnar styloid process, *J Hand Surg* (1990) **15B**:352–4.
6   Palmer AK, Werner FW, The triangular fibrocartilage complex of the wrist—anatomy and function, *J Hand Surg* (1981) **6A**:153–62.
7   Drewniany JJ, Palmer AK, Injuries to the distal radioulnar joint, *Orthop Clin North Am* (1986) **17**:451–9.
8   Fikry T, Lamine A, Essadki B, et al, Les instabilites pyramido-lunaires: role de l'indice radio-styloidien, *Ann Chir Main* (1993) **12**:243–9.
9   Levy M, Fischel RE, Stern GM, et al, Chip fractures of the os triquetrum: mechanism of injury, *J Bone Joint Surg* (1979) **61B**:355–7.
10 Kauer JMG, The articular disc of the hand, *Acta Anat* (1975) **93**:590–604.

Commentary

Chapter 40

This extremely well described and documented
new syndrome is reported by the authors.
Another cause of ulnar wrist pain is detected.
Implications for triquetrolunate instabilities and
their treatment are also discussed. This long
styloid should be systematically looked for in
patients with ulnar pain.

PS

41

Classification of Kienböck's disease based on new imaging

Marteinn Magnusson and Thomas E Trumble

History

Avascular necrosis of the lunate was first described by Dr Robert Kienböck,[1] a Viennese radiologist, in 1910, shortly after the discovery of X-rays (Figure 1).

Anatomy

The lunate bone is semicircular in shape and only the dorsal side and part of the volar side are devoid of cartilage.

The vascularity of the lunate is based on vessels entering the bone through the volar and dorsal surfaces in close proximity to the insertion of wrist ligaments. It has been debated which side is the more important contributor for the overall vascularity of the lunate. Gelberman et al reported on both the extra- and intra-osseous vascularity of the lunate.[2] They showed that there was a consistent extraosseous volar blood supply, but that 93% of the lunates also had a dorsal blood supply. When the lunate was supplied from both sides there was always an intraosseous anastomosis between the two sides. They identified three patterns of intraosseous anastomosis resembling the letters Y (59%), I (31%) or X (10%). The anastomosis was always distal to the lunates midline and the proximal part of the bone had a terminal type of arterial supply. The patients with the I pattern and a single dorsal and volar vessel were thought to be at risk for avascular necrosis.

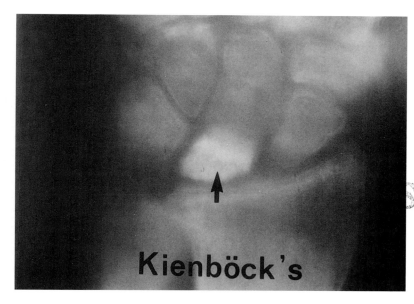

Kienböck's

Figure 1

Sclerotic lunate (arrow) with partial collapse in a patient with stage IIIA Kienböck's disease.

Etiology

It is simplest to state that the etiology of Kienböck's disease is unknown at this point in time. Many plausible theories have been put forward and are supported by observations of the risk factors for suffering this condition. However, no single risk factor is found in all cases.

Kienböck theorized that the changes in the lunate were secondary to changes in dorsal blood flow to the lunate after trauma.[1] He noted that the initial radiographs were normal and that the radiographic changes only materialized later in the course of the disease.

In 1928, Hulten described the association between a short ulna and Kienböck's disease.[3] His theory was that Kienböck's disease was secondary to the force concentration on a smaller area of the lunate. Trumble et al studied, in a biomechanical model, the effect of joint leveling procedures on the lunate loading and found that both radius shortening and ulnar lengthening of 2.0 mm resulted in a 70% reduction in the lunate load.[4]

In summary, the etiology of the avascular necrosis of the lunate is unclear. However, three factors are worth emphasizing:

(1) The lunate has a precarious extraosseous blood supply, sometimes just from one vessel. It also has a terminal type of intraosseous blood supply to the proximal pole.
(2) There is an increased incidence of ulnar minus variants among patients with Kienböck's disease.
(3) There is an environmental factor, highlighted by the fact that the disease is more common in heavy manual workers.

Symptoms

Typically the onset of symptoms is insidious and progressive. The patient complains of middorsal wrist pain that is aggravated by activity. The disease is most frequent in males in their third or fourth decade. Typically the patients are heavy manual workmen although the condition has also been identified in people without any history of heavy labor. There is sometimes a history of recent trauma to the wrist, but there is seldom a clear correlation with the trauma event and initiation of symptoms.

The exam reveals slight swelling and tenderness middorsal over the wrist with decreased flexion and extension, as well as decreased grip strength as compared to the unaffected side. Typically pronation and supination are unaffected. Only 20% of patients have bilateral findings and the dominant hand is more frequently involved.

Diagnosis

The process of diagnosing Kienböck's disease is changing. The diagnosis and staging of this disease have been based on changes seen in the lunate on X-ray films. In stage I the lunate has basically a normal appearance on radiographs, but a positive technetium (bone) scan.

It is important to realize that the increased density changes seen on radiographs in stage II of this disease represent a process of repair and collapse of trabecular architecture. The bone is already avascular and at this time is going through the process of bone resorption and attempted repair. It is at this stage that the bone is the weakest. Radioisotope bone scans may show abnormally high uptake in the midcarpal region in stage I but this study is not highly specific and confirmation with magnetic resonance imaging (MRI) is recommended.

As newer imaging modalities become readily available and we gain experience in interpreting the results, they become the new standard for clinical judgment of this disease. This will hopefully allow us to make a definitive diagnosis of Kienböck's disease earlier in the disease and this will also affect the treatment given. By being able to adequately treat patients in the early stages of Kienböck's disease, we can prevent the lunate collapse and thereby improve the outcome of this disabling condition.

Computerized tomograms (CT) of the wrist have been found to be more accurate in evaluation of the degree of sclerosis, compression fractures, lunate fragmentation and cyst formation than plain radiographs or conventional tomograms. This has proved to be especially useful in stages II and III of Kienböck's disease.

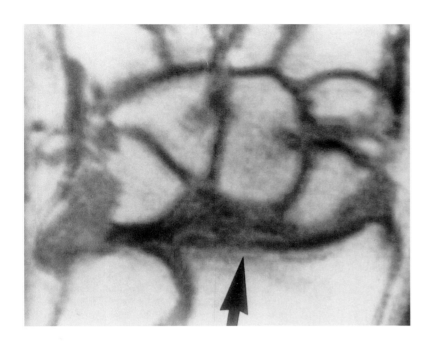

Figure 2

T1-weighted coronal magnetic resonance image which shows a decreased signal from the lunate (arrow), characteristic of osteonecrosis.

Evidence suggests that MRI may provide early and accurate diagnosis of osteonecrosis (Figure 2).[5] MRI is able to detect changes in the bone marrow of the lunate consistent with avascular necrosis and these changes precede the radiographic changes. Trumble et al provided the first convincing evidence that the loss of signal intensity on MRI correlated with histologic evidence of avascular necrosis.[6] They recommended CT to rule out acute fractures, intraosseous ganglions and other focal lesions which could displace the bone marrow and produce low signal intensity on MRI. They recommended that the interpretation of small focal artifacts as findings consistent with Kienböck's disease could be avoided by imaging the lunate in three planes (coronal, sagittal and transverse) with thin sections so that at least three images are available in each plane. Kienböck's disease was diagnosed by MRI if there were abnormal signal changes in approximately half of the lunate.

Classification

Lichtman presented a revised radiographic classification of Kienböck's disease.[7] Because the radiograph is not the best method to distinguish changes associated with avascular necrosis of bone we have added bone scans and MRI to modify Lichtman's classification. The bony changes, as seen on a radiograph, will always lag behind the true changes at the microscopic level.

Combined techniques for staging Kienböck's disease

Stage I

This stage is exemplified by normal or almost normal radiographs. A linear or a compression fracture may exist but the bone density is normal. Bone scintigraphy is usually positive. Magnetic resonance imaging shows abnormal signal changes in at least half of the lunate consistent with avascular necrosis.[6]

Stage II

In this stage the radiographs show an increased density of the lunate as compared to the neighboring carpal bones, but there is no sign of collapse. On MRI most of the bone marrow is abnormal and there can be an early sign of collapse (crescent sign).

Stage III

The hallmark of this stage is lunate collapse, scapholunate dissociation and proximal migration of the capitate as seen on radiographs and CT. The lunate is elongated in the sagittal plane. This stage is often divided into two subgroups based on concomitant rotation of the scaphoid. If there is no fixed rotation of the scaphoid, then this is grouped as IIIA. In group IIIB fixed rotation of the scaphoid is shown by a positive ring sign and an increased scapholunate angle on an anteroposterior view of the wrist.

Stage IV

This final stage of the disease is characterized by those changes seen in stage III, but now there are signs of generalized carpal arthritis.

References

1   Kienböck R, Über traumatische Malazie des Mondbeins un ihre Folgezustande: Entartungsformen und Kompressionsfrakturen, *Fortschr Rontgenstr* (1910) **16**:77.
2   Gelberman RH, Bauman TD, Menon J, et al, The vascularity of the lunate bone and Kienböck's disease, *J Hand Surg* (1980) **5**:272–8.
3   Hulten O, Über anatomische Variationen der Handgelenkknochen, *Acta Radiol* (1928) **9**:155–68.
4   Trumble TE, Glisson RR, Seaber AV, et al, A biomechanical comparison of the methods for treating Kienböck's disease, *J Hand Surg* (1986) **11A**:88–93.
5   Amadio PC, Hanssen AD, Berquist TH, The genesis of Kienböck's disease: evaluation of a case by magnetic resonance imaging, *J Hand Surg* (1989) **12A**:1044–9.
6   Trumble TE, Irving J, Histologic and magnetic resonance imaging correlations in Kienböck's disease, *J Hand Surg* (1990) **14A**:879–84.
7   Lichtman DM, Degnan CG, Staging and its use in the determination of treatment modalities for Kienböck's disease, *Hand Clin* (1993) **9**:409–16.

42

Kienböck's disease: Lunotriquetral fusion using vascularized bone graft

Takashi Masatomi, Kozo Shimada and Masakazu Murai

Introduction

There are many surgical treatments for Kienböck's disease. The concepts of the procedures may be classified into three categories. Decompression of the lunate is effective especially for ulnar minus variant cases and some early stage cases were reported which had shown remodelling of the lunate. Revascularization, such as grafting the vascular bundle, is indicated in early stage cases, but revascularization of the lunate may not be as successful. In advanced cases, it is necessary to reconstruct the new articulation at the wrist joint; treatment options include replacement of the lunate with a silastic implant or tendon anchovy,

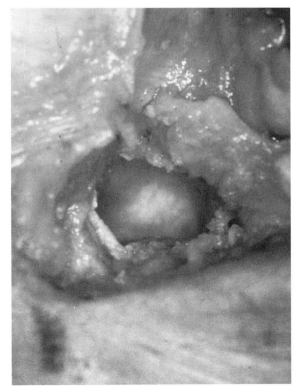

a

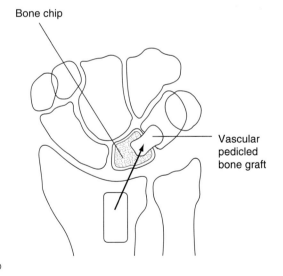

Bone chip

Vascular pedicled bone graft

b

Figure 1

Operative procedure. (a) Complete removal of the necrotic bone with a high-speed drill, preserving the subchondral bone and the articular cartilage of the lunate. (b) Grafting the cancellous bone chip from iliac bone and bridge grafting the vascularized bone of the radius.

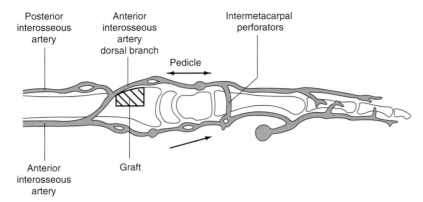

Posterior interosseous artery

Anterior interosseous artery dorsal branch

Intermetacarpal perforators

Pedicle

Anterior interosseous artery

Graft

a

Figure 2

The reverse dorsal interosseous vessels pedicled graft (RDIVPG). (a) The blood supply is based on the reverse flow through the inter-metacarpal perforators. (b) The vessels are found in the fourth compartment beside the posterior interosseous nerve. (c) Harvested bone block underneath the vessels (and posterior interosseous nerve). (d) The graft is elevated preserving the periosteum and the capsule with the vessels (and the posterior interosseous nerve). (e) Bleeding from the graft.

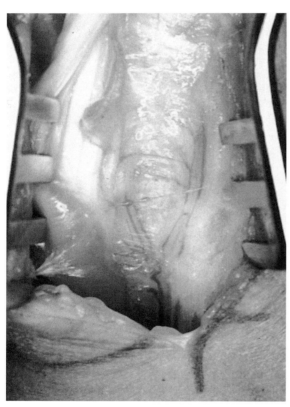

b

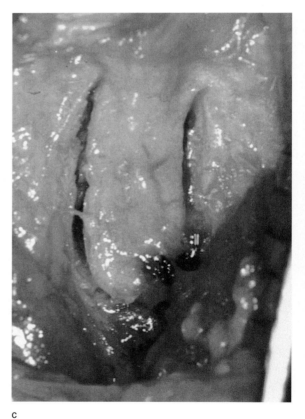

c

resection of the lunate, proximal row carpec-tomy, and peri-lunate carpal fusion.[1,2] A consensus therapeutic strategy has not been established, especially in the cases of ulnar zero or plus variant cases or advanced cases. In view of the fact that the lunotriquetral fusion has the least functional and kinematical deficits in the intercarpal fusions,[3,4] we aim to reconstruct carpal structure and revascularize the necrotic lunate by lunotriquetral fusion with vascularized bone graft for ulnar zero variant and/or advanced stage cases, stage III.

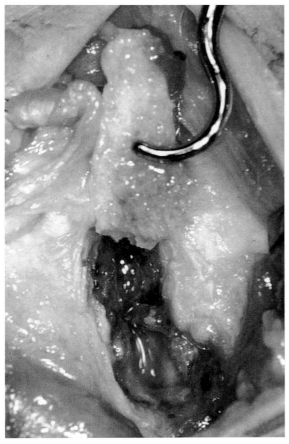

d

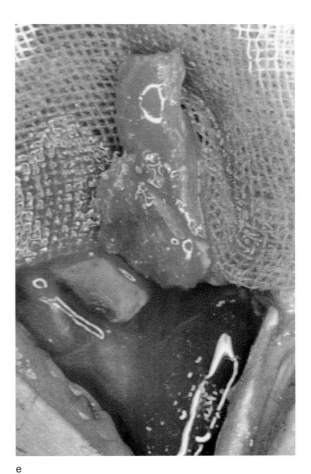

e

Technical aspects

First, we apply an external fixator to maintain carpal height and decompress the lunate during the immobilization. Second, we approach the lunate dorsally or volarly, and curette the necrotic bone completely with a high-speed drill, preserving the subchondral bone and the articular cartilage (Figure 1a). The cortical wall and articular cartilage at the lunotriquetral joint are removed and cancellous bone chips from iliac bone are grafted. The vascular pedicled bone graft is elevated from the distal radius. Our current preferences for a vascularized bone graft are either a pronator quadratus pedicled bone graft[5,6] or reverse dorsal interosseous vessels pedicle graft (RDIVPG), which we have newly

established. The pedicled bone is grafted as the bone bridge between the lunate and the triquetrum (Figure 1b). The pedicle of RDIVPG is the dorsal branch of the anterior interosseous artery and its blood supply is based on reverse flow through the intermetacarpal perforators (Figure 2a).

The pedicle should be elevated with a broad capsular flap, so the dorsal capsulotomy on approaching the lunate has to be performed ulnarly with the utmost care. It is easy to find the vessels in the fourth compartment beside the posterior interosseous nerve (Figure 2b). We sever the vessels proximally together with the posterior interosseous nerve after careful hemostasis. We harvest the bone block underneath the vessels (Figure 2c). The graft is elevated, preserving the periosteum and the capsule with the vessels and turned over (Figure 2d). When the air tourniquet is off, bleeding from the graft is confirmed (Figure 2e). The advantages of the RDIVPG are that: the volar ligaments of the wrist are not touched; it is easier to elevate the graft than a pronator quadratus pedicled graft; and we can perform neurectomy of the posterior interosseous nerve automatically which is effective for pain relief. The pedicled bone graft and carpal bones are fixed with a 1.2 mm Kirschner wire (Figure 3). The external fixator is removed at 8 weeks after operation and active range-of-motion exercise is begun.

Pros and cons compared to classical techniques

Decompression methods, such as radial shortening or wedge osteotomy, ulnar lengthening, or shortening of both radius and ulna, are easier and show relatively good clinical results.[7] However, revival of the lunate is not certain and remodelling is seen only in some early stage cases. So deformity of the wrist joint articulation still remains in advanced cases and might lead to osteoarthritic changes in the future. Decompression is recommended only for early stage cases, up to stage II, especially with the ulnar minus variant. The

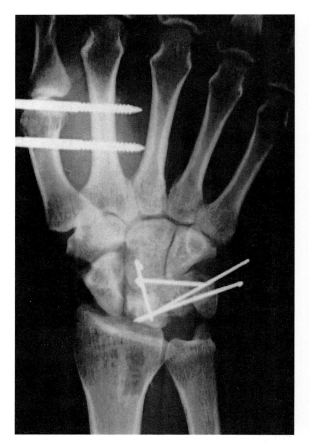

Figure 3

The pedicled bone graft and carpal bones are fixed with a 1.2 mm Kirschner wire.

Table 1   Results—numbers in parentheses are postoperative.

Case	Sex	Age	Side	Stage	Graft	Follow-up (months)	DF	VF	Grip (%)	SI (%)	Pain
1	M	23	R	III	PQ	34.0	30(50)	40(50)	36.0(80.0)	40.1(44.0)	none
2	F	60	L	II	PQ	26.1	15(45)	20(40)	40.0(55.0)	50.5(50.2)	none
3	M	28	L	III	PQ	24.8	40(40)	50(55)	70.3(79.3)	39.7(41.0)	none
4	M	27	L	III	RDIVPG	19.7	45(50)	50(50)	72.8(75.3)	38.9(40.3)	none
5	M	43	L	III	RDIVPG	15.2	35(50)	20(45)	30.8(60.5)	41.5(42.0)	none
6	M	28	L	I	RDIVPG	14.6	45(45)	40(60)	65.5(78.8)	51.1(50.8)	none
7	M	33	R	II	RDIVPG	14.2	45(50)	50(50)	68.2(75.8)	50.8(50.5)	none
8	M	51	R	III	RDIVPG	13.0	45(45)	40(45)	60.8(68.1)	38.4(40.3)	slight at HW
9	M	27	R	III	RDIVPG	12.5	45(40)	30(45)	56.0(75.2)	39.9(45.6)	none
10	F	54	R	III	RDIVPG	8.0	20(55)	20(45)	25.6(50.8)	41.6(40.4)	slight at HW
average		37.4				18.2	36.5(47.0)	36.0(48.5)	52.1(62.3)	43.3(44.5)	

PQ, pronator quadratus pedicle graft; RDIVPG, reverse dorsal interosseous vessels pedicle graft; DF, dorsiflexion; VF, volar-flexion, SI, Ståhl's index; HW, hard work.

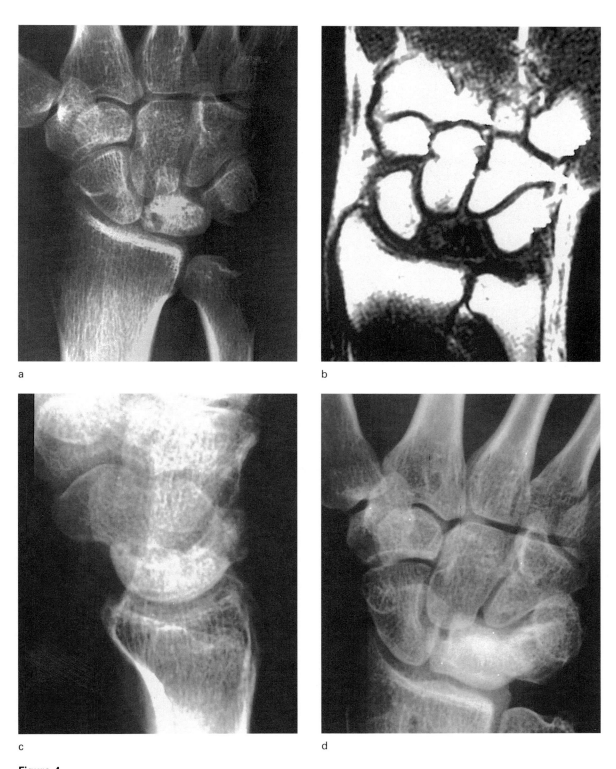

a

b

c

d

Figure 4

Case 1, a 23-year-old male glass worker. (a,b) Preoperative, stage III: DISI deformity is seen on the lateral view of a plan radiograph (c). (d) Postoperative, 24 months. *Continued*

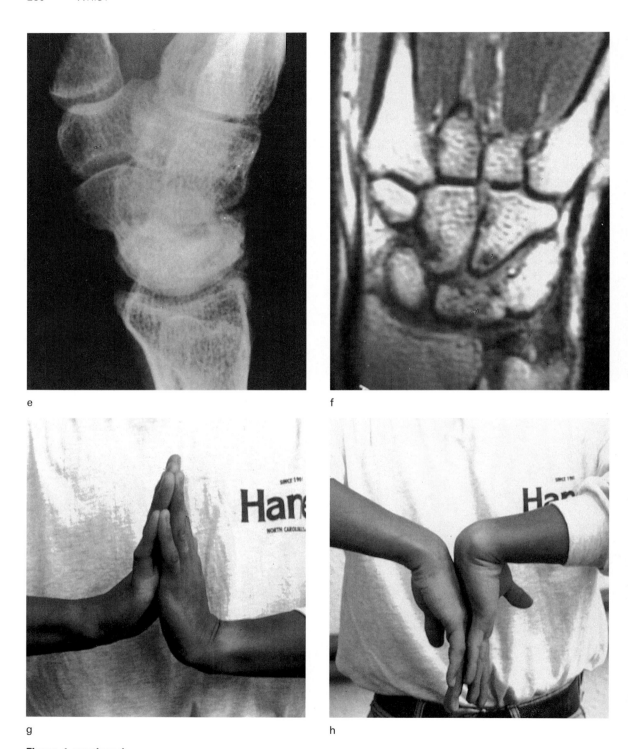

e

f

g

h

Figure 4 *continued*

Lunotriquetral fusion is complete and (e) DISI deformity is corrected on a plain radiograph. (f) The intensity at the lunate was recovering, as shown on MRI. (g,h) Range of motion at the wrist (28 months postoperatively).

efforts to revascularize by vascular bundle grafting or vascularized bone grafting only to necrotic lunate are ineffective; moreover the deformed lunate cannot be expected to recover its height, even after revascularization. Other procedures performed in advanced cases, such as removal of the lunate, proximal row carpectomy, or perilunate intercarpal fusion, leave the articulation of the wrist abnormal and destroy the carpal kinematics, which are fears associated with osteoarthritis. Our procedure has the potential to revive the necrotic lunate by complete removal of necrotic bone followed by cancellous bone graft, and to double vascularization from the triquetrum as well as the pedicled bone graft. It is theoretically possible to reconstruct an almost normal carpal structure by recovery of lunate height; a minimal kinematic deficit by lunotriquetral fusion. This procedure could, therefore, be applied to advanced stages.

Results

We operated on 10 cases of Kienböck's disease (stage I: 1, stage II: 2 and stage III: 7) (Table 1). The mean age at operation was 37.4 years (range 23–60 years). There were eight males and two females. The mean follow-up was 18.2 months. In three cases of stage III, the Ståhl's index was decreased 7% within 1 month of removal of the external fixator, but further collapse was not seen. Except for one case with the shortest follow-up (8 months), all had roentgenographical union. The range of motion of the wrist was increased after operation but resulted in almost half the range of normal motion. The preoperative wrist pain completely disappeared in all cases but two, who had slight pain on hard work. All cases returned to their former activities. The intensity of MRI at the fused lunate showed improvement in four cases at follow-up more than one and a half years after operation (cases 1–4) (Figure 4).

Indications

Our procedure aims to revascularize the lunate and reconstruct the carpal structures at the same time. The requisite condition, therefore, is complete decompression at the radiolunate articulation. Ulnar zero variant is indicated for this procedure, and ulnar minus variant cases should undergo radial shortening or wedged osteotomy combined with our method. Advanced cases without osteoarthritic change, stage III, are good indications for this procedure. We tried to reconstruct the carpus even in cases with a fragmented lunate. The efficacy of our procedure is not completely elucidated because of the relatively short follow-up, but we are sure that advanced cases are the best indications for our procedure, in view of our preliminary results.

References

1 Graner O, Lopes EJ, Carvalho BC, et al, Arthrodesis of the carpal bones in the treatment of Kienböck's disease, painful united fractures of the navicular and lunate bones with avascular necrosis, and old fracture-dislocation of carpal bones, *J Bone Joint Surg* (1966) **48A**:767–74.

2 Duparc J, Christel P, Traitment chirurgical des nécroses du semi-lunaire par arthrodese intercarpienne, *Ann Chir* (1978) **32**:565–9.

3 Simmons BP, McKenzie WD, Symptomatic carpal coalition, *J Hand Surg* (1985) **10A**:190–3.

4 Delany TJ, Eswar S, Carpal coalitions, *J Hand Surg* (1992) **17A**:28–31.

5 Kawai H, Yamamoto K, Pronator quadratus pedicled bone graft for old scaphoid fractures, *J Bone Joint Surg* (1988) **70B**:829–31.

6 Leung PC, Hung LK, Use of pronator quadratus bone flap in bony reconstruction around the wrist, *J Hand Surg* (1990) **15A**:637–40.

7 Rock MG, Roth JH, Martin L, Radial shortening osteotomy for treatment of Kienböck's disease, *J Hand Surg* (1991) **16A**:454–60.

Commentary

Chapter 41

It is absolutely right that a new classification based on the results of new imaging techniques should be established for Kienböck's disease. Unfortunately, the authors do not report the type of MRI sequences (T1, T2) which were used for diagnosis. Moreover, the injection of gadolinium (forbidden in the United States) enhances some areas of the condensed lunate and this gives an idea of whether lunate revascularization is possible after unloading procedures. This is important for surgical indications.

PS

Chapter 42

Revascularization by limited carpal arthrodesis with adjacent bones and by a vascularized graft have been proposed. It seems logical to combine two types of revascularization procedures for Kienböck stage II when the bone contour is preserved. It helps in the healing of the lunotriquetral arthrodesis, which has a 20% pseudarthrosis rate with a normal lunate and certainly more with devascularized bone.

PS

43
Ganglia treated by arthroscopy

Didier Fontes

Introduction

Ganglia of the wrist are the most frequent tumors of the hand. The nature of this tumor had been recognized by Hippocrates who named it ganglion, which meant a lump filled with mucus. Nevertheless the origin of the ganglion still remains controversial. In 1882 Volkmann considered the ganglion to be a prolapse of synovial tissue; in 1893 Ledderhose first proposed the tumor to arise from degenerative processes of periarticular tissues secondary to injury. In fact histopathologic examinations have indicated that the ganglion develops from connective tissue by myxoid degeneration and disintegration of collagen fibres.[1-3]

The origin is probably not unambiguous. Angelides and Wallace[1] described the relationship of a ganglion with the scapholunate ligament as either direct, with a large capsular and ligamentous basis of implantation (Figure 1) or with a long subtendinous pedicle. Clinical, anatomical and arthroscopic findings have supported this theory;[4-10] but Razemon[2] and Soren[3] believe that the myxoid degeneration of the dorsal articular capsule (Figure 2) is the site of origin of ganglia.

Despite a large cuff excision of the surrounding dorsal joint capsule, as proposed by Razemon,[2] most authors have reported a high rate of recurrence (10–25%).[3,11] It is generally believed that the ganglion may arise from any part of the joint capsule and the failure to remove this portion of the capsule will result in a recurrence. The systematic exploration and excision of the portion of the joint capsule that attaches to the scapholunate ligament seems to be important in order to decrease significantly the recurrence rate.

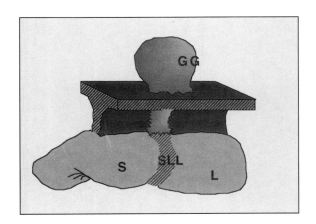

Figure 1

The theory of the origin of dorsal ganglia of the wrist in the scapholunate interosseous ligament, according to Angelides and Wallace.[1] S, scaphoid; L, lunate; SLL, scapholunate ligament; GG, ganglion.

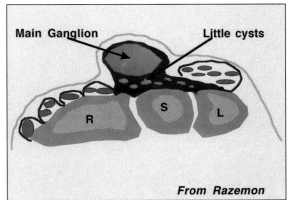

Figure 2

Razemon's theory of the origin of dorsal ganglia in myxoid degeneration of the joint capsule.[2] R, radius; S, scaphoid; L, lunate.

Despite the expected benignity of ganglion excision, classical surgical procedures often result in intolerable complications such as wrist stiffness, infection, neuroma formation and aesthetically unacceptable scars. Histopathological and clinical considerations, associated with an excessive recurrence rate, have led to the development of a minimally invasive arthroscopic procedure of excision of dorsal ganglia of the wrist.[7,8,12,13]

Technical aspects

The arthroscopic procedure

The intervention can usually be performed under locoregional anaesthesia during a one-day hospitalization by a hand surgeon familiar with therapeutic wrist arthroscopy. Distraction of the hand is by means of a distracting tower.

Intraarticular exploration

Two radiocarpal portals are usually sufficient for a complete exploration and management of a dorsal ganglion:

- the 1-2 portal (between the first and second dorsal extensor compartments) for the introduction of the scope (diameter 2.7 mm);
- the 4-5 or 6-R portal for the instruments (suction punch and shaver) or the scope, which can be exchanged for a complete visualization of the dorsal aspect of the joint capsule.

Midcarpal exploration (ulnar and radial midcarpal portals) is sometimes necessary when the synovial basis of implantation is exceptionally large distally. We prefer to use portals far from the ganglion to avoid ganglion perforation when the procedure begins. Manipulation of the instruments is more difficult than usual with these distant portals, as they induce a more obtuse working angle.

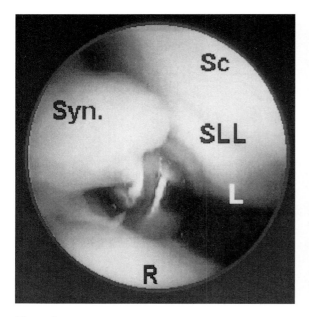

Figure 3

1-2 portal arthroscopic view of a focal hypertrophic synovium under a dorsal ganglion. Syn, synovium; Sc, scaphoid; SLL, scapholunate ligament; R, radius; L, lunate.

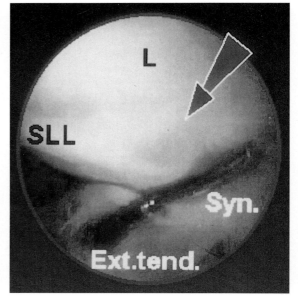

Figure 4

4-5 portal arthroscopic view of a dorsal cyst of the scapholunate ligament (arrow). SLL, scapholunate ligament; L, lunate; Syn, synovium; Ext. tend., extensor tendon.

Arthroscopic findings

We can distinguish two types of arthroscopic lesions:

- Characteristic lesions such as focal hypertrophic synovia are almost always present around the stoma of a dorsal ganglion (Figure 3), or single cysts or small clusters of cysts which can be located either on the dorsal aspect of the capsule joint (corroborating Razemon's theory[2]) or on the posterior part of the scapholunate interosseous ligament (Figure 4), thus supporting the theory of Angelides and Wallace;[1] both types of lesion can occur together.
- Associated lesions such as synovial cysts of carpal bones often arise in continuity with the ganglion through the scapholunate space, ligament tears and chondromalacia.

Arthroscopic synovectomy

This involves complete excision of the pathological synovium and cyst. The dorsal ganglion must collapse and it is important to excise all the synovium from the posterior margin of the radius to its attachment on the scapholunate ligament (Figure 5). To prevent recurrence of the ganglion it is necessary to debride all pathological associated tissue such as carpal bone synovial cysts (Figure 6) or ganglia of the scapholunate ligament (Figure 4). After complete excision, arthroscopic visualization of the extensor tendons is performed and, if the radiocarpal procedure is insufficient, a complement of midcarpal synovectomy must be done (Figure 7). All these procedures can be accurately performed by the use of soft tissue shavers or a suction punch. To avoid any damage to the scapholunate ligament and extensor tendons, perfect visualization of the dorsal aspect of the articulation is obtained by the use of a 70° scope.

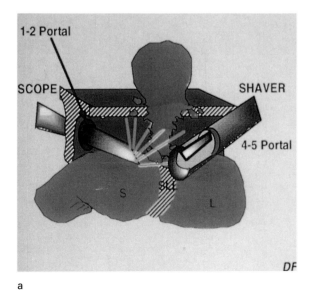

a

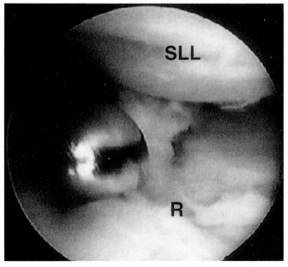

b

Figure 5

(a) Set-up and (b) 1-2 portal arthroscopic view of a complete excision of the dorsal joint capsule from the scapholunate ligament to the margin of the radius. S, scaphoid; L, lunate; SLL, scapholunate ligament; R, radius.

Postoperative management

The small cuts are closed with an absorbable suture and an aspirative drain is introduced through one arthroscopic portal, to be removed 3 hours after the procedure. A compressive bandage is applied for 1 hour. No splint or immobilization is necessary and the patient can immediately move the wrist gently, and may return to sedentary work 2 days after the intervention.

Pro and cons compared to classical techniques

Simple excision of the main cyst without its ligamentous or capsular attachments was abandoned because of an intolerably high recurrence rate (30–40%). Some years ago, radical excision of all the surrounding capsule and synovial attachments was recommended.[1,2] Despite such a procedure, recurrences were still reported,[7] and new problems such as postoperative stiffness joined the list of classical

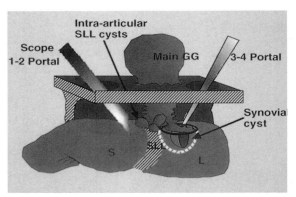

a

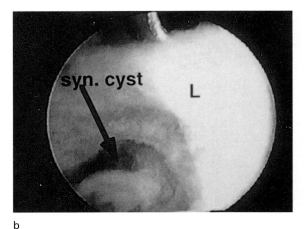

b

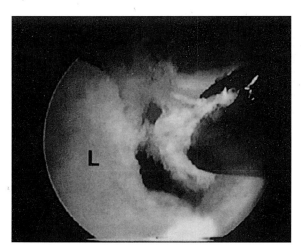

c

Figure 6

(a) Set-up; (b,c) 1-2 portal arthroscopic view of the excision of a synovial cyst of the lunatum through dorsal trephination. The synovial cyst is in direct continuity with a scapholunate ligament cluster of cysts and the dorsal ganglion. S, scaphoid; L, lunate; SLL, scapholunate ligament; GG, ganglion; Syn. cyst, synovial cyst.

complications including infection, neuromas and unaesthetic scars.

Improved understanding of the pathophysiology of the cyst, together with the development of minimally invasive procedures led Whipple[13] and Ostermann[12] to conceive a new approach for the treatment of dorsal ganglia of the wrist. Radiocarpal and midcarpal arthroscopy provides detailed information on the origin of the ganglion, so enabling more accurate excision of the synovitis and its associated lesions. In the author's experience focal hypertropic synovium is almost always present inside the joint and can be associated with scapholunate ligament cysts;[7,8] arthroscopy highlights the presence of such cysts, which might otherwise be missed during a classical open procedure. In addition, some pain in the dorsal aspect of the wrist has been attributed to occult scapholunate ligament ganglia,[9] revealed by arthroscopy[14] and excised.[7,8]

This new technique seems interesting, not only for the absence of scars and classical complications, but above all for the minimization of the recurrence rate secondary to a more accurate and complete excision of pathological tissues.

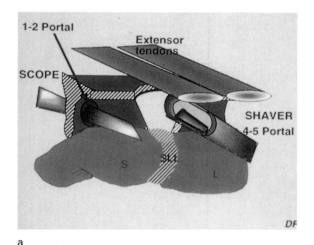

a

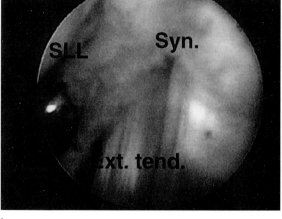

b

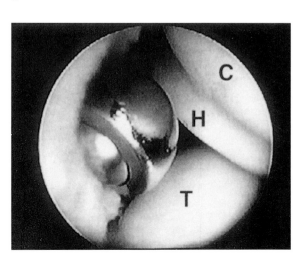

c

Figure 7

(a) Set-up; (b,c) radiocarpal and midcarpal exploration of a large dorsal ganglion, the extensor tendons must be exposed. S, scaphoid; L, lunate; SLL, scapholunate ligament; Syn, synovium; Ext. tend., extensor tendon; C, capitum; H, hamatum; T, triquetrum.

Results

Between 1990 and 1994 we performed 280 wrist arthroscopies, 32 of which were indicated for dorsal ganglia (11.4% of our indications). There were 18 females and 14 males, 16 right wrist and 16 left wrist. The mean age was 34 years (range 14–77 years). The mean duration of the ganglion was 9 months.

For 50% of the patients the origin of the ganglion was attributed to trauma. Discomfort and pain were indications for excision for 63% of the patients, but 75% experienced aesthetic problems. In 14 cases (44%) a previous treatment had failed:

- three attempts of 'crushing'
- four aspirations
- four aspirations with corticoid injections
- three previous classical surgical procedures

Arthroscopic exploration and management

Radiocarpal exploration was systematic in our series, but a complement of midcarpal arthroscopy was necessary for 12 cases (37.5%). We have observed a constant hypertrophic dorsal synovium lesion and treatment consisted of the excision of all pathological tissue to expose the extensor tendons (see Fig. 7). Associated lesions were frequent and noted in 13 cases (40.6%):

- five triangular fibrocartilage complex (TFCC) tears (Palmer classification 1A, 1B, 1D, 2A)
- two chondromalacia lesions (radius, scapho-trapezo-trapezoid joint)
- four scapholunate ligament lesions (three cysts, one partial tear)
- two carpal bone synovial cysts (lunatum (Figure 6) and scaphoid).

Each associated lesion has been followed by a specific treatment: unstable flaps of TFCC, cartilage and scapholunate ligament were debrided and cysts of the scapholunate ligament and carpal bone synovial cysts were excised arthroscopically according to the original technique described by the author.[7,8]

It was noted that the three recurrences following a previous surgical procedure were systematically associated with some cysts of the dorsal part of the scapholunate ligament in direct continuity with the dorsal recurrent synovitis (Figure 4). Those small intraarticular cysts had probably not been previously investigated and excised, which led to recurrence of the dorsal ganglion.

Assessment of the results

The first goal of the surgical treatment is to excise the ganglion definitively. The principal aim of assessment, therefore, is to look for an unexpected recurrence. The general criteria of assessment were rated according to the Mayo Clinic wrist score:

- pain (25, 20, 15, 0)
- functional status (25, 20, 15, 0)
- motion (25, 20, 15, 10, 5, 0)
- grip strength (25, 15, 10, 5, 0)

The results were graded as follows:

Excellent	91–100 points
Good	80–90 points
Fair	65–79 points
Poor	< 65 points

Results compared to the literature

After a follow-up period of 18 months for the more recent cases of our series of 32 patients, we have observed only one recurrence, in a 42-year-old male patient who presented with a ganglion of the anatomical snuff-box. Arthroscopic excision of the dorsoradial synovitis had been necessarily limited because of the proximity of the radial artery, so this case was probably not a good indication.

In terms of the Mayo Clinic wrist score, 90% of the isolated dorsal ganglia obtained an excellent or good result. The fair results in our series were due to concurrent pathologies such as radius malunion or chondrocalcinosis. Ostermann obtained similar results with a series of 38 patients (28 females and 10 males) who presented with an isolated dorsal ganglion.[12] Trauma was related in 22% of cases and indication was discomfort for 68% and cosmetic for 77% of cases. Radiographs were normal in all cases (no carpal bone synovial cysts). Arthroscopic portals were 6-R for the scope and 3-4 for the shaver. The ganglion had an intraarticular extension in 63% of cases. Many associated lesions were observed (42%), especially scapholunate ligament disorders. After a follow-up of 16 months Ostermann reported no recurrence and normalization of mobility and grip strength.

Indications

The complaints elicited by a ganglion depend essentially on its location and size and sometimes on its anatomical relationship to neighbouring structures (tendons, posterior interosseous nerve, radiocarpal articulation, etc). The desire for removal of this cosmetically disturbing deformity primarily leads the patients to seek medical treatment. A ganglion of shorter duration (<4 months) may be burst by firm compression. However, this crushing is often painful and ineffective, and the ganglion may recur.

For ganglia of longer duration aspiration of the intraganglionic fluid can be practised, which may be followed by injection of steroid medication. However, complete evacuation of the fluid is almost always impossible and the steroid medication is of little benefit against degenerative changes of the joint capsule, which usually lead the ganglion to recur (in 65% of the cases for Ostermann[12] and in 50% of the author's cases).

Thus the decision of most physicians to treat the ganglia by excision appears reasonable. However, despite the radical excision advocated by some authors,[1,2] the ganglion recurs in a high percentage of cases. This may be explained on the basis of failure to expose and thus remove all degenerative tissue.

If a ganglion occurs on a part of the body where scarring would be aesthetically unacceptable, then use of a procedure which would produce a better cosmetic result, at lower risk, would appear to be justified. Soren proposed a subcutaneous dissection to open all cavities of the ganglion.[3] He obtained good results with a

low recurrence rate (< 2%) but this 'blind' procedure seems dangerous in other hands. The extensor tendons are particularly at risk because of the subcutaneous manipulation of a tenotome.

Thus arthroscopic excision of ganglia as proposed by Whipple,[13] Ostermann[12] and Fontes[7,8] seems to be a suitable procedure for their treatment. This technique is very rewarding for dorsal ganglia located at the radiocarpal projection of the scapholunate space because of the requirement for only too small aesthetic portals without the necessity of complementary midcarpal exploration. The scope improves visualization of the degenerative tissue, facilitating its excision and avoiding any lesion of extensor tendons, interosseous ligaments and cartilage. Scarring and postoperative problems are minimized and the recurrence rate seems to decrease significantly compared to other procedures.

This original technique is a minimally invasive, cosmetic and logical alternative to the open excision of dorsal ganglia. It enables an exhaustive articular exploration to investigate and treat associated or previous lesions such as scapholunate ligament cysts. However, larger multicentric series with longer follow-up are needed for a full evaluation of the real rate of recurrence.

References

1   Angelides AC, Wallace PF, The dorsal ganglion of the wrist: its pathogenesis, growth and microscopic anatomy, and surgical treatment, *J Bone Joint Surg* (1976) **1**:228–35.

2   Razemon JP, Traitement chirurgical des kystes dits synoviaux du poignet avec exérèse capsulaire – à propos de 300 observations, *Ann Chir Main* (1983) **2**:230–43.

3   Soren A, Pathogenesis, clinic and treatment of ganglion, *Arch Orthop Traumat Surg* (1982) **99**:247–52.

4   Berger RA, The scapholunate ligament, *J Bone Joint Surg* (1982) **7**:87–90.

5   Crawford GP, Taleisnik J, Rotatory subluxation of the scaphoid after excision of dorsal carpal ganglion and wrist manipulation – a case report, *J Bone Joint Surg* (1983) **8**:921–4.

6   Duncan KH, Lewis RC Jr, Scapholunate instability following ganglion cyst excision, *Clin Orthop Rel Res* (1988) **228**:250–3.

7   Fontes D, Traitement arthroscopique des kystes synoviaux du poignet, *Lett Rhumatol* (1995) **209**:16–18.

8   Fontes D, Therapeutic interest of wrist arthroscopy – a series of 280 cases. *6th Congress of the IFSSH* (Monduzzi Editore: Bologna, 1995) 723–8.

9   Gunther SF, Dorsal wrist pain and the occult scapholunate ganglion, *J Hand Surg* (1985) **10A**:697–703.

10 Hixson ML, Microvascular anatomy of the radioscapholunate ligament of the wrist, *J Hand Surg* (1990) **15A**:279–82.

11 Le Viet D, Les kystes dits synoviaux du poignet et de la main. *Cahier d'enseignement de la Société Française de Chirurgie de la Main* (Expansion Scientifique Française: Paris, 1991) **3**:49–59.

12 Ostermann L, Arthroscopic management of the wrist ganglions (oral communication). *Wrist Advanced Winter Course* (Zermatt 1994)

13 Whipple TL, *Arthroscopic Surgery: The Wrist* (JB Lippincott: Philadelphia, 1992).

14 Viegas SF, Intraarticular ganglion of the dorsal interosseous scapholunate ligament: a case for arthroscopy, *Arthroscopy* (1986) **2**:93–5.

44

Arthro-CT for assessment of scapholunate ligament injuries

Isabelle Pigeau, Constantin Sokolow, Philippe Saffar and Philippe Valenti

Introduction

The long-term result of carpal ligament injuries is osteoarthritis (70% of wrist osteoarthritis results from wrist instability). Consequences such as this may be avoided by early diagnosis and treatment.[1] Many procedures have been recommended for the investigation of scapholunate (SL) ligament injuries. They may be divided in two types: dynamic and static investigations.

Dynamic investigations provide direct or indirect assessment of carpal and radioulnar bones and their ligament constraint:[1]

- Dynamic series: flexion, extension, radial and ulnar deviation radiographs
- Provocative tests: make a fist, anterior and posterior drawer maneuver at midcarpal joint, traction, and compression radiographs
- Cineradiography and cinearthrography[2]
- Arthroscopy,[3] which provides a direct visualization of cartilage and ligaments with the possibility of wrist movement: however, there are limitations in the visualization of the posterior part of the joint space.

Static examinations demonstrate the bone contours and dissociations:

- Plain radiographs: posteroanterior, lateral, oblique and specific views
- Arthrography[4-6] has important limitations due to overlapping bone contours and articular recesses, which result in contrast overlaps
- Magnetic resonance imaging (MRI)[7,8] is a promising technique because ligaments and cartilage are demonstrated without contrast injection; it is the only technique to show

extrinsic ligaments.[9] However, for interosseous ligaments, MRI seems to be currently less sensitive than arthroscan, which employs CT (arthro-CT)
- Arthro-CT combines arthrography and computed tomography: a small number of papers have mentioned this type of examination.[10] It seems to be currently the most sensitive imaging modality for the study of wrist ligaments and cartilage,[11,12] due to its ability to perform millimetric and contiguous slices and avoid overlaps (Figure 1).

Arthro-CT has been evaluated in 55 patients in assessment of the SL ligament. Results were compared with arthrography and surgical findings.

Materials and methods

In the period 1990–96, 520 arthro-CTs were performed for the assessment of ligament, bone, and/or cartilage injuries, mainly after traumatic injuries or in various pathologies (such as scaphoid nonunion, Kienböck's disease, and intraosseous ganglia). For this study we selected patients who underwent tricompartmental arthrography, arthro-CT, and then SL ligament exploration by surgery or arthroscopy, within a maximum delay of 2 months after radiographic examination. The first 150 arthro-CTs, performed between 1990 and 1992, were not included because the technique has been improved since then. We did not include cases in which arthro-CT was unable to show the complete radiocarpal or midcarpal joints; this involved 10 postoperative studies.

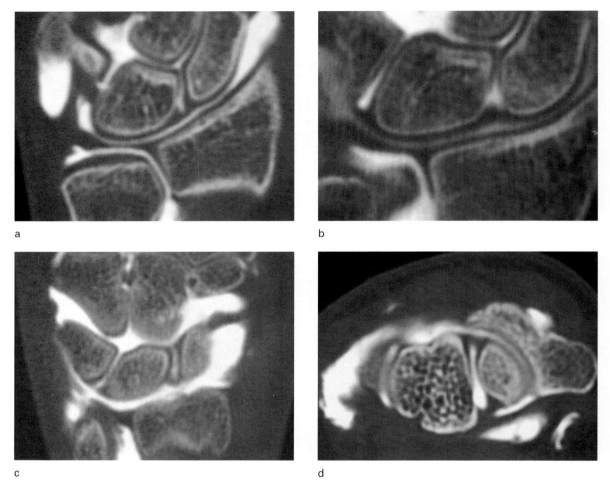

a

b

c

d

Figure 1

Normal scapholunate ligament, previously explored by arthroscopy. Arthro-CT: successive anterior, proximal, and posterior scans (a, b and c), axial scan (d). The normal successive anterior, proximal, and posterior parts of the ligament are well demonstrated on successive coronal slices. Lunotriquetral, TFCC ligaments, and cartilage (radioscaphoid, radiolunate, scaphocapitate, lunocapitate, distal ulna) are also depicted. The axial scan demonstrates the distal anterior and posterior parts of the scapholunate ligament.

Thus 55 cases were selected: 36 males and 19 females; 13 cases were postoperative examinations. The average age was 42.7 years. Exploration was performed by arthrotomy in 43 cases, arthroscopy in 6 cases. Six patients underwent both investigations. Artho-CT included a standard arthrography followed as soon as possible by CT examination (General Electric). Delay between the two examinations did not exceed 20 minutes. After that time there is a contrast dilution and an intracartilage diffusion which make interpretation impossible. This is particularly true in cases of neurosympathetic dystrophy, synovitis, or postoperative study. This disadvantage can be reduced by the use of 0.5 ml adrenaline, mixed with the contrast medium. Arthrography was performed under fluoroscopic control. In order for the examination to be considered complete, all three joints (midcarpal, radiocarpal, and distal radioulnar) had to be filled by contrast.

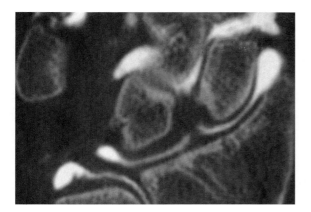

Figure 2

Stretched scapholunate ligament (anterior and coronal scan). The anterior part of the scapholunate ligament is obviously stretched, and measures 7 mm. There is no leakage and this is consistent with fibrosis and a scarred ligament tear (posttraumatic case). This stretched aspect was confirmed by arthrotomy.

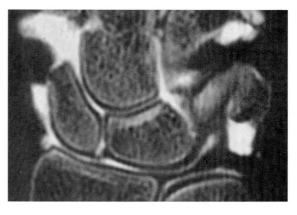

Figure 3

Thin scapholunate ligament (proximal and coronal scan). The proximal part of the scapholunate ligament is obviously thin but there is no tear. At arthroscopy a thinned ligament was also seen.

Preliminary results from our study showed that arthro-CT was able to visualize a significant number of small tears which were missed by single compartment arthrography.[10] These tears became obvious when injection was performed on both articular surfaces of the ligament, probably because the tear behaved like a door which can only be opened in one direction. Our normal procedure is to inject in the midcarpal joint, followed by the radioulnar and radiocarpal joints when these two joints were not filled by a leakage from the midcarpal joint.

Radiographs were taken during each injection and after motion. Tomography was performed when injection was finished. The patient was in the prone position, and the flexed elbow and wrist were firmly immobilized above the head. Arthro-CT was performed in the coronal, sagittal and axial planes, with 1 mm thick and contiguous slices. The coronal study analyzed the SL ligament from the volar to the dorsal plane, to visualize its successive anterior, proximal, and posterior parts. The axial plane studied the anterior and posterior parts, in their distal aspects. The sagittal plane was useful for cartilage study or triangular fibrocartilage complex (TFCC) assessment.

Surgical exploration demonstrated 28 SL ligaments in continuity and 27 tears. The results were analyzed as follows:

- If the ligament was in continuity, was it of normal appearance or was it stretched, thinned, or with an irregular surface?
- If there was a ligament tear, was it limited or complete? The site of the tear (anterior, proximal, or posterior part of the ligament) and extension (involving one, two, or all parts of the ligament) were indicated. The presence and status of the remaining ligament were examined.
- In all cases, associated tears of lunotriquetral ligament and/or TFCC were reported.

Arthro-CT findings were compared with results from arthrography and surgical data.

Results

Comparisons between arthro-CT and surgery (Table 1)

Ligaments in continuity at surgery

Of the 28 ligaments found to be in continuity at surgery, 15 were normal, 8 were stretched, 4 had an irregular surface, and 1 was thinned. The arthro-CT results correlated in 23 cases: 15 normal

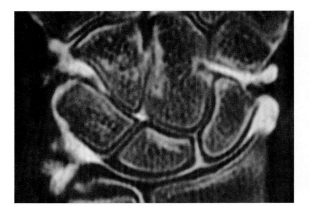

Figure 4

A complete tear of the scapholunate ligament (proximal and coronal scan). The tear involves the proximal part of the ligament, and also the anterior and posterior parts (not shown). There is no remaining ligament. The cartilage and TFCC are intact. There is an associated complete lunotriquetral tear, with a remaining ligament attached to the lunate bone.

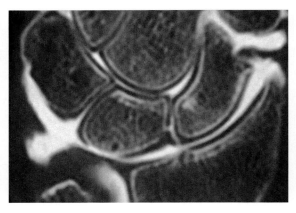

Figure 5

A complete tear of the scapholunate ligament (proximal and coronal scan). The tear involves the proximal part of the ligament, and also the anterior and posterior parts (not shown). This is a complete tear, but the ligament stump remains attached to the lunate bone, which allows a direct suture. The cartilage and TFCC are intact. There is an associated complete lunotriquetral tear, with no remaining ligament. Cartilage wear on the superomedial part of the lunate is evident.

ligaments, 6 stretched (Figure 2), 1 with an irregular surface due to postoperative fibrosis, and 1 thinned (Figure 3). In 8 cases of stretched ligaments, radiographs showed a diastasis. Arthro-CT showed a stretched ligament in 8 cases but continuity in 6 cases. Arthro-CT was not correlated in 5 cases: 3 which presented with an irregular surface and 2 which were stretched.

In two cases of stretched ligament, explored by arthroscopy, arthro-CT showed posterior limited tears, 2 mm thick. A leakage was obvious on arthrography, from the midcarpal to the radiocarpal joint, not explained by a lunotriquetral tear on arthro-CT or arthroscopy.

In the three cases with an irregular surface, arthro-CT showed two posterior tears and one anterior limited tear, less than 2 mm thick. One was related to a fold at arthrotomy and was diagnosed by arthro-CT as a posterior limited tear. There was a leakage on arthrography from the midcarpal to the radiocarpal joint, which could also be explained by a lunotriquetral tear, well demonstrated by arthro-CT and surgery. The second case presented with postoperative adhesions but was in continuity at arthrotomy.

Arthro-CT showed a limited anterior tear. A leakage was obvious on arthrography, not explained by a lunotriquetral tear on arthro-CT. The lunotriquetral ligament was not seen at surgery. The third case, with a very irregular surface at arthrotomy, was considered an anterior limited tear on arthro-CT. Arthrography showed a leak from the midcarpal to the radiocarpal joint. The lunotriquetral ligament was normal on both arthro-CT and arthrotomy.

Ligaments torn at surgery

27 ligaments were torn at surgery: 20 were complete and 7 were limited tears. Arthro-CT correlated in 26 cases: 19 complete and 7 limited tears. Of the 19 complete tears, arthro-CT and surgery both detected the presence of a remaining ligament, attached to the lunate bone in four cases (Figures 4 and 5), and to the scaphoid bone in one case. One complete tear explored by arthrotomy was interpreted on arthro-CT as a limited posterior-proximal tear (Figure 6). In fact, the remaining ligament had been misdiagnosed as an intact anterior part.

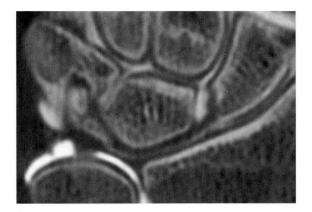

a

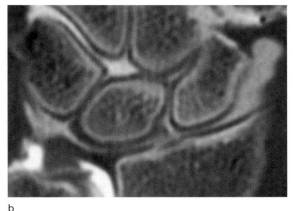

b

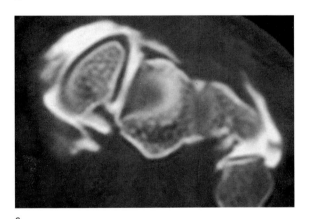

c

Figure 6

A limited posterior tear of the scapholunate ligament, successive proximal (a), posterior coronal (b) and axial (c) scans. Arthro-CT demonstrates an intact anterior and proximal part of the ligament (a), but a limited posterior tear (b), also nicely demonstrated on the axial view (c). A ligament stump remains attached to the lunate bone, with irregular margin, but a direct suture was possible at surgery. There is also a small posterior limited lunotriquetral tear. The TFCC and cartilage are intact.

Of the seven limited tears, arthro-CT and surgery correlated for the site in six cases: five involving the posterior part, one involving the anterior and proximal. In one case, arthroscopy demonstrated a proximal tear when arthro-CT described a posterior one.

If surgery is considered as the gold standard, sensibility and specificity are 95% and 100% for the diagnosis of continuous or torn ligaments, respectively; 100% and 88% for limited tears; and 100% and 100% for normal ligament.

Comparisons between arthro-CT and arthrography

Ligaments in continuity on arthro-CT

Twenty-three ligaments were in continuity on arthro-CT: 15 normal ligaments, 6 stretched, 1 with an irregular posterior surface due to postoperative fibrosis, and 1 thinned. Arthrography correlated in the cases of 14 ligaments in continuity (8 normal and 6 stretched). However, arthrography could not demonstrate an irregular posterior surface nor a thinned ligament. In 9 cases arthrography was unable to assess the continuity of the SL ligament. There was a leakage on arthrography, but the SL ligament was in continuity on arthro-CT and at surgery. The leakage was explained on arthro-CT by lunotriquetral tears.

Ligaments torn on arthro-CT

Arthro-CT showed 26 tears: 19 complete and 7 limited. Arthrography correlated in 21 cases (19 complete and two limited). Nevertheless, even though arthrography was able to demonstrate

Table 1 A comparison of arthro-CT and surgery.

	Complete tear	Limited tear	Ligament in continuity
Arthro-CT	19	13	23
Surgery	20	7	28

the SL site of the leakage in 19 complete tears, this method could not determine the nature of the tear (limited or complete), its extension or the status of the remaining ligaments. In two cases of limited tears, the precise site of the leakage (anterior, proximal, or posterior) could not be determined. Arthrography did not correlate with arthro-CT in five cases of limited tears: the leakage to the radiocarpal joint was obvious, but the site between the lunotriquetral and SL ligaments was uncertain.

Associated tears

Arthro-CT demonstrated 13 lunotriquetral and 11 TFCC tears. Tears were also shown on surgery in 9 cases of lunotriquetral and 8 cases of TFCC exploration.

Discussion

Arthro-CT scan is our method of choice for wrist ligament and cartilage examination, due to its ability to perform millimetric and contiguous slices in the required planes, avoiding overlaps. Articular distension created by injection facilitates the detection of very small ligament and/or cartilage injuries. A very precise and complete assessment of ligament and/or cartilage injuries is necessary to establish either a conservative or surgical treatment, and to define the surgical strategy: type of approach and stabilization (primary or secondary suture, or reattachment, capsulodesis, or limited carpal arthrodesis). Moreover, it is essential to determine the site of the tear, since the biomechanical role of each part of the ligament differs.[13] The proximal membranous part has no biomechanical role. A tear in this zone results in leakage during arthrography but does not have a bad prognosis. Conversely, the posterior part of the SL is biomechanically important: tears are followed by static or dynamic instability.

There are other interesting findings: limited posterior tears are more frequent than isolated anterior ones. The remaining ligament is in most cases (four out of five) attached to lunate bone. This study demonstrates that arthro-CT has significant advantages compared to arthrography. Arthrography was the standard,[2,4,5] but it has important limitations, as bone contours and articular recesses cause contrast overlaps. A ligament tear may be identified by a leakage at its site during injection or after wrist motion, but extension of this tear cannot be assessed by this method. No information is given about the status of the remaining ligament. Moreover, a ligament tear may be diagnosed but other smaller associated tears can be obscured when the injection is complete because of an articular recess overlap. For the same reason, small cartilage injuries can be missed.

The major disadvantage of arthrography is its inability to determine precisely the site of the leakage: it only visualizes the proximal part of the ligament which does not have an important biomechanical role. The anterior and posterior parts are not depicted in their lower portion, even by tomography.

In this study, arthro-CT correlated well with surgical findings (48 of 55 cases). They did not correlate in seven cases. Two cases were absolute failures of arthro-CT. One of the failures was due to a fold, interpreted as a 2 mm anterior limited tear; the leakage on arthrography could be also related to a lunotriquetral tear. In another case, arthro-CT diagnosed a limited proximal and posterior tear when arthrotomy showed a complete tear: the remaining ligament, anteriorly positioned, was misdiagnosed as an intact anterior part of the ligament.

Five cases reflected more discrepancies than failure since arthrotomy and arthroscopy also have their own limits: respectively, the anterior and posterior part of the ligament can be blinded. This could explain why arthro-CT showed an anterior or posterior limited tear when surgery demonstrated a ligament in continuity or when there is a leakage on arthrography which is not explained by a lunotriquetral tear. Results for sensibility and specificity are thus questionable since surgical findings might not reflect the gold standard. Nevertheless, these results show that there is no discordance for the normal ligament, very good results for complete tears and some discordance in cases of limited tears. Whereas the posterior part of the ligament is easily analyzed, the anterior part is more difficult since it is larger, with oblique oriented fibers, as also reported by Berger et al.[13]

The principal disadvantage of arthro-CT is its static aspect. Arthroscopy is certainly a more appropriate technique to assess ligament competence. Nevertheless, arthro-CT in combination with a dynamic radiographic series resolves most of the diagnostic problems. Arthroscopy should be reserved for therapeutic indications or when physical and radiological findings do not correlate. Arthro-CT also has some technical limitations for postoperative studies: wrist stiffness may make it impossible to perform a standard right coronal plane analysis. Semicoronal study is generally possible but analysis of the ligament is less precise. Intraarticular postoperative fibrosis is the principal limitation of the technique when the contrast is not able to diffuse homogeneously in the articular cavity. Conversely, hemosiderin deposits or material for bone fixation cause almost no artefacts with arthro-CT, as they do with MRI.

In comparison with arthroscopy, arthro-CT is a minimally invasive technique and is also less expensive. In comparison with arthrography, arthro-CT is more expensive (50–70%), but arthro-CT corrects many of the false results of arthrography and, moreover, provides additional information essential for treatment selection.

Conclusion

Arthro-CT has become the most sensitive imaging modality for the study of wrist ligaments and cartilage. This technique helps to determine treatment and surgical strategy and provides insights to pathophysiology. Ligament competence is quite well determined by a combination of arthro-CT and dynamic radiography. Arthroscopy should be reserved for treatment or when physical and radiological findings do not correlate.

Our series are still limited. Anatomic correlation and the results of a prospective study, still in progress, are needed to evaluate the true sensitivity and specificity of arthro-CT.

References

1   Saffar Ph, *Les traumatismes du Carpe. Anatomie, Radiologie et Traitement Actuel* (Springer-Verlag: Paris, 1989).

2   Saffar Ph, Sokolow C, Mathoulin C, et al, Cine-arthrography of the wrist in carpal instability. In: Brunelli G, Saffar Ph, eds, *Wrist Imaging* (Springer-Verlag: Paris, 1992) 109–31.

3   Bour C, Merle M, Wrist arthroscopy: In: Brunelli G, Saffar Ph, eds, *Wrist Imaging* (Springer-Verlag: Paris, 1992) 133–9.

4   Gilula LA, Hardy DC, Totty WB, et al, Fluoroscopic identification of torn intercarpal ligaments after injection of contrast material, *AJR* (1987) **149**:761–4.

5   Quinn SF, Pittman CC, Belsole RS, Digital subtraction wrist arthrography: evaluation of the multiple compartment technique, *AJR* (1988) **151**:1173–4.

6   Metz VM, Mann FA, Gilula LA, Three-compartment wrist arthrography: correlation of pain site with location of uni- and bidirectional communications, *AJR* (1993) **160**:819–22.

7   Zlatkin MB, Chao PC, Osterman AL, et al, Chronic wrist pain: evaluation with high-resolution MR imaging, *Radiology* (1989) **173**: 723–9.

8   Gundry CR, Kursunoglu-Brahme S, Schwaighofer B, Is MR better than arthrography for evaluating the ligaments of the wrist? In vitro study, *AJR* (1990) **154**:337–41.

9   Pigeau I, Frija G, Seeman I, et al, Advantages of MRI in the study of the wrist ligaments. In: Brunelli G, Saffar Ph, eds, *Wrist Imaging* (Springer-Verlag: Paris, 1992) 173–82.

10 Quinn SF, Belsole RS, Greene TL, et al, Work in progress: postarthrography computed tomography of the wrist: evaluation of the triangular fibrocartilage complex, *Skeletal Radiol* (1989) **17**:565–9.

11 Pigeau I, Sokolow C, Saffar Ph, et al, Apport de l'arthro-CTner dans les lésions ligamentaires du poignet (ligaments interosseux et triangulaire). Comparaison avec l'arthrographie conventionnelle. Communication au Ier Congrès Européen de Chirurgie de la main. Bruxelles 26–30 May 1993.

12 Pigeau I, Sokolow C, Saffar Ph, et al, Apport de l'arthroscanner dans le bilan préchirurgical des lésions ligamentaires du poignet. Communication à la Société Française de Chirurgie de la Main, Paris, 8–11 December 1993.

13 Berger RA, Blair WF, Crowninshield RD, et al, The scapholunate ligament, *J Hand Surg* (1982) **7**:87–91.

Reconstruction of the scapholunate ligament using a vascularized flap of the interosseous membrane

Frédéric A Schuind, Sinna Alemzadeh, Fabienne Dhaene and Véronique Feipel

Introduction

The scapholunate interosseous ligament connects the scaphoid and the lunate bones by spanning the proximal, dorsal and palmar margins of the scapholunate joint. This interosseous ligament complex, particularly its strongest dorsal region, composed of collagen fascicules oriented in a parallel fashion, has been demonstrated to be a critical structure for maintaining carpal stability.[1,2] Disruption or elongation of the scapholunate ligament is associated with the clinical condition termed dorsal intercalated segmental instability, characterized by widening of the space between the scaphoid and the lunate, palmar flexion of the scaphoid, and lunotriquetral dorsiflexion. This causes a redistribution of the force transmission through the wrist. Chronic instability therefore leads to degenerative changes and secondary osteoarthritis.[3–6]

Treatment of chronic scapholunate dissociation remains difficult. The results of scapholunate interosseous ligament reconstruction by dorsal capsulodesis or by tendon ligamentoplasty are unpredictable. Limited wrist arthrodesis is a demanding procedure, with potential pitfalls and frequent complications, and has important consequences on the kinematics of the wrist.[7]

We had the idea to use the interosseous membrane of the forearm as a vascularized ligamentous flap to reconstruct the disrupted scapholunate membrane. The surgical technique that will be reviewed in this chapter, has already been published.[8] We present here an original anatomical study, demonstrating the feasibility of the surgical procedure, and then discuss our preliminary clinical results.

Anatomical study

Materials and methods

Sixteen preserved upper extremity cadaver specimens (8 male, 8 female) were used. The vascular anatomy of the interosseous vessels was studied. All measurements were expressed with the radial styloid as reference landmark. The external diameter of the vessels was measured using a precision vernier.

Results

The interosseous membrane is vascularized by the anterior interosseous artery. The artery contributes to the vascularization of the volar and dorsal aspects of the forearm.[9–11]

The origin of the interosseous arteries was, in most cases, the common interosseous artery. This always originated in the ulnar artery, under the elbow, except in one case (6.3%) where the common interosseous artery originated directly in the brachial artery in the upper part of the arm. In three cases (18.8%) there was no common interosseous artery, in the sense that both posterior and anterior interosseous arteries originated directly in the ulnar artery.

The common interosseous artery had a mean diameter of 2.7 mm (median 2.7 mm, standard deviation 0.9 mm, range 1.8–3.6 mm). After a mean distance of 7.5 mm (median 5 mm, SD 6.9 mm, range 2–27 mm), the common interosseous artery divided in its two terminal branches, the anterior and the posterior interosseous arteries.

At its origin, which was situated at a mean distance of 178.3 mm from the radial styloid (median 175 mm, SD 16.9 mm, Range 158–205 mm), the anterior interosseous artery had a mean external diameter of 1.8 mm (median 1.6 mm, SD 0.4 mm, range 1.4–2.8 mm). The mean diameter of the posterior interosseous artery at its origin from the common interosseous artery was 1.8 mm (median 2.0 mm, SD 0.5 mm, range 1.1–2.5 mm).

The anterior interosseous artery, always accompanied by two veins, descended within the volar aspect of the forearm, applied on the interosseous membrane, inbetween the flexor pollicis longus and the flexor digitorum profundus. The artery contributed to the vascularization of the volar and dorsal aspects of the forearm. We counted a mean of 18.2 collateral branches originating from the anterior interosseous artery within the forearm (median 18, SD 2.9, range 15–27). Among these branches, an average of 9.8 (median 9.5, SD 2.1, range 6–14) perforated the membrane, for the vascularization of the interosseous membrane and of the dorsal forearm.

At the distal third of the forearm, the artery was located on the volar aspect of the forearm interosseous membrane, deep to the pronator quadratus in most of the cases. The proximal border of the pronator quadratus was situated at 64.5 mm, on average, from the radial styloid (median 65 mm, SD 12.4 mm, range 30–85 mm). At this level the artery had an average external diameter of 1.2 mm (median 1.1 mm, SD 0.3 mm, range 0.7–1.8 mm) and was sometimes already partially covered by fibres of the interosseous membrane. Under the proximal border of the muscle, at an average of 64.2 mm from the radial styloid (median 63 mm, SD 9.6 mm, range 45–76 mm), the anterior interosseous vessels, still comprising one artery and two veins, perforated the interosseous membrane.

In all our cases, and in 95% of those reported by Hu et al,[9] a medial branch arose which anastomosed with the posterior interosseous artery.[12,13] The artery, which had now a mean diameter of 0.8 mm (range 0.5–1 mm), participated in the dorsal vascular network of the wrist.

Surgical technique

After ligature of the anterior interosseous vessels proximally, the surgical procedure consists of transferring to the scapholunate interval a rectangular interosseous membrane island flap, based on the retrograde blood flow through the anterior interosseous vessels, supplied by the dorsal vascular network of the wrist and/or by the medial anastomosis with the posterior interosseous vessels (Figures 1–3).

The distal third of the forearm and the wrist are approached through a longitudinal incision centred just ulnar to Lister's tubercle. The extensor retinaculum is opened as a radially-based flap. Arthrotomy confirms the scapholunate ligament rupture and the impossibility of secondary repair.

The dissection is carried out through the intermuscular space, between the long finger extensor and the wrist and thumb extensor muscles (Figure 3f). The distal part of the anterior interosseous artery is exposed as well as its medial anastomosis with the posterior interosseous artery. The location of this anastomosis determines the point of rotation of the flap, as the dorsal vascular network of the wrist can be compromised by the transcapsular approach to the carpal bones. The interosseous membrane is opened at the proximal border of the flap. The anterior interosseous vessels, at this site volar to the membrane, are then ligated and attached to the membrane. The flap is then raised, turned (Figure 3h) and attached to the lunate and to the scaphoid bones. It is important to align the fibres of the membrane perpendicular to the interosseous space and to avoid compression of the vascular pedicle (Figure 3i). For the fixation we use mini Mitek anchors (Mitek Surgical Products Inc, Norwood, MA, USA) inserted within the lunate and the scaphoid.

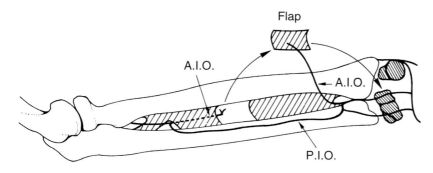

Figure 1

Schematic drawing of the surgical procedure (AIO: anterior interosseous artery, PIO: posterior interosseous artery).

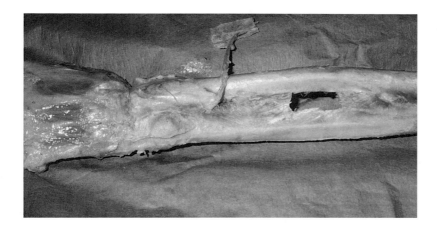

Figure 2

Dissection of the interosseous membrane and of the island flap in a preserved cadaver specimen.

Before the sutures are tightened, the carpal bones are anatomically reduced by means of one Kirschner wire (Figure 3j).

The retinacular flap is relocated under the extensor tendons. The wrist is then immobilized by a plaster cast for at least 6 weeks. Physiotherapy is then instituted until acceptable functional recovery is achieved.

Further details concerning the surgical procedure have been reported elsewhere.[8]

Clinical experience

We were very careful and our clinical experience is therefore limited. After we operated on the first case we waited for 2 years in order to assess the results before operating on other patients.

Our first case, reported previously,[8] has by now a follow-up duration of 35 months, and the subjective and objective results are satisfactory. The results were also good in the more recent cases (Figure 3). However, some lengthening of the ligamentoplasty was observed in all cases. At the time of ligament repair, one patient presented already with some radioscaphoid osteoarthritis. After the successful reconstruction of the scapholunate membrane, the patient went back to work but continued to complain of pain at the degenerated radioscaphoid joint. As the patient undertook heavy work we finally decided to perform a total wrist fusion. After the arthrotomy, we found a strong and healed ligament spanning the proximal, dorsal and palmar margins of the scapholunate joint. Histologically, the ligament was found to be well vascularized and strongly anchored to the scaphoid and

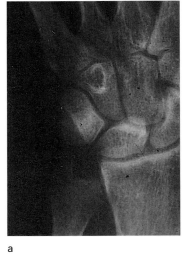

a

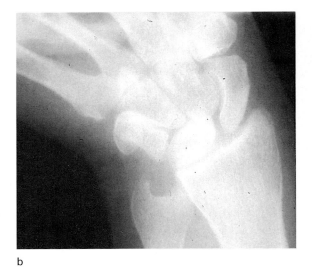

b

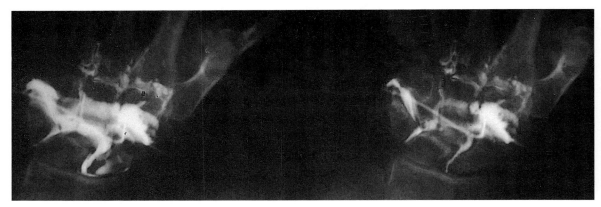

c

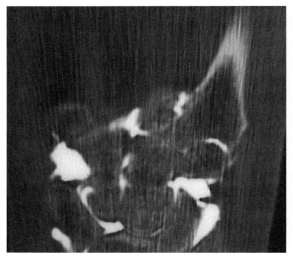

d

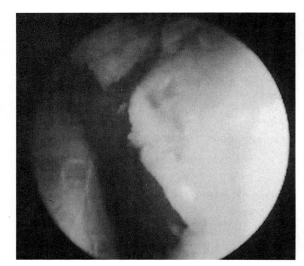

e

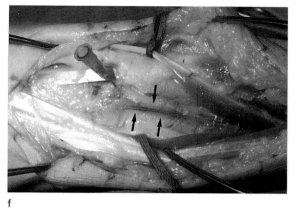

f

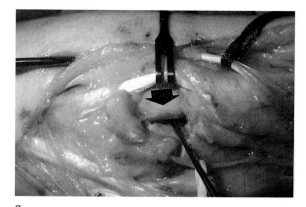

g

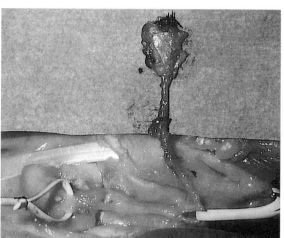

h

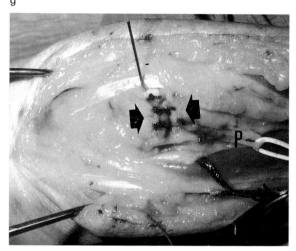

i

Figure 3

Clinical case of scapholunate disruption in a 44-year-old patient. (a–d) The preoperative dynamic radiographs, arthrography and arthro-CT clearly demonstrate an abnormal gap between the scaphoid and lunate. (e) Arthroscopic confirmation of the scapholunate tear (midcarpal view). (f) Operative views. The needle is inserted within the radiocarpal joint and the distal part of the interosseous vessels is clearly visible (arrows). (g) After arthrotomy, the disruption of the scapholunate membrane is evident, and the scaphoid and lunate bones can easily be separated from each other (arrow). (h) The interosseous membrane flap has been isolated on its nutrient vessels. (i) After scapholunate repair (arrows), the preserved pedicle (P) is clearly visible). (j) Radiological results: ligament fixation using Mitek anchors, scapholunate fixation using Mitek anchors, scapholunate fixation using a Kirschner wire.

j

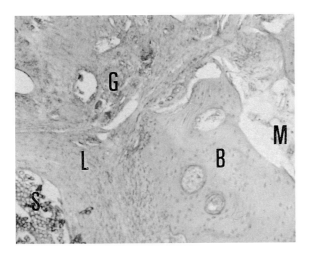

Figure 4

Histological section 1 year after scapholunate repair using the vascularized interosseous membrane flap. The viability of the ligament (L) is preserved. The ligament (L) is strongly anchored to the scaphoid bone (B). M: bone marrow S: broken suture material (Ticron) with foreign body granulomatous reaction (G). (Courtesy of Professor JL Pastels, Brussels.)

lunate bones. There was some granulomatous reaction to broken suture material (Figure 4).

Discussion

The best treatment of chronic scapholunate dissociation is probably direct repair of the torn ligament, particularly of its dorsal part. Even several months after the injury, there is sometimes sufficient ligament to perform a direct reapproximation of the structure. However, in most cases, a satisfactory repair is impossible. In these cases, reconstruction using tendon graft augmentation has been recommended. However, such procedures lose effectiveness with time, possibly because of the differences in material properties between normal ligament and tendon.[14] The interosseous membrane, on the other hand, behaves like a ligament, linking the radius to the ulna.[15] It is easily possible to show that the interosseous

fibres follow the normal arrangement of the original scapholunate ligament. The flat appearance of the scapholunate membrane can also be restored. Whether important or not, the communication between the radiocarpal and midcarpal joints may be closed. Moreover, because it is possible to keep the vascularization to the interosseous membrane flap, one can hope that the transfer will not undergo necrosis, with loss of its mechanical properties over time. This may be especially important if one considers the well known precarity of the osseous vascularization to the scaphoid and lunate bones. Further clinical experience and biomechanical studies are needed to delineate, in the future, the precise indications of this new technique.

References

1   Berger RA, Blair WF, Crowninshield RD, et al, The scapholunate ligament, *J Hand Surg* (1982) **7A**:87–91.
2   Berger RA, Imaeda T, Berglund L, et al, The anatomic, constraint and material properties of the scapholunate interosseous ligament: a preliminary study. In: Schuind F, An KN, Cooney WP, et al, eds, *Advances in the Biomechanics of the Hand and Wrist* (Plenum: London, 1994) 9–16.
3   Green DP, Carpal dislocations and instabilities. In: Green DP, ed, *Operative Hand Surgery* (Churchill Livingstone: New York, 1993) 861–928.
4   Linscheid RL, Dobyns JH, Beabout JW, et al, Traumatic instability of the wrist: diagnosis, classification, and pathomechanics, *J Bone Joint Surg* (1972) **54A**:1612–32.
5   Viegas SF, Patterson RM, Contact pressures within wrist joints. In: Schuind F, An KN, Cooney WP, et al, eds, *Advances in the Biomechanics of the Hand and Wrist* (Plenum: London, 1994) 137–51.
6   Watson HK, Ballet FL, The SLAC wrist: scapholunate advanced collapse pattern of degenerative arthritis, *J Hand Surg* (1984) **9A**:358–65.
7   McAuliffe JA, Dell PC, Jaffe R, Complications of intercarpal arthrodesis, *J Hand Surg* (1993) **18A**:1121–8.
8   Schuind F, Scapholunate reconstruction using a vascularized flap of the interosseous membrane, *J Orthop Surg Tech* (1996) **9**:21–6.
9   Hu W, Martin D, Baudet J, The anterior interosseous retrograde island flap. Anatomic study and clinical applications. (Abstract) In: *First Congress of the Federation of the European*

Societies for Surgery of the Hand, Brussels, May 1993 (Longman: London, 1993) 15.

10 Pahl S, Schmidt HM, Klinische Anatomie der interossären Arterien des Unterarmes, *Mikrochir Plast Chir* (1994) **26**:246–50.

11 Schmidt HM, Lanz U, *Chirurgische Anatomie der Hand* (Hippokrates: Stuttgart, 1992).

12 Masquelet AC, Penteado CV, Le lambeau interosseux postérieur, *Ann Chir Main* (1987) **6**:131–9.

13 Zancolli EA, Angrigiani C, Posterior interosseous island forearm flap, *J Hand Surg* (1988) **13B**:130–5.

14 Kuhlmann JN, Luboinski J, Laudet C, et al, Properties of the fibrous structures of the wrist, *J Hand Surg* (1990) **15B**:335–41.

15 Hotchkiss RN, An KN, Siwa DT, et al, An anatomic and mechanical study of the interosseous membrane of the forearm: pathomechanics of proximal migration of the radius, *J Hand Surg* (1989) **14A**:256–61.

Commentary

Chapter 43

This technique is difficult and time consuming and should be reserved for skilled wrist arthroscopists. The 1-2 portal is not a usual one and a good intraarticular visualization is not easy. However, it is logical to remove ganglia at their roots.

PS

Chapter 44

The combination of arthrography and immediate postarthrography CT imaging adds important detail to the arthrographic study, specifically in delineating the size and shape of defects. Some drawbacks, however, remain. Without direct inspection of probing of cartilage, ligaments and bone, flaps, chondromalacia and lax ligaments are difficult to identify. In contrast to direct inspection via arthroscopy or open surgery, both false positives and false negatives exist. Granted, it is not always clear what the 'gold standard' might be; our understanding of carpal instability remains incomplete. Yet I believe that both arthro-CT and arthroscopy have a place in our diagnostic armamentarium. In cases where the diagnosis seems likely on clinical grounds, and an arthroscopic surgical solution is a possibility if the diagnosis is confirmed, I would favor arthroscopy over arthro-CT. Where the diagnosis is less clear, and in particular if any bony pathology is suspected, then I would favor arthro-CT evaluation.

PCA

Chapter 45

We are anxious to know the long-term results of this interesting technique, because the problem of scapholunate ligament repair by soft tissue techniques has not been resolved.

PS

46

Vascularized pedicle grafts from the dorsal distal radius: Design and application for carpal pathology

Allen T Bishop

Introduction

The blood supply to the distal dorsal radius is robust and constant, provided by a series of longitudinal vessels which demonstrate consistent spatial relationships to surrounding anatomic landmarks. We have recently described the anatomy of the vascular supply of the distal radius in some detail.[1] By demonstrating the extraosseous vessels and their nutrient artery size and intraosseous course, this study has made possible the design of several pedicled vascularized bone grafts based on distal anastomotic connections which will reach the carpus for clinical use. These grafts are easily harvested through the same operative field used for carpal exposure, with minimal additional morbidity. They provide living bone based on a reverse-flow arteriovenous pedicle analogous to the radial forearm flap.[2] This bone may be used to aid or accelerate fracture healing, replace bone deficiency, or aid in direct revascularization of ischemic bone.

Anatomy

Dorsal blood supply

Four extraosseous vessels contribute nutrient vessels to the distal radius and ulna (Figure 1). The anterior interosseous artery divides into anterior and posterior divisions proximal to the distal radioulnar joint. Its posterior division and

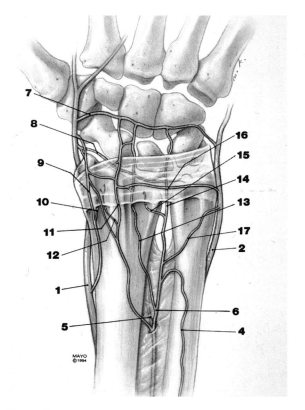

Figure 1

Blood supply of distal radius (dorsal aspect): 1, Radial artery; 2, ulnar artery; 4, posterior interosseous artery; 5, anterior division, anterior interosseous artery; 6, posterior division, anterior interosseous artery; 7, dorsal intercarpal arch; 8, dorsal radiocarpal arch; 9, 1,2 ICSRA; 10, 2nd EC br, 1,2 ICSRA; 11, 2,3 ICSRA; 12, 2nd EC br, 2,3 ICSRA; 13, 4th ECA; 14, 5th ECA; 15, 4th EC br, 5th ECA; 16, dorsal supraretinacular arch; 17, dorsal oblique artery of the distal ulna.

Table 1

Artery supplying nutrient arteries	Number of nutrient arteries [mean (range)]	Nutrient artery internal diameter (mm) [mean (range)]	Distance from nutrient artery penetration to RC joint (mm) [mean (range)]	Nutrient arteries that penetrate cancellous bone (%)
1,2 ICSRA	3.2 (0–9)	<0.10 (<0.05–0.15)	15 (4–26)	6
2nd EC br of 1,2 ICSRA	1 (1)	0.16 (0.14–0.19)	21 (17–28)	57
2,3 ICSRA	1.8 (0–5)	0.11 (0.07–0.19)	13 (3–24)	22
2nd EC br of 2,3 ICSRA	1.4 (1–4)	0.19 (0.09–0.28)	18 (14–32)	48
4th ECA	3.2 (1–6)	0.16 (0.07–0.29)	11 (3–19)	45
4th EC br of 5th ECA	1.2 (1–2)	0.15 0.15	10 (6–12)	43
dRCa	2.6 (0–7)	0.18 (0.14–0.29)	4 (1–12)	79
ODA distal ulna	3.3 (0–9)	0.20 (0.11–0.27)	11 (1–18)	42

Note: br = branch, EC = extensor communis, ECA = extensor compartment artery, dRCa = dorsal radiocarpal arch, ODA = oblique dorsal artery of distal ulna.

the radial artery are the primary sources of orthograde blood flow to the distal radius.

The four vessels supplying nutrient arteries to the dorsal radius are best described by their relationship to the extensor compartments of the wrist and the extensor retinaculum. Two of the vessels are superficial in location, lying on the dorsal surface of the extensor retinaculum between the first and second, and second and third dorsal compartments. Because of their location, they have been named the 1,2 and 2,3 intercompartmental supraretinacular arteries (1,2 and 2,3 ICSRA) (Figure 1).[1]

Two deep vessels also provide nutrient vessels to the dorsal distal radius. They lie on the surface of the radius in the floor of the fourth and fifth dorsal compartments. They are consequently named the fourth and fifth extensor compartment arteries (4th and 5th ECA) (Figure 1).[1]

The 1,2 intercompartmental supraretinacular artery (1,2 ICSRA) (Figure 1, Table 1) originates from the radial artery approximately 5 cm proximal to the radiocarpal joint. Its position superficial to the retinaculum and directly on the bony tuber-

cle between the first and second extensor compartments make its dissection and use as a vascularized pedicled graft to the scaphoid fairly straightforward. However, its arc of rotation is short, and its nutrient artery branches small in number and caliber.

The 2,3 intercompartmental supraretinacular artery (2,3 ICSRA) (Figure 1, Table 1) originates proximally from the anterior interosseous artery or the posterior division of the anterior interosseous artery. Like the 1,2 ICSRA, the 2,3 ICSRA is easily based as a retrograde pedicle for a vascularized bone graft because of its position superficial to the retinaculum (Figure 1). Because of its midaxial dorsal position, its arc of rotation reaches the entire proximal carpal row. Its nutrient arteries are somewhat larger and more likely to supply cancellous bone than those of the 1,2 ICSRA, particularly if a proximal branch to the floor of the second compartment is included. It is potentially useful for Kienböck's disease.

The fourth extensor compartment artery (4th ECA) (Figure 1, Table 1) lies directly adjacent to the posterior interosseous nerve on the radial aspect

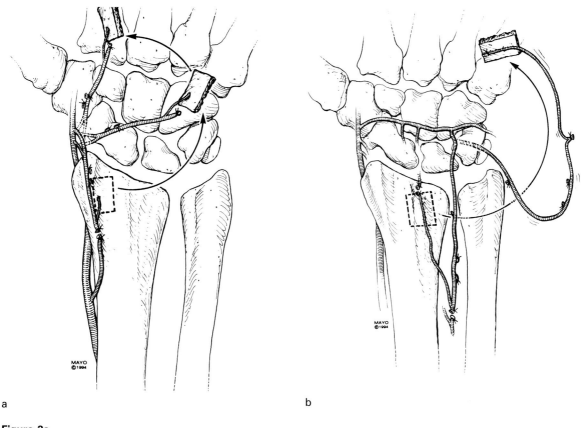

a   b

Figure 2a

(a) Modified 1,2 ICSRA graft. (b) 4th plus 5th ECA graft.

of the fourth extensor compartment. The 4th ECA is the source of numerous nutrient vessels to the floor of the fourth compartment that frequently penetrate cancellous bone (Table 1). The vessels entering more distally tend to supply primarily cortical bone, whereas those more proximal are more likely to penetrate cancellous bone.

The fifth extensor compartment artery (5th ECA) (Figure 1, Table 1) is generally the largest of all the dorsal vessels supplying nutrient branches (mean 0.49 mm internal diameter). It is located in the radial floor of the fifth extensor compartment, passing mostly through the 4,5 septum in one third of specimens.[1] It is perhaps most useful as a large conduit of retrograde flow from the intercarpal arch to other vessels with

more consistent nutrient branches. Its large diameter and multiple anastomoses allow creation of a vascular pedicle that can reach almost anywhere in the hand (Figure 2b).

Distal anastomoses

A series of arches across the dorsum of the hand and wrist provide anastomoses with these inter-compartmental and compartmental arteries. These include the dorsal intercarpal arch (dICa), dorsal radiocarpal arch (dRCa), and dorsal supra-retinacular arch (Figure 1).

The dICa does not contribute nutrient arteries to the distal radius or distal ulna except indirectly through arteries with which it connects. It is an important part of several potential grafts because of its anastomotic connections. The arch can be used as a source of retrograde arterial flow allowing proximal vessel ligation and graft mobilization.

The dRCa contributes significantly to the dorsal distal radius via small nutrient arteries. Because of its close proximity to the radius and location on or deep to the superficial joint capsule, it has limited usefulness as a potential source of retrograde arterial flow due to limited arc or rotation and difficult dissection.

A dorsal supraretinacular arch (Figure 1) provides anastomoses between the arteries running parallel to the radial and ulnar diaphyses. It is not a single artery but, rather, an anastomotic network of small vessels connecting the dorsal arteries. Because of its small caliber vessels, it is not of great utility in providing retrograde bone graft pedicle blood flow.

Technical aspects: elevation of vascularized bone grafts

1,2 ICSRA graft

Grafts based upon a retrograde 1,2 ICSRA pedicle were originally described by Zaidenberg et al for scaphoid nonunion.[3] It is important to note that the vessel lies superficial to extensor retinaculum, and is thus easily visible after retraction of the skin and subcutaneous tissues (Figure 3). It is not useful for other carpal bones due to its limited arc of rotation.

The 1,2 ICSRA is visualized on the surface of the extensor retinaculum, and dissected carefully towards its distal anastomosis with the radial artery. The first and second dorsal compartments are opened at the graft elevation site to create a cuff of retinaculum containing the vessels and their nutrient branches. The center of the graft should be 1.5 cm proximal to the radiocarpal joint to include the nutrient vessels. A graft of appropriate dimension, including the vessel and cuff of retinaculum, is raised using osteotomes. The graft is transposed beneath the radial wrist extensor tendons to reach the nonunion site, where it is gently impacted into position with the vessels

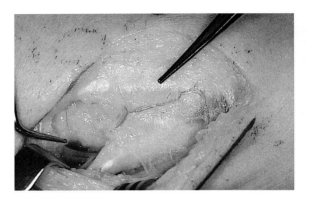

Figure 3

1,2 ICSRA in a clinical case.

and cortical bone lying on the dorsal surface of the bone. Initial stability is provided by Kirschner wire or compression screw fixation. The pedicle may be prolonged by including the branch to the second extensor compartment when present, increasing its arc of rotation (Figure 2a).

2,3 ICSRA graft

The 2,3 ICSRA allows elevation of a vascularized graft from the dorsal tubercle of the distal radius via its distal anastomosis to the dorsal intercarpal arch. Its placement is ideal for the lunate or the proximal scaphoid pole. Elevation is performed similarly to the 1,2 ICSRA, and is likewise technically relatively simple because of its superficial location. Protection of the distal pedicle is crucial, however, and its dissection and mobilization must be performed prior to joint capsulotomy to preserve its integrity. The graft should be centered 13 mm proximal to the radiocarpal joint, in order to include its nutrient vessels. In Kienböck's disease, the graft is oriented to allow the dorsal radial cortex and attached vessels to enter the lunate oriented vertically (ligated proximal vessel placed deeply into lunate), using the underlying graft cortical bone as a strut to help prevent lunate collapse during revascularization.

4th ECA graft

A fourth extensor compartment artery graft based on retrograde flow from the intercarpal arch may also be useful. Its arc of rotation consistently reaches the lunate. The nutrient arteries are numerous and large, but some may penetrate and supply bone too near the radiocarpal joint to make their inclusion desirable. Nevertheless, there are almost always one or more nutrient vessels penetrating the floor of the fourth extensor compartment a sufficient distance from the radiocarpal joint to make a graft based on the 4th ECA and the intercarpal arch potentially useful.

4th plus 5th ECA graft

In most cases, I now prefer to use the 5th ECA as the source of retrograde blood flow (Figure 2b). Its large diameter provides optimal blood flow to the bone graft. Other important advantages are the very long pedicle this design creates, and the ulnar location of the 5th ECA. It is therefore relatively protected from injury with wrist capsulotomy and carpal bone exposure.

Bone graft harvest requires identification of the 5th ECA by opening of the fifth dorsal compartment. The vessel is easily visualized on the radial aspect of the compartment with retraction of the extensor digiti minimi tendon. It is traced proximally to its origin from the anterior interosseous artery. The 4th ECA and 2,3 ICSRA origins should be identified and included with the distally-based 5th ECA pedicle, the anterior interosseous artery. This creates a lengthy pedicle with retrograde flow from the 5th ECA, continuing in an orthograde fashion into the other vessels. A bone graft is then raised based on one or both of these vessels. Figure 2b demonstrates the use of bone based on the 4th ECA nutrient vessel.

Indications

Vascularized bone grafts from the dorsal distal radius are potentially useful in scaphoid fractures and avascular necrosis, and in Kienböck's disease.

Pros and cons compared to classical techniques

Scaphoid fracture

Vascularized bone grafting offers the advantages of a supply of living bone with no need for creeping substitution and a reduced risk of stress fracture. It may allow revascularization of an ischemic proximal pole, and has been demonstrated to result in shorter healing times than those expected with conventional grafts.[4] However, in chronic nonunions with a significant 'humpback' deformity and bone loss, the radius graft may not be of sufficient size or structural quality to provide adequate reconstruction.

Kienböck's disease

In Kienböck's disease, conventional treatment is directed at altering loads placed on the avascular lunate.[5,6] For example, various intercarpal fusions, joint leveling by radial shortening or ulnar lengthening, or capitate shortening have been shown to be useful. Vascularized bone grafts offer a potential solution to the primary problem, that of deficient blood supply, while also permitting expansion of the lunate height by placement of a corticocancellous bone graft. They are a particularly appealing option in ulnar neutral or positive variance, when joint leveling cannot be done. Possible problems associated with vascularized grafts include structural weakening of the lunate with revascularization, possibly worsening the extent of carpal instability and subsequent arthritis, and inability to use a graft in advanced cases with extrusion of a volar or dorsal fragment or associated with degenerative arthritis. In such cases, salvage by lunate excision and intercarpal fusion is preferable.

Results

Kienböck's disease

We have reviewed the results of nine vascularized grafts obtained from the radial metaphysis in patients with Kienböck's disease, using the reverse-flow pedicles described above.[1] These included grafts based on the 2,3 ICSRA in two patients, 4th ECA in four, 5th plus 4th ECA in two, and palmar radiocarpal arch in one. The procedure was used without joint leveling in four patients who had ulnar neutral or positive variance. Three patients with ulnar negative variance had a concomitant radial shortening. Eight out of nine patients had external fixation for temporary lunate unloading. Follow-up averaged 32 months (range 7–90).

Clinical results were very satisfactory. Pain was absent in six, and mild and occasional in three. With the use of a satisfaction scale of 0 (completely dissatisfied) to 5 (very satisfied), patients averaged 4.2 (range 2.5–5). Grip strength improved by 25%, ultimately measuring a mean of 86% of the opposite side (range 60–100%). Range of motion was not significantly different from preoperative status. Mean carpal height ratio (CHR), lunate index (LI), and scapholunate angle (SL) were unchanged from preoperative values. Only two patients were without collapse preoperatively, based on the CHR value. Both progressed postoperatively, although absolute numerical change was slight. Subjectively, lunate sclerosis resolved with time, but lunate fractures failed to heal in four out of five patients. MRI data demonstrated progressive signs of revascularization with time. Normalization of T2 values was seen first, generally by 18 months, followed by T1 values by 36 months.

Scaphoid nonunion

Fifteen patients with established scaphoid nonunions have been treated by vascularized bone grafting. All were males with an average age of 27.6 years (range 17–42). The time interval from injury to surgery averaged 36.2 months (range 3 months–10 years). Five patients had prior attempts at conventional autogenous bone grafting which failed. In six patients the fracture was located at the scaphoid waist and in seven patients in the proximal third. Six patients had radiographic or MRI suggestion of proximal fragment avascular necrosis. Six patients had early radiocarpal joint degenerative changes. In 14 patients, the 1,2 ICSRA was utilized as a vascularized pedicle for bone graft from the dorsal radial aspect of the radius. Twelve patients had the graft placed with a dorsal inlay technique. In three patients the graft was placed palmarly to correct scaphoid malalignment. Four patients had a concurrent partial radial styloidectomy. Five patients had supplemental nonvascularized bone graft from the distal radius. Fracture fixation included Herbert screw or Kirschner wire stabilization in the majority. Immobilization consisted of a long arm cast initially, followed by a short arm cast until healing was demonstrable by trispiral tomography.

Follow-up averaged 2.5 years (range 1–4 years). All patients achieved union. Time to union averaged 11.1 weeks (range 5.5–16 weeks), judged by bridging trabeculae on trispiral tomography. Subjectively 66% were very satisfied with the results of surgery. Seventy per cent had only occasional pain or discomfort with strenuous activity. Fifty-eight per cent had returned to their usual work and leisure activity with only mild limitations. There were no perioperative complications, but three patients, all with preoperative degenerative changes, had additional surgery: one styloidectomy, one dorsal neurectomy, and one complete wrist fusion. Eighty per cent demonstrated a postoperative range of motion average flexion/extension arc of at least 90° and an average ulnar/radial deviation arc of 42°. Scapholunate/capitolunate angles averaged 58.3°/8.8° respectively. The carpal height index averaged 0.54. Interscaphoid angulation averaged 23.6° posteroanteriorly and 24.6° laterally. The majority of patients enjoyed a functional range of motion. Radiographic measures of carpal alignment were within normal limits.

Conclusion

Vascularized bone grafts harvested from the dorsal distal radius are easily harvested on a retrograde pedicle based on the 1,2 and 2,3 ICSRA, and the 4th and 5th ECA. Grafts may be selected to reach any location in the carpus through the same incision used for carpal bone exposure. Our clinical experience in Kienböck's disease and scaphoid fracture has been generally satisfactory. Their use allows rapid, reliable union of established scaphoid nonunion, even with proximal location and avascular changes. Poorer clinical results may be expected when degenerative changes are present. Clinical results in Kienböck's disease have been gratifying as well, and MRI evidence of revascularization has been consistently found on follow-up studies.

References

1 Sheetz KK, Bishop AT, Berger RA, The arterial blood supply of the distal radius and its potential use in vascularized pedicled bone grafts, *J Hand Surg* (1995) **20A**:902–14.

2 Lin SD, Lai CS, Chiu CC, Venous drainage in the reverse forearm flap, *Plast Reconstr Surg* (1984) **74**:508–12.

3 Zaidenberg C, Siebert JW, Angrigiani C, A new vascularized bone graft for scaphoid nonunion, *J Hand Surg* (1991) **16A**:474–8.

4 Green DP, The effect of avascular necrosis on Russe bone grafting for scaphoid nonunion, *J Hand Surg* (1985) **10A**:597–605.

5 Rock MG, Roth JH, Martin L, Radial shortening osteotomy for treatment of Kienbock's disease, *J Hand Surg* (1991) **16A**:454–60.

6 Condit DP, Idler RS, Fischer TJ, et al, Preoperative factors and outcome after lunate decompression for Kienböck's disease, *J Hand Surg* (1993) **18A**:691–6.

Vascular bundle implantation and bone grafting for scaphoid nonunions with impaired vascularity

Diego L Fernandez and David M Lamey

The management of scaphoid non-unions with vascular compromise of the proximal fragment remains problematic. The unfavorable results reported in a number of studies using conventional autogenous nonvascularized bone grafting procedures[1-4] have led some authors to recommend alternative treatments such as excision of the proximal fragment with prosthetic[5,6] or allograft replacement,[7] or salvage procedures including resection arthroplasty and partial or total wrist arthrodesis.[5,8,9] Alternatively, several investigators have attempted to gain union in the presence of an avascular proximal segment by providing additional vascularity to the nonunion site, either through the implantation of a vascular pedicle[8,10] or by means of vascularized bone grafts.[11-18]

From 1981 to 1995 the senior author (DLF) has used a combination of implantation of a vascular bundle from the dorsal intermetacarpal artery between the first and second metacarpal into the proximal scaphoid fragment and an inlay corticocancellous iliac crest graft in 15 consecutive patients with nonunited scaphoid fractures associated with radiographic and clinical signs of impaired vascularity of the proximal segment. In addition to bone grafting and vascular bundle implantation all scaphoids, with the exception of one very small proximal pole, were internally fixed with Kirschner wires and immobilized in plaster until union was confirmed by trispiral tomography.

The presence of decreased vascularity was established by specific radiographic and clinical criteria. The radiographic criteria included an increase in the bone density, loss of the normal trabecular appearance, collapse of the subchondral bone, cystic changes, and deformity of the osseous segment. Clinically, a finding of sclerotic bone without visible punctate bleeding points after debridement of the proximal segment was required to confirm the diagnosis. Neither magnetic resonance, bone scans, nor intraoperative biopsy were used as further diagnostic measures in the patients treated.

Surgical technique

With the patient under general anesthesia and the iliac crest draped free, the scaphoid is exposed through an extensile dorsoradial exposure. The proximal part of the incision begins at Lister's tubercule and extends 4 cm obliquely distally parallel to the extensor pollicis tendon and ends at the dorsoulnar aspect of the base of the thumb. Following identification and protection of the sensory branches of the radial nerve an interval is developed between the extensor carpi radialis longus and brevis and the extensor pollicis longus. The wrist capsule is incised in the long axis of the scaphoid. The arterial nutrient branches arising from the radial artery are identified as they enter the dorsal ridge of the distal fragment and are protected throughout the whole procedure. Next the nonunion site is visualized and a careful debridement of the interposed fibrous tissue is performed with a scalpel, taking care to preserve and not to damage the joint cartilage. A small spreader clamp may be used to distract the nonunion site to visualize the nonunion surface of the proximal fragment. A sharp curette is employed to scrape off the sclerotic surface of the nonunion.

If the surface of the nonunion is very irregular, a small oscillating saw can be used to smooth off bony prominences. Next the surface of the proximal fragment is carefully inspected for bleeding points under magnification following the macroscopic intraoperative appreciation guidelines proposed by Green:[1]

'If the bleeding points were numerous and imparted a slightly pinkish hue to the bone, vascularity was considered good; if the points were sparse but present, vascularity was graded fair or poor; if there were absolutely no punctate bleeding points, the proximal pole was considered totally avascular.'

Usually the punctate bleeding points are seen even with the tourniquet inflated. However, if the surgeon is in doubt whether or not a small red spot is in fact a vessel, the tourniquet may be released and the surface observed under continuous irrigation of saline solution while the bleeding from the surrounding soft tissues is blocked with a sponge. Having confirmed the absence of adequate vascularity of the proximal pole fragment associated with white dense sclerotic bone, the central portion of the proximal fragment is excavated with power drills and burrs for subsequent insertion of an iliac peg graft. The size of this cavity should not exceed 5 mm in diameter. A rectangular trough is prepared on the dorsoradial aspect of the distal fragment by use of a mini-oscillating saw and small chisels. The most distal transverse cut of the trough is cut slightly obliquely into the depth of the scaphoid in order to provide a trapezoidal surface to lock the graft in place.

Once the trough on the distal fragment and a cylindrical central cavity in the proximal fragment have been prepared, the scaphoid is now reduced and the length, width, and depth of the graft are measured in millimeters. Next a corticocancellous peg graft is cut off the iliac crest in accordance with the measurements of the scaphoid defect using power tools and small chisels. Additional cancellous chips are obtained with a curette and the wound is closed. The scaphoid fragments are slightly separated with a spreader clamp and the graft is inserted first to

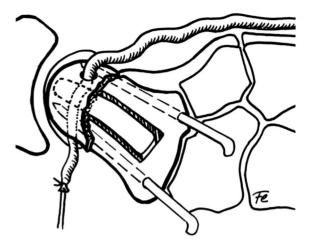

Figure 1

Schematic representation of the procedure. Notice central strut corticocancellous graft, Kirschner wire position, and the vascular pedicle across the proximal scaphoid pole. (Reproduced with permission from Fernandez and Eggli.[19])

the proximal central cavity and then reduced into the trough of the distal fragment. Care is taken to insure that the cortical surface of the graft lies dorsoradially and that the nonunion surface is not distracted by an oversized graft. Additional cystic cavities and the nonunion site may be packed with free cancellous bone chips before the peg graft is reduced into the distal fragment.

Depending on the size of the proximal fragment, one or two Kirschner wires are used to stabilize the nonunion. If the proximal fragment is very small, less than one-third of the size of the scaphoid, a single Kirschner wire (1.0–1.2 mm) is inserted parallel to the peg graft in the most radial aspect of the scaphoid (Figure 1). The Kirschner wires are inserted with a power drill with image intensifier control without entering the scaphotrapezoidal joint and directed to the proximal pole of the scaphoid. Pin placement should not jeopardize the point of entry of the vascular bundle which is planned slightly ulnar to the center of the proximal pole close to the scapholunate junction. If the proximal fragment is large enough a second Kirschner wire may be inserted on the most ulnar aspect of the scaphoid, with care taken not to violate the scaphocapitate joint.

The skin incision is then extended distally to the second dorsal web space, and the extensor tendons to the index finger are retracted ulnarwards. The dorsal intermetacarpal artery and its venae comitantes are identified between the first and second metacarpal. The vessels lie underneath a thin layer of aponeurosis that cover the interosseous muscles. This fascial layer is split longitudinally to the level of the second web space, and the vascular bundle is carefully dissected from proximal to distal, with care taken to elevate the artery and its venae comitantes together with a thin layer of perivascular areolar tissue. Small collateral branches found during dissection are ligated and cut. The vascular bundle is prepared up to the level of the web space, and at this point the vessels are ligated with a 5-0 monofilament suture and transsected. Once the intermetacarpal artery and venae comitantes have been freed from the base of the second metacarpal to the level of the web space, a pedicle of 5–6 cm long is produced that easily reaches the proximal pole of the scaphoid or the lunate for revascularization purposes.

Following elevation of the vascular bundle, a hole is drilled with a 2.7 mm drill bit across the proximal pole of the scaphoid. The drill hole has to be carefully placed just ulnar to the iliac peg graft and is usually begun close to the scapholunate junction and directed slightly obliquely in a radial volar direction. Then the vascular bundle is passed through the drill hole from dorsal to palmar. The passage is facilitated by attachment of a fine reabsorbable suture to the end of the pedicle and a straight needle is used to guide the suture and the vascular pedicle through the bone; care is taken to insure that a proper tension to the pedicle is given, so that kinking of the artery is avoided. Once the suture has been retrieved through the palmar skin just radial to the tendon of the flexor carpi radialis, a small skin incision is performed and the suture is tied over the palmar antebrachial fascia. Next the tourniquet is released and the course of the vascular pedicle is checked for bleeding and kinking, and a careful hemostasis is performed. The wrist capsule is closed with interrupted sutures at the proximal aspect of the arthrotomy; however, at the point of entry of the vascular pedicle the capsule is left open to prevent constriction of the vascular pedicle.

In those instances in which a previous surgical procedure had been performed through a palmar approach, the original incision is utilized to approach the scaphoid nonunion. Previous placed screws are removed and the screw channel and adjacent osteolytic cavities are curetted out. Under fluoroscopic control the screw channel is enlarged to approximately 4–4.5 mm diameter by the use of progressively thicker drill bits and burrs. A corticocancellous peg graft also obtained from the iliac crest is inserted in the channel from distal to proximal with a rounded impactor, and internal fixation of the scaphoid is performed with two 1.0–1.2 mm diameter Kirschner wires. Implantation of the vascular bundle is then performed as described above through a separate dorsal incision.

Postoperatively a thumb spica cast that includes the elbow is applied for 4 weeks followed by a short navicular cast for another 4 weeks. At 8 weeks, the cast is removed and bone healing is evaluated with standard radiographs as well as anteroposterior tomograms of the scaphoid. Prior to radiographic assessment the Kirschner wires were removed through stab incisions under local anesthesia. The nonunion was considered to be healed if there was tomographic evidence of the bridging bony trabeculae at the nonunion site (Figure 2). Thereafter the patient was encouraged to use the hand for activities of daily living; however, for strenuous activities a removable wrist brace was recommended for another 4 weeks. For those patients in which tomographic evidence of union was uncertain, wrist immobilization was continued for another 2 weeks in a short thumb spica cast, at which time anteroposterior tomograms of the scaphoid were repeated.

Results

Detailed information on the outcome of the first 11 cases treated with this procedure has been reported elsewhere.[19] In this series there were 10 men and 1 woman. The average duration of nonunion was 14 months (range 6–33 months). Six patients had had previous unsuccessful operative attempts to obtain union. Eight nonunions were in the proximal one-third and three at the waist of the scaphoid. Union was

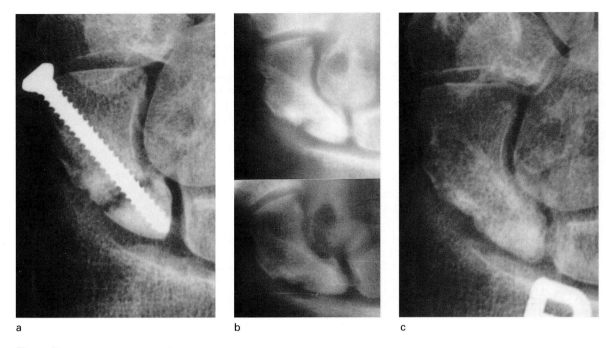

a   b   c

Figure 2

Radiographs of a scaphoid nonunion that failed to heal with interpositional grafting and lag screw fixation. (a) Notice vascular compromise of the proximal segment. (b) Tomograms at 10 weeks reveal disappearance of the nonunion gap and persistence of the vascular pedicle channel. (c) Radiograph at late follow-up show a healed nonunion.

achieved in 10 patients at an average of 10 weeks postoperatively.

According to the wrist-scoring system of the Mayo Clinic, at an average of 5 years (range 2.5–11 years), three patients had a grade of excellent, three good, three fair, and two poor. Four patients had subsequent reconstructive procedures: radial styloidectomy, styloidectomy and resection of osteophytes, radioscapholunate arthrodesis, and total wrist arthrodesis were performed in one patient each.

In the period between 1992 and 1995 four subsequent scaphoid nonunions with evidence of vascular compromise of the proximal fragment were managed in the same manner accounting at the time of writing for a total of 15 patients. There were four men with an average age of 22.6 years (range 20–25 years); the average duration of the pseudarthrosis was

12 months (range 8–21 months); three nonunions were at the proximal third and one at the waist. Two of them had previous failed Russe procedures, one failed internal fixation, and one very proximal pole nonunion failed to heal with conservative treatment (see Figure 3).

The criteria to establish healing were the absence of pain with tomographic evidence of bridging bony trabeculae at the nonunion site. Restoration of normal bone density equal to that of the neighboring carpal bones as well as reappearance of normal cancellous trabecular structure on plain radiographs were considered signs of revascularization. Irregular areas of patchy sclerosis in the proximal pole were interpreted as a sign of partial revascularization. Persistent pain and a visible gap in both plain roentgenograms and tomograms was considered a failure.

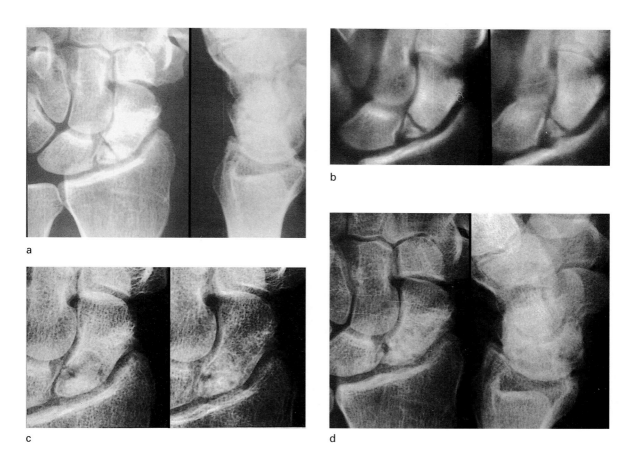

Figure 3

(a) Plain radiographs and (b) tomograms of a very proximal scaphoid nonunion with avascular proximal pole. (c) Radiographs at 8 and 12 weeks show slow incorporation of the graft. (d) Radiographs at 2 years show irregular patchy sclerosis, disappearance of the nonunion gap, and persistence of the vascular channel close to the scapholunate junction.

Radiographic evidence of union was present at an average of 9 weeks postoperatively (range 8–10 weeks) in three patients while in one, although the graft seemed to have incorporated with disappearance of the pseudarthrosis gap, at 2 years the proximal two-thirds of the scaphoid showed areas of increased patchy sclerosis, that was interpreted as partial revascularization. Nevertheless the patient was free of pain and refused a planned magnetic resonance study of his wrist (see Figure 3).

Discussion

The use of vascular bundle implantation is a measure that may provide direct capillary ingrowth to avascular bone. Its clinical use has gained popularity in the treatment of the early stages of Kienböck's disease, with or without curettage of the central necrotic areas of the lunate, producing radiographic disappearance of sclerotic zones and cystic changes in 74% of 27 cases followed up to 3 years by Tamai and coworkers.[20] Bochud and Büchler could assess partial revascularization with follow-up magnetic resonance imaging in 22 patients treated for Stage 3 Kienböck's disease with vascular bundle implantation.[21]

The advantages of the procedure are its simplicity and the shorter operative time, since there is no need of complex vascular dissection of arterial pedicles or microvascular reconstruction. Furthermore, manipulation of a free iliac peg graft is easier to accommodate than a graft that is attached either to muscle or to a vascular pedicle. Insertion of a smaller free iliac graft needs a smaller trough, and more cartilage surface of the scaphoid can be preserved; therefore the possibility of late arthritic changes is reduced.

The vascular pedicle used seems to be of sufficient dimensions and was a constant finding in all patients. However, if the dorsal intermetacarpal vessels are not of sufficient caliber, the dorsal branch of the anterior interosseous artery and vein of the distal forearm can be used alternatively. This artery emerges dorsally through the interosseous membrane in the posterior aspect of the distal forearm and crosses the wrist at the radioulnar joint level. It provides nutrient branches to the lunate and capitate and anastomoses distally with the dorsal carpal arch.

Conclusion

We believe that the acceptable results in our series lie in the fact that both factors that govern the healing of a nonunion (stability and vascularity) were addressed simultaneously. The following details of this combined technique may have been equally important to achieve union and revascularization in a relatively short period of time:

(1) the use of an internal central strut graft of autologous corticocancellous bone provides axial stability and an indirect pathway for capillary invasion from the distal fragment;
(2) rotational and shearing micromotion is controlled by Kirschner wire fixation;
(3) the peripheral subchondral areas that may retain patchy areas of viable bone are left in place;

(4) vascular bundle implantation provides direct capillary ingrowth and remodels residual necrotic areas of the proximal pole following debridement.

In view of the lack of experimental models, biopsy material, or comparison with similar series, the authors postulate that ultimate revascularization and healing of the nonunion is most probably obtained through a double source of capillary ingrowth: (a) direct, through the vascular pedicle and (b) indirect, through incorporation and revascularization of the inlay graft from the viable cancellous bone of the distal fragment. Internal fixation provides a mechanical neutral environment which also plays a role in undisturbed bone healing.

References

1   Green DP, The effect of avascular necrosis on Russe bone grafting for scaphoid nonunions, *J Hand Surg* (1985) **10A**:597–605.
2   Hull WJ, House JH, Gustillo RB, et al, The surgical approach and source of bone graft for symptomatic nonunion of the scaphoid, *Clin Orthop* (1976) **115**:241–7.
3   Mulder JD, The results of 100 cases of pseudarthrosis in the scaphoid bone treated by the Matti-Russe operation, *J Bone Joint Surg* (1968) **50B**:110–15.
4   Schneider LH, Aulicino P, Nonunion of the carpal scaphoid: the Russe procedure, *J Trauma* (1982) **2**:315–19.
5   Herbert TJ, *The fractured scaphoid* (Quality Medical Publishing Inc: St Louis, 1990) 121–38.
6   Zemel NP, Stark HH, Ashworth CR, et al, Treatment of selected patients with an ununited fracture of the proximal part of the scaphoid by excision of the fragment and insertion of a carved Silicone-Rubber Spacer, *J Bone Joint Surg* (1984) **66A**:510–17.
7   Carter PR, Malinin TI, Abbey PA, et al, The scaphoid allograft: a new operation for treatment of the very proximal scaphoid nonunion or for the necrotic fragment scaphoid proximal pole, *J Hand Surg* (1989) **14A**:1–11.
8   Carozzella JC, Stern PJ, Murdock PA, The fate of failed bone graft surgery for scaphoid nonunions, *J Hand Surg* (1989) **14A**:800–806.
9   Fernandez DL, Scaphoid non-union: current approach to management. In: Nakamura R, Linscheid RL, Miura T, eds, *Wrist Disorders*, (Springer Verlag: Tokyo, 1992) 156–64.

10 Hori Y, Tamai S, Okuda H, et al, Blood vessel transplantation to bone, *J Hand Surg* (1979) **4A**:23–33.

11 Braun RM, Viable pedicle bone grafting in the wrist. In: Urbaniak JR, ed, *Microsurgery for major limb reconstruction*, (CV Mosby: St Louis, 1987) 220–29.

12 Brunelli F, Mathoulin Ch, Saffar Ph, Description d'un greffon osseux vascularisé prélevé au niveau de la tête du deuxième métacarpien, *Ann Chir Main* (1992) **11**:40–45.

13 Guimberteau JC, Panconi B, Recalcitrant nonunion of the scaphoid treated with a vascularized bone graft based on the ulnar artery, *J Bone Joint Surg* (1990) **72A**:88–97.

14 Kawai H, Yamamoto K, Pronator quadratus pedicled bone graft for old scaphoid fractures, *J Bone Joint Surg* (1988) **70B**:829–31.

15 Kuhlmann JN, Mimoun M, Boabighi A, et al, Vascularized bone graft pedicled on the volar carpal artery for non-union of the scaphoid, *J Hand Surg* (1987) **12B**:203–10.

16 Leung PC, Hung LK, Use of pronator quadratus bone flap in bony reconstruction around the wrist, *J Hand Surg* (1990) **15A**:637–40.

17 Pechlaner S, Hussl H, Künzel H, Alternative Operationsmethode bei Kahnbeinpseudarthrosen, *Handchirurgie* (1987) **19**:302–5.

18 Zaidenberg C, Siebert JW, Angrigiani C, A new vascularized bone graft for scaphoid nonunion, *J Hand Surg* (1991) **16A**:474–8.

19 Fernandez DL, Eggli S, Non-union of the scaphoid: revascularization of the proximal pole with implantation of a vascular bundle and bone-grafting, *J Bone Joint Surg* (1995) **6A**:883–93.

20 Tamai S, Yajima H, Mizumoto S, et al, Treatment of Kienböck's disease with vascular bundle implantation. in: *Book of Abstracts of the 45th Annual Meeting of the American Society for Surgery of the Hand* (American Society for Surgery of the Hand: Toronto, 1990):3–69.

21 Bochud RC, Büchler U, Kienböck's disease, early stage 3—height reconstruction and core revascularization of the lunate, *J Hand Surg* (1994) **19B**:466–78.

48
Vascularized bone graft for scaphoid nonunion

Carlos Zaidenberg

Despite improved internal fixation devices and advances in bone carpentry, many scaphoid fractures and pseudoarthroses fail to unite.[1] Even when healing is obtained with a conventional bone graft, the healing time is prolonged. Transplantation of living bone into regions of nonunion and avascular necrosis allows faster revascularization and more reliable bone healing than conventional nonvascular bone grafts. A vascularized autogenous bone graft does not require replacement by creeping substitution. It is more resistant to resorption and maintains its original size and structure, avoiding collapse.[2] A vascularized bone graft clearly presents an advantage over applying nonvascularized bone to a nonvascularized bed (neither of which can produce living bone).[3]

A number of vascularized bone graft sources for use in the carpus have been reported. Braun proposed using the volar distal radius,[3,4] reportedly vascularized by a periosteal blood supply derived from direct muscle attachment. Kuhlmann et al described a vascularized bone graft harvested from the medial aspect of the radial epiphysis pedicle upon the radial branch of the volar carpal arch.[5] Guimberteau and Panconi described the use of a pedicle graft derived from the ulnar diaphysis and based upon the ulnar artery.[6] A free vascularized bone graft based upon a corticocancellous graft from the iliac crest was reported by Pechlander and Hussl.[7] Hori et al described the use of a vascular bundle transplantation as a potential source of blood vessel proliferation and new bone formation.[8]

Encouraged by previous reports in the literature concerning vascularized bone grafts,[3,4] we began in 1984 to study the distal radius as a possible donor site for vascularized island bone grafts. We reported a definite pattern of irrigation in the distal radius in injected fresh cadavers.[9] As a result of this anatomical study a vascularized island bone graft was proposed for the treatment of scaphoid nonunion. The results of our first seven consecutive cases were reported in the Argentinian Congress of Hand Surgery held in Mar del Plata, Argentina in 1988, and later published in 1991.[10] At the present time, our clinical series covers 60 patients who underwent a vascularized bone graft from the distal radius for the treatment of scaphoid nonunion and avascular necrosis of the proximal pole.

Anatomy

An anatomical study was performed on 50 fresh wrists of cadaveric specimens injected with colored latex (Elbio Cozzi technique) through a catheter placed in the brachial artery. The limbs were preserved in 5% formaldehyde and were dissected under 4× magnification. This technique allows visualization of vessels of diameter less than 0.1 mm after the adventitia has been stripped off. The dissection focused on the distal radius.

The radial artery and the anterior interosseous artery contribute to the irrigation of the distal radius bone through epiphyseal–metaphyseal branches. No osseous branches to the distal radius were found to arise from the ulnar artery. The vascularization of the distal radius may be classified into volar and dorsal. With reference to the volar aspect, an anastomotic network is

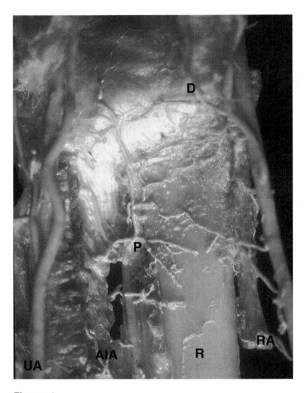

Figure 1

Irrigation of the palmar aspect of the distal radius. AIA = anterior interosseous artery; D = distal volar anastomosis (palmar carpal arch); P = proximal volar anastomosis; R = radius; RA = radial artery; UA = ulnar artery.

observed between the radial and the anterior interosseous arteries (Figure 1). We have observed that two volar anastomoses are consistently present between these two arteries, with variable diameters. The proximal volar anastomosis between the radial and the anterior interosseous arteries is placed underneath the medial portion of the pronator quadratus muscle (P on Figure 1). The distal anastomosis is located at the level of the distal fibers of the same muscle (palmar carpal arch) (D on Figure 1). These arterial anastomoses give off muscular branches to the pronator quadratus muscle and periosteal branches to the distal radius, which are completely independent from the muscular ones.

Several osseous branches (7–9) arising from the distal radial artery were consistently observed in our dissections. These branches are very short (5–10 mm in length) and small in diameter (0.2 mm). They enter the radius bone through the lateral volar edge. At the dorsal aspect of the distal radius, the blood supply showed a quite distinct pattern, separate from that of the palmar irrigation (Figure 2). Vascularity is derived principally from septal vessels which course between compartments.

The first septal vessel, as an ascending irrigation branch of the radial artery, courses under the floor of the first compartment.[10] This vessel lies supraretinacular on the septal portion. When

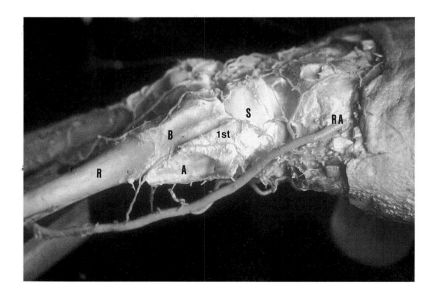

Figure 2

Irrigation of dorsoradial aspect of the distal radius; course of dorsoradial aspect of the first septal artery. A = first compartment; B = second compartment; R = radius; RA = radial artery; S = scaphoid; 1st = first septal artery.

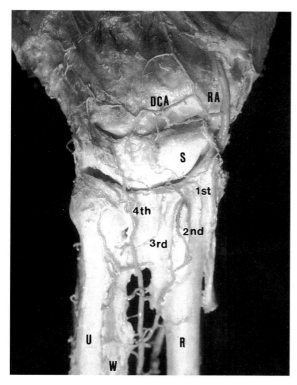

Figure 3

Irrigation of the dorsal aspect of the distal radius. DCA = dorsal carpal arch; R = radius; RA = radial artery; S = scaphoid; U = ulnar; W = dorsal branches of the anterior interosseous artery; 1st = first septal artery; 2nd = second septal artery; 3rd = third septal artery; 4th = fourth septal artery.

the first septal artery leaves proximal to the septal portion, it lies within the periosteum. At the end it is connected to a proximal branch from the radial artery. The second septal artery, originates as a dorsal branch of the anterior interosseous artery and passes along Lister's tubercle (Figure 3). Anastomoses with the transverse carpal arch and vessels of the radiocarpal capsule were variably present. The third septal artery is also a dorsal branch of the anterior interosseous artery. This vessel lies within the third dorsal compartment. Distal anastomoses were not observed. The fourth septal artery, another of the dorsal branches of the anterior interosseous artery, lies between the fourth and fifth dorsal compartments. Distal anastomoses were always complete with the transverse carpal dorsal arch.

Surgical procedure

Under axillary block anesthesia, the patient is placed in a supine position with the hand pronated on the operating table. A 5 cm long oblique incision is made on the dorsoradial aspect of the wrist, parallel to and inferior to the extensor pollicis longus (Figure 4). The incision is carried down to the vein level. Care must be taken to avoid injury to branches of the dorsal

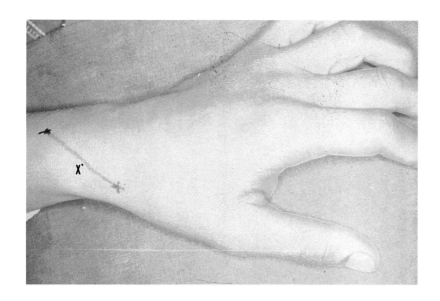

Figure 4

Dorsal approach. X' = oblique incision, parallel to the extensor pollicis longus.

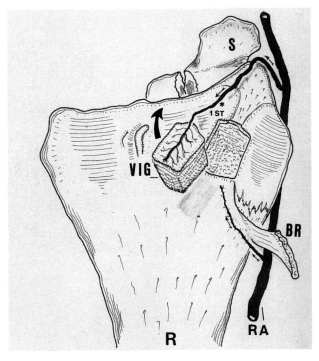

Figure 5

Vascularized bone graft. BR = brachioradialis tendon; DR = distal radius; RA = radial artery; S = scaphoid; VIG = vascularized island graft; 1st = first septal artery.

sensory branch of the radial nerve. The dorsal vein of the thumb is retracted ulnarly. As the first septal artery is located underneath this vein, it becomes completely exposed once the vein is retracted.

The next step is the scaphoid exposure through a transverse incision over the capsule of the radiocarpal joint. This maneuver facilitates the visualization of the proximal and middle portion of the scaphoid. The nonunion is approached and the sclerotic bone ends are freshened. A bed is prepared for receiving the bone island graft, which is harvested from the distal radius at the level of the first dorsal septum underlying the first septal artery. The extensor retinaculum is divided, and the first dorsal compartment containing the extensor pollicis brevis and the abductor pollicis longus tendons is retracted palmarly.

The extensor carpus radialis and the extensor pollicis longus are reflected ulnarly. The longitudinal course of the irrigating vessel is easily identified over the distal radius (Figure 5), and dissected proximally up to its origin on the radial artery, sectioning the floor of the first compartment. This maneuver allows easy rotation of the pedicles of the island graft to the scaphoid (Figure 6). The bone graft is secured in place with

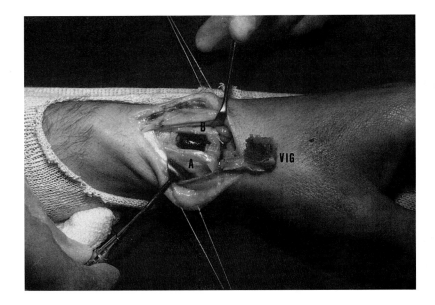

Figure 6

Intraoperative dissection: vascularized island graft rotated to the carpus. A = first compartment; B = second compartment; VIG = vascularized island graft.

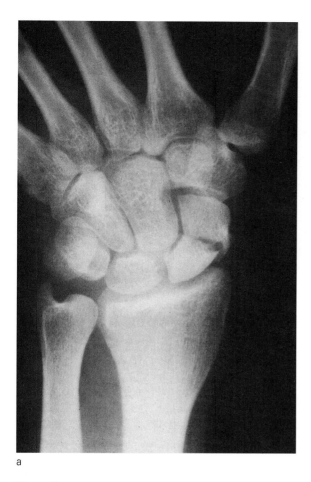

a

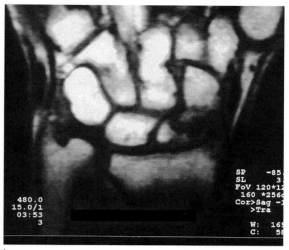

b

Figure 7

(a) Posteroanterior radiograph of the left wrist of a 29-year-old student, with failure of the Matti–Russe procedure 2 years previously. Note the opacity of the proximal portion of the scaphoid. (b) MRI shows significant bone loss from the scaphoid. Next page: (c) Posteroanterior radiograph of the left wrist: intraoperative with Kirschner wire fixation intact. (d) Posteroanterior radiograph showing revascularization of the proximal segment at 8 weeks after surgery.

two Kirschner wires, after a complete reduction of the fracture has been achieved. A short arm cast is applied for 1 month.

Discussion

There is no standard method for the treatment of scaphoid nonunion. Difficult cases of scaphoid

nonunion may be efficiently treated with vascularized bone grafts from the distal radius which allow revascularization of avascular segments. Several procedures for harvesting vascularized bone grafts from the distal radius have been reported.[3,4,7,8]

The anatomical basis for the pronator quadratus periosteal vascular contribution to the volar distal radius has not been anatomically confirmed. As a conclusion of our anatomical studies and clinical experience, we believe that vascularized bone grafts from the volar aspect of the distal radius can be safely obtained without pronator quadratus muscle, based on the periosteal metaphyseal–epiphyseal branches of the radial or anterior interosseous arteries. Free vascularized bone grafts from distant donor sites may be indicated when a local vascularized island bone graft is unavailable, as in cases with previous surgery of the dorsal radial aspect of the radius.

In our experience, the dorsal approach provides an excellent exposure of the middle and proximal third of the scaphoid, and we use this approach in all our cases. Even for the proximal pole, the graft insertion is performed at the dorsal aspect of the scaphoid without difficulty.

Initially, we used vascularized bone graft from the distal radius for the treatment of avascular necrosis of the proximal pole. Subsequently, the indications have been extended to scaphoid

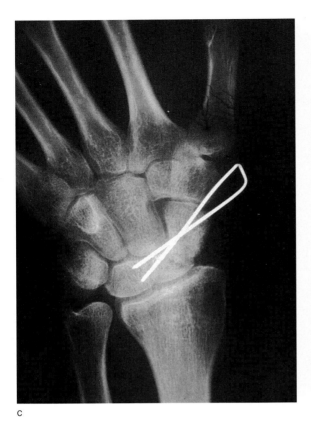

c

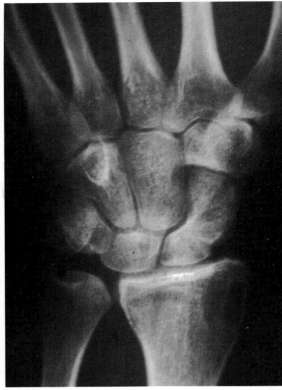

d

nonunion with significant shortening and/or angular deformity. Preoperative diagnosis is based on MRI (Figure 7a–d) which clearly indicates the amount of bone loss. In our series of 60 consecutive cases treated with vascularized bone grafts, healing occurred between the sixth and ninth postoperative weeks (average 7.8 weeks).

References

1 Osterman L, Mikuliks M, Scaphoid nonunion, *Hand Clin* **14**:437–55.

2 Weiland A, Hotchkiss A, Vascularized bone grafts. In: Green DP, ed, *Operative Hand Surgery*, 3rd edn (Churchill Livingstone: New York, 1993). ch. 30.

3 Hastings H, Zaidenberg C, Vascularity of the distal radius: Clinical implications for harvesting bone grafts. In: Vastamaki M, ed, *Current Trends in Hand Surgery* (Excerpta Medica: Amsterdam 1995): 167–76.

4 Braun RM, Viable pedicle bone grafting in the wrist. In: Urbaniak J, ed, *Microsurgery for Major Limb Reconstruction*. (Mosby: New York, 1987).

5 Kuhlmann JN, Mimoun M, Boabighi A, Baux S, Vascularized bone graft pedicle on the volar carpal artery for nonunion of the scaphoid, *J Hand Surg* (1987) **12B**:203–10.

6 Guimberteau JC, Panconi B, Recalcitrant nonunion of the scaphoid treated with a vascularized bone graft based on the ulnar artery, *J Bone Joint Surg* (1990) **72A**:88–97.

7 Pechlander S, Hussl H, Kunzel KH, Alternative operations methoden bei kahnbein pseudoarthrosen. Eine prospektive studie, *Hand Chir Mikrochir Plast Chir* (1987) **19**:302–5.

8 Hori Y, Tamai S, Okuda H, et al, Blood vessel transplantation to bone, *J Hand Surg* (1979) **4**:123–33.

9 Zaidenberg C, Irrigacion de la extremidad inferior del radio. Estudio anatomico. Actas de la Sociedad Rioplatense de Anatomia, *Capitulo* (1995) **1**:165–73.

10 Zaidenberg C, Siebert J, Angrigiani C, Vascularized bone graft for scaphoid nonunion, *J Hand Surg* (1991) **16A**:474–8.

Commentary

Chapter 46

Following up on the pioneering work of Zaidenberg, Allen Bishop and coworkers have defined a series of vascularized bone graft donor sites from the distal radius which are nicely outlined in this report. The report also reviews clinical applications and preliminary results. These vascularized bone grafts from the distal radius appear to be a very worthwhile addition to our surgical armamentarium.

PCA

Chapter 47

The results of Doctor Fernandez's work have recently been published in the *Journal of Bone and Joint Surgery*. Here Doctor Fernandez outlines the details of his approach and under-lines its advantages of ease and relative predictability. Alternatives include vascularized bone grafting, as discussed by Zaidenberg, and of course conventional bone grafting techniques.

PCA

Chapter 48

Most scaphoid fractures heal, and most scaphoid nonunions respond to conventional bone grafting techniques. However, there are some situations where scaphoid fractures do not heal when we wish or how we wish. Further, there are certain fracture patterns where this is more of a problem, particularly those involving the proximal portion of the scaphoid. In this article Doctor Zaidenberg reviews a powerful tool, vascularized bone grafting, to help solve the difficult problem of nonunion of difficult scaphoid fractures.

PCA

New methods for the diagnosis and treatment of reflex sympathetic dystrophy

David S Ruch, Thomas L Smith, Beth P Smith, Gary G Poehling and L Andrew Koman

Introduction

Reflex sympathetic dystrophy (RSD) is initiated by trauma, is exacerbated by circumstance (such as constrictive dressings or casts), and is produced by incompletely understood pre-existing, acquired, congenital and/or genetic factors. The diagnosis is based upon clinical criteria which must include pain associated with trophic change(s), autonomic dysfunction, and impaired function. Abnormalities of the sympathetic nervous system are central to the dystrophic process, and current concepts support 'sympathetically maintained pain' as a preferred descriptor of the process.[1,2] Traditionally, clinical criteria have been used to diagnose RSD, and treatment has been based upon empiric guidelines. The purposes of this chapter are:

(1) to present new techniques and instruments that convert subjective complaints and functional impairment into objective information,
(2) to outline methods that define and categorize dystrophic pathophysiology, and
(3) to formulate treatment strategies based upon physiologic staging.

Sympathetic/autonomic control

Objective evaluation of sympathetic/autonomic control is a prerequisite for the diagnosis of sympathetically maintained pain. The magnitude of peripheral sympathetic activity may be determined by evaluation of the regulation of microvascular blood flow and/or sudomotor function, both being evaluations that provide objective criteria for the categorization of autonomic function. In patients with sympathetically maintained pain, the autonomic regulation of peripheral blood flow is abnormal and nutritional deprivation secondary to this abnormal regulation may produce pain. Therefore, the appropriateness of sympathetic activity may be determined by the evaluation of microvascular perfusion, thermoregulation, and nutritional flow before, during, and after a stress eliciting sympathetic activity. Under normal circumstances, total blood flow is 80–95% thermoregulatory and 5–20% nutritional. In pathologic states such as RSD, an inappropriate distribution of flow caused by abnormal autonomic regulation is common, and segmental nutritional deprivation may produce pain and/or fibrosis.[3]

Cold stress testing with digital temperature measurements and laser Doppler fluxmetry

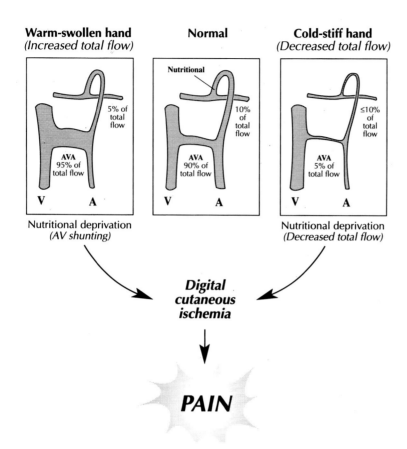

Warm-swollen hand
(Increased total flow)

Normal

Cold-stiff hand
(Decreased total flow)

5% of total flow

AVA 95% of total flow

V   A

Nutritional deprivation
(AV shunting)

Nutritional

10% of total flow

AVA 90% of total flow

V   A

≤10% of total flow

AVA 5% of total flow

V   A

Nutritional deprivation
(Decreased total flow)

***Digital
cutaneous
ischemia***

PAIN

Figure 1

Patients with RSD can be classified according to physiologic staging mechanisms based upon total flow and presence or absence of normal nutritional flow. (Reproduced from the *Bowman Gray Orthopaedic Manual*, Koman LA, ed, (Orthopaedic Press: Winston-Salem, NC, 1996) with permission of the Department of Orthopaedic Surgery, Wake Forest University).

allows the reproducible evaluation of variations in digital blood flow. Vital capillaroscopy provides a direct measurement of nutritional blood flow.[4] Quantitative analysis of thermoregulatory and nutritional flow allows the physiologic staging of sympathetically maintained pain (Figure 1) and a direct evaluation of the effects of intervention[5] (Figure 2).

Sympathetic blockade

Relief after sympathetic blockade (such as stellate ganglion block) has been considered presumptive support of the diagnosis of RSD and is consistent with the concept of sympathetically maintained pain (SMP). The role of peripheral neurotransmitters and receptors in the etiology and potentiation of SMP by (1) abnormal

patterns of microvascular perfusion and segmental tissue ischemia and/or (2) central sensitization from sympathetic receptor-mediated efferents independent of microvascular transmission is consistent with diminished pain following sympathetic blocks or sympathetic drugs.[6] If SMP is a receptor disease, then a decrease in pain after administration of phentolamine—a mixed alpha$_1$ and alpha$_2$ blocking agent—provides objective evidence of receptor-mediated sympathetic effects and supports the clinical diagnosis.

Although transient pain relief following the intravenous injection of 5–30 mg phentolamine is considered positive evidence of SMP,[7] one must remember that other neurotransmitters and/or receptors may also be involved in the process. The majority of reports suggest that 50–80% of patients with a strong clinical history of RSD and SMP report decreased pain (positive response)

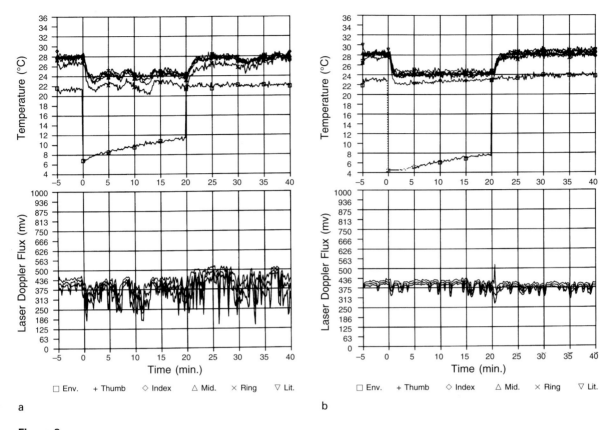

a   b

Figure 2

Isolated cold stress testing and laser Doppler fluxmetry (LDF) evaluations demonstrate the effects of continuous autonomic blockade on digital microvascular perfusion. Test results before a block are demonstrated in (a). The consistency of digital temperatures and the elimination of fluctuations in LDF measurements during the cooling and rewarming phases of the test during continuous blockade confirm 'adequate' autonomic bloackade (b). (Reproduced from the *Bowman Gray Orthopaedic Manual*, Koman LA, ed, (Orthopaedic Press: Winston-Salem, NC, 1996) with permission of the Department of Orthopaedic Surgery, Wake Forest University).

after intravenous administration of phentolamine. Furthermore, patients who do not improve after phentolamine may benefit from autonomic blockade.

Stress testing

Endurance testing with computerized equipment is used infrequently in the evaluation of RSD. However, this commonly available equipment, which is designed for either upper or lower extremity testing, may provide quantitative measures of extremity function with a greater sensitivity than is possible by static evaluations.

Stress is an important component of dynamic testing when indirect physiologic measurements such as digital temperature, laser Doppler fluxmetry, or plethysmography are utilized. For example, although digital temperature measurements provide an indirect monitor of total digital blood flow, these measurements have little diagnostic value in the absence of stress.[3] However, the simultaneous evaluation of extremity perfusion by temperature and laser Doppler fluxmetry before, during, and after stress, provides reproducible physiologic data.

Physiologic staging

The physical findings of RSD are dependent upon the extent of the altered extremity physiology, which may be either acute or chronic. Acute events are reversible without residual damage, while chronic conditions often include irreversible structural damage (that is arthrofibrosis). Sympathetic activity alone does not produce pain, and pain in the absence of cellular damage requires a somatosensory processing defect, a secondary subcritical cellular insult, or both.

Patients with persistent extremity pain, which is disproportionate to identifiable cellular damage, may be categorized as having sympathetically maintained pain (SMP) or sympathetically independent pain (SIP), the type being based upon responses to specific interventions that affect the sympathetic nervous system. SMP, present in the early stages of RSD, may over time become sympathetically independent.[8] In general, patients with SIP do not respond to traditional management protocols for RSD. SMP patients will have identifiable residual pathologic diagnoses—'trigger events'—in less than 50% of cases (i.e. neural injury).

Abnormalities in receptor sensitivity may be postulated from an estimation of autonomic function based upon microvascular events that are associated with SMP. The role of abnormal receptor sensitivity in RSD is supported by the rapid diminution or elimination of pain follow-ing sympatholytic medications.[5,6,7] More significantly, abnormalities in nutritional flow provide a common mechanism for pain in the 'hot-swollen' extremity and the 'cold-atrophic-stiff' extremity (Figure 1). If specific receptor abnormalities can be identified and specific flow dynamics during painful events can be defined, then specific treatment protocols can be devised to increase total flow and/or nutritional flow. For example, the patient with (1) a warm-swollen-edematous hyperalgesic extremity, (2) increased total blood flow, and (3) nutritional deprivation will be characterized by elevated digital temperatures, increased laser Doppler fluxmetry measure-

ments, and decreased capillary flow and may benefit from topical clonidine, an alpha$_2$ agonist, and phenytoin, a membrane stabilizer.[9] Without knowledge of such specific receptor involvement, indirect measures and postulated receptor control mechanisms must be relied upon. However, in the future, direct analysis of receptor subtype dysfunction may determine interventional strategies in reversible types of RSD.

Newer treatment strategies

Management of dystrophic focus

An initiating or contributory neural event is identifiable in approximately half of all patients with RSD. When recognized, the neural injury should be managed concurrently with the dystrophic process. However, in some cases, it may be necessary to treat the dystrophic response before the specific nerve injury can be identified. For example, a peripheral nerve injury may not be detectable clinically in a patient with a swollen, hyperalgesic extremity until the diffuse hyperalgesia is treated.

Recent reports suggest efficacy in the early aggressive management of an identifiable peripheral nerve lesion and RSD.[10] Principles of management include:

(1) reduction of the dystrophic response,
(2) identification of the neural injury,
(3) repair of the nerve or management of the neuroma (including minimum tension of the repair sites, optimization of the neural bed/environment, and avoidance of further neural damage), and
(4) postoperative pharmacologic and mechanical protection.

Parenteral medication

Intravenous regional blockade

Currently, in the United States, bretylium tosylate is the only FDA-approved intravenous sympathetic blocking agent. For a modified Bier block technique, 1–1.5 ml/kg of bretylium tosylate is mixed with 40–50 ml of 0.5% lidocaine and injected intravenously distal to a suprasystolic inflated tourniquet. Although the sympathetic inhibition produced by bretylium tosylate is theoretically less than guanethidine, bretylium tosylate is often effective in relieving SMP.[9]

Continuous autonomic blockade

The use of continuous 3- to 7-day paravertebral sympathetic ganglion block, brachial plexus block, peripheral nerve block, or epidural block may be necessary to break a dystrophic cycle.[10,11] Three to seven days of continuous blockade are usually sufficient.[11] The adequacy of sympathetic blockade may be assessed by bedside laser Doppler fluxmetry which is distinctive in the absence of autonomic control (Figure 2).

Clonidine

Clonidine, an alpha$_2$ adrenergic agonist, has received recent attention in the treatment of RSD. Used as a transdermal patch, clonidine has effectively relieved pain in patients with edema and hyperalgesia in the area surrounding its application.[6,12] Clinical trials to evaluate clonidine as a topical cream are in the early phase of evaluation, and second and third phase trials to evaluate epidural clonidine for refractory RSD are in progress.

Conclusion

Reflex sympathetic dystrophy is a complex pain process that is best treated by early and aggressive management. Objective estimations of symptom(s) and function combined with quantitative analysis of physiologic status facilitate evaluation and guide management. Physiologic staging provides a systematic approach to treatment and, if possible, correction of an underlying dystrophic focus may effect a 'cure'.

References

1   Amadio PC, Mackinnon SE, Merritt WH, et al, Reflex sympathetic dystrophy syndrome: consensus report of an ad hoc committee of the American Association of Hand Surgery on the definition of reflex sympathetic dystrophy syndrome, *Plast Reconstr Surg* (1991) **87**:371–5.

2   Mersky H, ed, Classification of chronic pain: descriptions of chronic pain syndromes and definitions of pain terms, *Pain* (1986) **26**:S3–S29.

3   Koman LA, Smith BP, Smith TL, Stress testing in the evaluation of upper extremity perfusion, *Hand Clin* (1993) **9**:59–83.

4   Kurvers HAJM, Jacobs MJHM, Beuk RJ, et al, Reflex sympathetic dystrophy: evolution of microcirculatory disturbances in time, *Pain* (1995) **60**:333–40.

5   Koman LA, Smith TL, Poehling GG, et al, Reflex sympathetic dystrophy, *Curr Opin Orthop* (1993) **4**:85–8.

6   Raja SN, Meyer RA, Campbell JN, Peripheral mechanisms of somatic pain, *Anesthesiology* (1988) **68**:571–90.

7   Arner S, Intravenous phentolamine test: diagnostic and prognostic use in reflex sympathetic dystrophy, *Pain* (1991) **46**:17–22.

8   Schwartzman RJ, Reflex sympathetic dystrophy, *Curr Opin Neurol Neurosurg* (1993) **6**:531–6.

9   Czop C, Koman LA, Smith TL, The pharmacological approach to the painful hand, *Hand Clin* (1996) **12**:633–42.

10 Jupiter JB, Seiler JG III, Zienowicz R, Sympathetic maintained pain (causalgia) associated with a demonstrable peripheral-nerve lesion, *J Bone Joint Surg* (1994) **76A**:1376–83.

11 Hobelman CF Jr, Dellon AL, Use of prolonged sympathetic blockade as an adjunct to surgery in the patient with sympathetic maintained pain, *Microsurgery* (1989) **10**:151–3.

12 Davis KD, Treede RD, Raja SN, et al, Topical application of clonidine relieves hyperalgesia in patients with sympathetically maintained pain, *Pain* (1991) **47**:309–17.

Commentary

Chapter 49

Hand surgeons are faced with many problems whose solutions are not surgical. Probably the most vexing is reflex sympathetic dystrophy. This condition has been plagued by difficulties of definition as well as difficulties of patient management. In this brief but excellent review Doctors Ruch et al outline for us the current state of knowledge regarding diagnosis, evaluation, and treatment.

PCA

50

Current classification of congenital hand deformities based on experimental research

Toshihiko Ogino

Introduction

Swanson et al[1] reported a classification of congenital hand deformities based on the concept of embryological failure. Further updating and modification of this classification was reported by Swanson and colleagues.[2,3] In this classification, there are seven categories as follows:

(1) Failure of formation of parts.
(2) Failure of differentiation of parts.
(3) Duplication.
(4) Overgrowth.
(5) Undergrowth.
(6) Congenital constriction band syndrome.
(7) Generalized skeletal abnormalities.

Kino induced constriction band syndrome in animal experiments with amniocentesis.[4] Bleeding inside the hand plate might cause this syndrome. On the other hand, clinical manifestations of congenital constriction band syndrome support the concept of local compression by the amniotic band. Although constriction band syndrome may not be caused by a single factor, this syndrome does appear after the formation of the digital radiations. The appearance of constriction ring, acrosyndactyly and amputation are quite different from each other; however these anomalies are classified together in Swanson's system.

Investigations into the teratogenic mechanisms of ulnar and radial deficiencies have been reported.[5,6] Longitudinal deficiency (except for central deficiency) is not caused by localized damage of the limb bud but by a deficit of mesenchymal cells due to damage before limb bud formation.[7] On the other hand, it has been supposed that polydactyly, syndactyly and central deficiency (typical cleft hand) may derive from a common teratogenic mechanism.[8,9] In Swanson's classification, polydactyly is classified into duplication, syndactyly into failure of formation of parts and typical cleft hand into failure of formation of parts. However, in the author's experience, some cases cannot be clearly classified into polydactyly, syndactyly or cleft hand; in other cases, polydactyly, syndactyly and cleft hand are associated in various combinations. Ogino induced these congenital deformities in rat fetuses.[10] The clinical features of these deformities in rats were the same as those in clinical cases, as were the critical periods of these deformities. The findings suggest that these congenital deformities may appear when the same teratogenic factor acts on an embryo at a particular developmental period and that they should belong to the same teratogenic entity, that is, failure of induction of digital rays.[11]

In Swanson's classification, brachysyndactyly is classified into undergrowth and transverse deficiency into failure of formation of parts, and there is no item of atypical cleft hand. The severe type of brachysyndactyly resembles atypical cleft hand and the severe type of atypical cleft hand resembles transverse deficiency. Many cases are difficult to assign to brachysyndactyly, atypical cleft hand or transverse deficiency. Blauth and Gekeler have suggested that these deformities have developed as morphological variants of symbrachydactyly.[12] Experimental research has failed to demonstrate that these anomalies belong to the same category. However, clinical studies have suggested that the essential feature of symbrachydactyly seemed to be reduction of the digital rays which represented an arrest of formation in the limb anlage. Many authors agree with Blauth and Gekeler and propose that brachysyndactyly, atypical cleft hand and transverse deficiency should be classified into the same category.[13,14]

However, there is no item of triphalangeal thumb in Swanson's classification. There are two types of triphalangeal thumb: opposable and nonopposable. Nonopposable thumb is classified into radial deficiency. Ogino et al thought that opposable triphalangeal thumb might arise as a result of incomplete fusion of the duplicated thumb.[15] On the basis of these clinical and experimental studies, the author has modified the classification of congenital hand deformities proposed by the International Federation of Societies for Surgery of the Hand, as will be described in the following section.

Classification of congenital hand deformities

Category I Failure of formation of parts (arrest of development)

This category includes transverse deficiency, longitudinal deficiency, phocomelia, absent tendons or muscles and absent nail or skin. In this classification, transverse deficiency is synonymous with symbrachydactyly as reported by Blauth and Gekeler.[12] Longitudinal deficiency includes radial and ulnar deficiencies which are considered to be caused by deficit of mesenchymal cells.

A Transverse deficiencies (so-called symbrachydactyly)

This category includes short-webbed finger to amputation-like deformities. The anomaly belonging to this category usually has unilateral affection, hypoplasia of the adjacent digits and/or whole affected limb, and sometimes pectoral muscle absence is associated in every type.

(1) Peripheral hypoplasia type. While in short-webbed finger, hypoplasia of the phalanx appears predominantly in the middle phalanges, in this type it appears predominantly in the distal phalanges. Therefore, in this type, hypoplasia of the distal phalanx or aplasia of the distal phalanx and absence of nails are common clinical features. Syndactyly is not usually associated in this type.

(2) Short-webbed finger type. Short fingers and syndactyly are essential clinical features of this type. Brachymesophalangy, absence of the middle phalanx and/or absence of two phalanges including the middle phalanges in a single finger ray are commonly observed.

(3) Didactyly type. All phalanges of one or more central finger rays are missing. In the most severe form, all phalanges of the central three finger rays are missing.

(4) Monodactyly type. All phalanges of the ulnar four digital rays are missing. There are one or two phalanges in the thumb.

(5) Adactyly type. All phalanges are missing.

(6) Metacarpal type. All or some part of the metacarpals are missing.

(7) Carpal type. All or some part of the carpals are missing.

(8) Forearm type. All or some part of the forearm bones are missing.

(9) Upper arm type. All or some part of the humerus is missing.

B Longitudinal deficiencies

(1) Radial deficiencies. Here deformities of the hand and of the forearm appear in various combinations. They are therefore categorized as a combination of hand deformity according to Blauth and Gekeler's classification and forearm deformities:
  • Dysplasia of the radius:
     hypoplasia
     partial absence
     total absence.
  • Deformities of the hand:
     five-fingered hand (nonopposable triphalangeal thumb)
     hypoplastic thumb: Blauth's grade: 1, 2, 3 (A and B), 4, 5.

(2) Ulnar deficiencies. Here deformities of the hand, forearm and elbow occur in various

combinations. Therefore, deformities must be expressed as a combination of hand deformity, forearm deformities and elbow deformities:

- Dysplasia of the ulna:
  hypoplasia
  partial absence
  total absence.
- Deformities of the hand:
  hypoplasia of the little finger
  absence of the fifth digital ray
  absence of the fourth and fifth digital rays
  absence of the third, fourth and fifth digital rays
  absence of the second, third, fourth and fifth digital rays.
- Dysplasia of the elbow:
  contracture of the elbow joint
  humero-radial synostosis
  radial head dislocation.

C Phocomelia

The major manifestation of complete phocomelia is absence of the humerus and forearm bones, that of proximal type is absence of the humerus and that of distal type is absence of the forearm bones.

D Absent tendons or muscles

E Absent nail and skin

Category II Failure of differentiation of parts

As in Swanson's classification, the basic unit of the hand and arm develops but the final form is not completed.

A Synostosis

(1) Humero-ulnar synostosis.
(2) Humero-radial synostosis.
(3) Radio-ulnar synostosis.
(4) Carpal coalition.
(5) Metacarpal synostosis.

B Radial head dislocation

C Symphalangism

This includes ankylosis of the PIP joint, that is a proximal type, ankylosis of the DIP joint, that is a distal type, and combination of proximal and distal types.

D Contracture

(1) Soft tissue:
  a Arthrogryposis multiplex.
  b Pterygium cubitale.
  c Trigger digit.
  d Clasped thumb.
  e Windblown hand.
  f Camptodactyly (without other anomalies). There are two types: in the single digit type, only one digit is involved, usually the little finger. In the multiple digit type several digits are involved.
  g Aberrant muscles.
  h Muscle contracture.
  i Swan-neck deformity.
  j Isolated nail deformity without other anomalies.
(2) Skeletal:
  a Clinodactyly without shortening of the digit.
  b Kirner's deformity.
  c Delta bone.
  d Madelung's deformity.

E Tumorous conditions

These include:

a Hemangioma.
b Arteriovenous fistula.
c Lymphangioma.
d Neurofibromatosis.
e Juvenile aponeurotic fibroma.

Category III Duplication

A Thumb polydactyly

This can be subclassified according to Wassel's classification, but there are other types, such as floating thenar muscle hypoplasia and radially deviated types.

B Polydactyly of the little finger

(1) Floating type.
(2) Others.

C Opposable triphalangeal thumb (without other anomalies)

D Mirror hand

Category IV Failure of induction of digital rays

Manifestations of abnormal segmentation of the digital rays in the hand plate due to failure of induction of digital rays are included in this category. Cleft of the palm means a deep, V-shaped excessive interdigital space. It is usually associated with absence of the central finger rays. When the index finger seems to be missing, triphalangeal thumb is frequently associated. When only a single digit is preserved, it is necessary to distinguish it from the monodactyly type of symbrachydactyly: hypoplasia of the carpal bone or hypoplasia of the forearm bones do not occur even in the most severe type of typical cleft hand (when four digits are absent), but always occur in severe symbrachydactyly. Clinodactyly and camptodactyly are sometimes associated with cleft hand. In such cases, associated clinodactyly and camptodactyly should not be classified into other categories. Cleft hand complex means a combination of the manifestations in this category and it can be expressed as a combination of cutaneous syndactyly, cleft of the palm, camptodactyly, osseous syndactyly, central polydactyly, triphalangeal thumb and absence of the central finger rays.

A Soft tissue

(1) Cutaneous syndactyly.
(2) Cleft of the palm.
(3) Camptodactyly.

B Skeletal

(1) Osseous syndactyly.
(2) Central polydactyly.
(3) Cleft hand (absence of central finger rays).
(4) Triphalangeal thumb.
(5) Cleft hand complex.

Category V Overgrowth

A Macrodactyly

B Hemihypertrophy

Category VI Undergrowth

(1) Microcheiria.
(2) Brachydactyly.
(3) Clinodactyly with shortening of the digit.
(4) Micronychia.

Category VII Constriction band syndrome

(1) Constriction ring.
(2) Lymphedema.
(3) Acrosyndactyly.
(4) Amputation type.

Category VIII Generalized skeletal abnormalities and syndromes

Category IX Others

(1) Unclassifiable cases.
(2) Others.

References

1   Swanson AB, Barsky AJ, Entin MA, Classification of limb malformations on the basis of embryological failures, *Surg Clin North Am* (1968) **48**:1169–79.

2   Swanson AB, A classification for congenital limb malformations, *J Hand Surg* (1976) **1A**:8–22.

3   Swanson AB, Swanson GG, Tada K, A classification for congenital limb malformations, *J Hand Surg* (1983) **8A**:693–702.

4   Kino Y, Clinical and experimental studies of the congenital constriction band syndrome, with an emphasis on its etiology, *J Bone Joint Surg* (1975) **57A**: 636–43.

5   Ogino T, Kato H, Clinical and experimental studies on ulnar ray deficiency, *Handchir Mikrochir Plast Chir* (1988) **20**:330–7.

6   Kato H, Ogino T, Minami A, Ohshio I, Experimental study of radial ray deficiency, *J Hand Surg* (1990) **15B**:470–6.

7   Ogino T, Kato H, Histological analysis of myleran induced oligodactyly of longitudinal deficiency. *Handchir Mikrochir Plast Chir* (1988) **20**:271–4.

8   Miura T, Syndactyly and split hand, *Hand* (1978) **10**:99–103.

9   Ogino T, Clinical and experimental study on the teratogenic mechanisms of cleft hand polydactyly and syndactyly, *J Jpn Orthop Assoc* (1979) **53**:535–43.

10 Ogino T, Teratogenic relationship between polydactyly syndactyly and cleft hand, *J Hand Surg* (1990) **15B**:201–9.

11 Ogino T, Kato H, Clinical and experimental studies on teratogenic mechanisms of congenital absence of longitudinal deficiencies, *Cong Anom* (1993) **33**:187–96.

12 Blauth W, Gekeler J, Zur Morphologie und Klassifikation der Symbrachydaktylie, *Handchir Mikrochir Plast Chir* (1986) **18**:161–95.

13 Ogino T, Minami A, Kato H, Clinical features and roentgenograms of symbrachydactyly, *J Hand Surg* (1989) **14B**:303–6.

14 Buck-Gramcko D, Symbrachydactylie, classification et traitement chirurgical. In: Gilbert A, Buck-Gramcko D, Lister G, eds, *Les Malformations Congenitales du Membre Superieur*, (Expansion Scientifique Française: Paris, 1991) 98–106.

15 Ogino T, Ishii S, Kato H, Opposable triphalangeal thumb. Clinical features and results of treatment, *J Hand Surg* (1994) **19A**:39–47.

51

An approach for radial hypoplasia

David M Evans

Introduction

Radial hypoplasia is expressed in varying degrees of severity, and includes mild hypoplasia of the thumb at one extreme, and complete absence of the thumb with absence of the radius at the other. Absence of the radius necessarily involves a deformity of the wrist, since there is no proximal articular surface to support the carpal bones. This deformity, often called radial club hand, consists of severe radial deviation of the whole hand and carpus. It places the hand in a mechanically inefficient position, slackening the long flexor and extensor tendons, but in the presence of elbow stiffness, which may be part of the abnormality, the radially deviated position of the wrist may prove to be the only position in which the hand can be brought to the mouth. This situation should be recognized before any attempt at wrist correction is made.

Centralization or radialization

Sayre, in 1893, described a procedure to straighten the wrist by centralization of the ulna in the carpus, and current techniques are based on this principle.[1] There is often some tendency for the deformity to recur, and Buck-Gramcko has added the idea of radialization,[2] in which the ulna is brought over to the ulnar side and balanced with tendon transfers.

Distraction devices

Another area of developing interest is the use of external distraction devices to alleviate soft-tissue constraints which limit the extent to which correction can be achieved,[3] especially in older children. The full value of this additional technical exercise is not yet fully proven, but Nanchahal and Tonkin believe that it facilitates the surgical correction of the radial angulation at the wrist.[3] These authors found that five out of six limbs treated by preoperative distraction could be radialized, but without distraction five out of six required centralization with carpal resection.

Soft-tissue tension

The factors affecting correction are tension in the skin and the structures on the palmar aspect of the wrist, which become radially placed structures as a result of the absence of the radius. The most important tight structure found here is the median nerve, and in older children in whom early correction has not been available this nerve can be tight enough to prevent full correction, or to suffer temporary or even permanent conduction block if too much tension is imposed on it. Whether or not a major nerve trunk can safely be elongated by gradual distraction under these circumstances has yet to be demonstrated.

Tension in the skin is found on the radial aspect of the wrist during straightening, and is associated with redundancy of the skin on the ulnar side. Various incisions have been used, some of which have dealt with the skin redundancy, but few with the radial tension. Lamb[4] and Buck-Gramcko[2] used an S-shaped incision with excision of redundant skin, although Lamb preferred separate ulnar and radial incisions when soft-tissue release was required. Manske et al described a transverse incision with skin excision.[5]

a

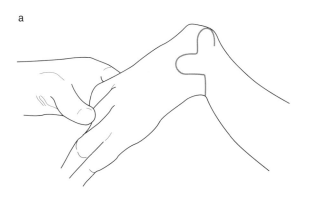

b

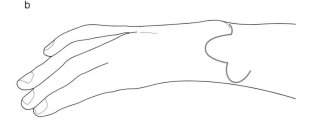

Figure 1

(a,b) The design of the bilobed flap for correction of radial club hand. The radial side of the wrist is below, and the incision starts there, in order to relax tension as the deformity is corrected. The two flaps are long and wide enough to fit the defect that this and the dorsal flap create.

The bilobed flap

Evans et al have described the use of a bilobed flap which transfers redundant skin from the ulnar side of the wrist to the radial side (Figure 1).[6] The technique is illustrated in a challenging case requesting correction of an untreated deformity at the age of 17 (Figure 2). The design of the incision starts at the point of greatest tension at the ulnar side of the wrist, where a transverse incision 2–3 cm in length runs just on to the dorsum. The incision turns distally to form a gothic arch the same length and width as the first incision (Figure 3), and from the radial side of this flap another similar flap is designed to run at 90° to the first around the ulnar side of the wrist, where the skin is loose. The flaps are raised beneath subcutaneous fat, preserving terminal superficial nerve branches if possible,

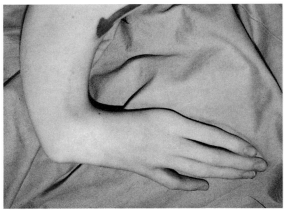

Figure 2

The right wrist of a 17-year-old boy with an uncorrected radial club hand.

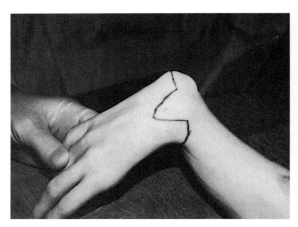

Figure 3

The design of the skin incisions.

and this approach gives excellent access across the wrist for a centralization or radialization procedure to be carried out (Figure 4). Care is needed to protect the median nerve in the first (radial) incision. After correction and stabilization of the deformity the flaps readily fall into their new position (Figure 5), and in fact they rotate little because the wrist rotates beneath them. The flap from the ulnar side replaces the first flap on the dorsum of the hand, and here there is some risk of marginal necrosis if there is any tension; subcuticular suturing of the flap tips is advisable.

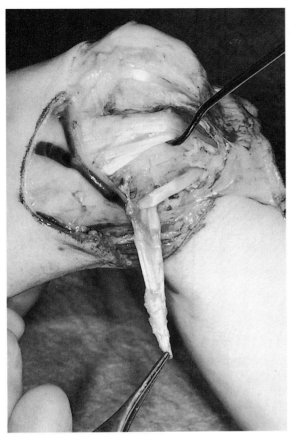

Figure 4

The wide exposure provided by this technique, allowing access to the whole wrist for release and stabilization, here by centralization.

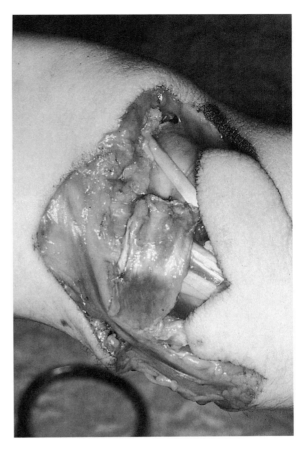

Figure 5

After stabilization the two flaps lie ready to be sutured in place.

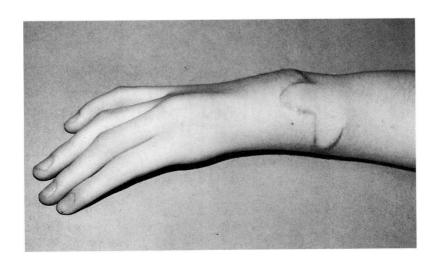

Figure 6

The result 3 months later. The intramedullary pin is still in place, and was removed subsequently.

The dorsal flap turns radially and relaxes tension on the radial side of the wrist (Figure 6).

The success of the procedure depends largely on the skeletal correction and rebalancing of the wrist, but use of this bilobed flap helps to achieve this by giving good access and ease of skin closure without tension.

References

1   Sayre RH, A contribution to the study of club hand, *Trans Am Orth Assoc* (1894) **6**:208–16.

2   Buck-Gramcko D, Radialization as a new treatment for radial club hand, *J Hand Surg* (1985) **10A**:964–8.

3   Nanchahal J, Tonkin MA, Pre-operative distraction lengthening for radial longitudinal deficiency, *J Hand Surg* (1996) **21B**:103–7.

4   Lamb DW, The treatment of radial club hand, *Hand* (1972) **4**:22–30.

5   Manske PR, McCarroll HR, Swanson K, Centralization of the radial club hand, *J Hand Surg* (1981) **6A**:423–33.

6   Evans DM, Gateley DR, Lewis JS, The use of a bilobed flap in the correction of radial club hand, *J Hand Surg* (1995) **20B**:333–7.

52

Longitudinal radial deficiency

Michael A Tonkin

Introduction

Radial longitudinal deficiency (radial club hand) may be divided into four types according to the degree of radial hypoplasia or aplasia:[1]

Type 1: short radius with abnormal distal physeal growth.
Type 2: short radius with abnormal proximal and distal physeal growth.
Type 3: partial radial absence.
Type 4: total radial absence.

Type 1 deficiency rarely requires treatment. Although lengthening a short radius is feasible, centralization has become the main method of treatment of type 2, 3 and 4 deficiencies.[2–6]

Surgical correction must attend to the absence of radial support of the carpus and shortening of the soft tissues across the concavity of the deformity. These include skin, musculotendinous structures and the median nerve. It is the last of these that may determine the degree of correction possible. The radial nerve innervated muscles (especially brachioradialis, extensor carpi radialis longus, extensor carpi radialis brevis and the extrinsic thumb extensors and abductor) are absent or hypoplastic, and often fibrotic with poor excursion. Flexor carpi radialis and the finger flexors cross the concavity. These and extensor digitorum communis are also tight and may compromise placement of the carpus over the end of the ulna.

Most have advised resection of a central portion of the carpus, with the ulna placed within it, to allow correction and maintain stability.[4] Some also shave off the distal end of the ulna.[1,6] Watson has achieved correction without skeletal shortening.[7] Buck-Gramcko champions radialization, in which the carpus is placed to the ulnar side of the ulna and is maintained in position by releasing the tight radial structures and reinforcing the action of extensor carpi ulnaris.[8] A portion of carpus is not excised.

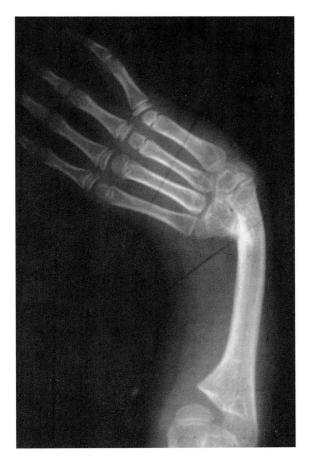

Figure 1

Recurrence of deformity, with short forearm and physeal closure following centralization.

Replacement of the absent or deficient radius is an attractive concept. Nonvascularized fibular and metacarpal replacement have not been successful in maintaining the corrected position.[9] Similarly, results of vascularized fibular transfer with an intact epiphysis have been disappointing, with premature physeal closure frequent.[10] The early results of Vilkki's vascularized metatarsophalangeal joint transfer are encouraging, with support of the carpus achieved and growth of the transferred bone preventing recurrence of deformity in the short term (personal communication). The metatarsal is joined to the ulna and the proximal phalanx to the metacarpal. It is too soon to know the rate of growth of the 'new radius' and whether it will keep pace with the growth of the ulna, or tether it and tend to increase the deformity. It is this recurrence of deformity that presents one of the major problems, together with the shortened forearm that follows surgery (Figure 1). The following approach aims to overcome or minimize these complications.

Surgical management

Preoperative

Splinting and stretching exercises are instituted from birth. Undoubtedly it is difficult to apply splints effectively to a newborn with significant deformity.[11] This should not prevent the attempt.

Distraction

After 3 months of age, provided that the general health of the child allows, a decision is made as to whether soft tissue distraction is appropriate. This is employed if the hand cannot be reduced onto the end of the ulna. My preference is to use the Kessler device.[12] However this device allows distraction mainly in the longitudinal plane, with little preferential lengthening on the radial side. In fact this deficiency within the device is useful. If it is not possible to passively correct the position of the hand such that parallel wires may be placed through the metacarpals and the ulna

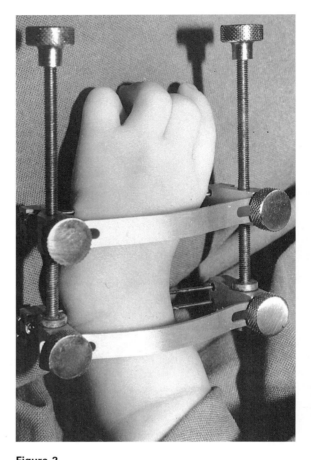

Figure 2

Kessler distraction in place.

to allow application of the distractor, then a formal soft tissue release of the radial structures is indicated. Short skin may be attended to at the same time by creating a Z-plasty within a longitudinal incision placed at the apex of the concavity on the radial side. This allows visualization of the abnormal musculature, the median nerve, its branches and accompanying vessels. The brachioradialis, radial extensors and, oftimes, the flexor carpi radialis are divided distally. Fibrotic tissue is excised. If any or all of these musculotendinous units are considered of appropriate quality for subsequent tendon transfer to extensor carpi ulnaris, they are tagged for later identification. The integrity of these muscles is also an important determining factor in deciding whether centralization or radialization will be the better procedure to achieve wrist stability.

The distractor is applied in the corrected position under radiological control (Figure 2). Postoperative distraction is delayed for 1 week to allow the soft tissues to adapt to the corrected position and the wound to settle. Distraction is then commenced at a rate of between 0.5 and 1 mm per day according to skin tightness, development of finger contractures and as determined by the comfort of the child. Distraction is ceased or the rate is decreased if such complications arise. Distraction is continued over a 3-week period according to the degree of lengthening and correction of the deformity required. The distractor is then left in place for a further week prior to formal open realignment. At times it is necessary to remove the distractor and maintain the correction in plaster splints if pin tract infection intervenes and delays open surgery.

Surgical realignment

This is performed at about 6 months of age depending on the time of application of the distractor and the duration of distraction. If no previous release has been performed, I have used a lazy S incision to allow adequate mobilization of the carpus and attention to the radial musculotendinous unit. More recently Evans and colleagues have described a bilobed incision, which allows transfer of redundant ulnar skin to the radial concavity where there is a relative shortage[13] (see Chapter 51).

If a Z-plasty has previously been employed, then a longitudinal incision in the line of the ulna extending along the line of the third metacarpal is safe. The carpus is mobilized, protecting the finger and thumb extrinsic tendons and extensor carpi ulnaris (ECU). It is advisable to identify ECU proximally and distally and mobilize this separately before the distal end of the ulna is freed, to protect its blood supply. The carpus is transferred to the ulnar side of the ulna. If this is easily achieved, and if there are adequate radial musculotendinous units to transfer to ECU, then radialization as described by Buck-Gramcko is preferred (Figure 3).[8] However, if transfer of the carpus ulnarwards is difficult, and/or if there are

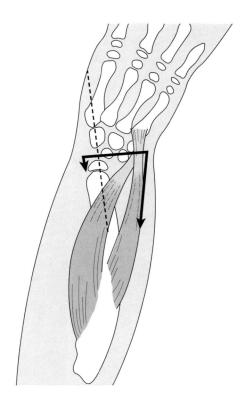

Figure 3

Radialization. (Reproduced with permission from Buck-Gramcko D, Congenital malformations. In: Nigst H et al, eds, *Hand Surgery* (Thieme: New York, 1988).

inadequate musculotendinous units to rebalance the wrist and maintain the position, then excision of a portion of carpus with formal centralization is advisable.[4]

Two Kirschner wires are used to maintain the carpus in position. These will be removed if radialization has been performed. It may not be necessary to remove them following centralization. The limb is placed in a long arm plaster for 4 weeks. Intermittent day and night splinting may be necessary until skeletal maturity.

I prefer to delay performing an osteotomy of the ulna. If radial bowing of the ulna is significant, correction is indicated because the deformity tends to increase, particularly if there is unequal tension present. However, I believe that the blood supply of the ulnar physis is at risk following simultaneous mobilization of carpus, distal end of ulna and midshaft ulnar osteotomy. Osteotomy can be performed at 2 years of age or later and may be combined with a forearm lengthening.

Discussion

The advantages of centralization are wrist stability, improved excursion of extrinsic tendons and improved appearance. However Vilkki has reviewed the long-term work of H.E. Heikel in Finland in the 1950s.[14,15] Recurrence of deformity occurred even with ankylosis of the ulnocarpal joint, presumably at the carpometacarpal joints. Intracarpal dissociation was also present. Vilkki has estimated that the average length of a normal ulna is 25 to 30 cm. In reviewing Heikel's patients who did not undergo surgical correction, he found an average ulnar length of 15–18 cm, or 60% of normal. This supports the findings of Lamb and others.[3,4] However in Heikel's centralization group the average length was 11.5 cm, or only 40% of normal growth. This is due to surgical shortening of the carpus, of the ulna at the time of ulnar osteotomy, and premature physeal closure.

The physis closes prematurely if damaged directly at the time of surgery or if its blood supply is interrupted. The physis is also in danger as a consequence of ulnocarpal fusion or of excessive tension on the physeal plate if the corrected position is not balanced adequately. Excessive tension on the radial aspect of the ulna may also lead to increasing radial deviation as the tight tissues tether longitudinal growth. The shortening and recurrence of deformity in Heikel's patients following centralization resulted in poorer function, with a decreased arm reach, in spite of the hand being placed on the end of the ulna, when compared with the untreated group. Perhaps the results of centralization have

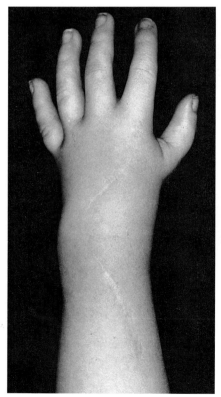

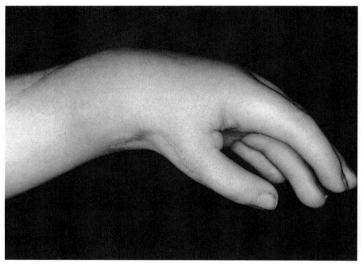

b

Figure 4

(a,b) Result after radialization.

a

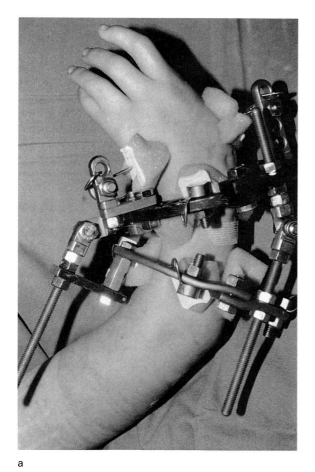

a

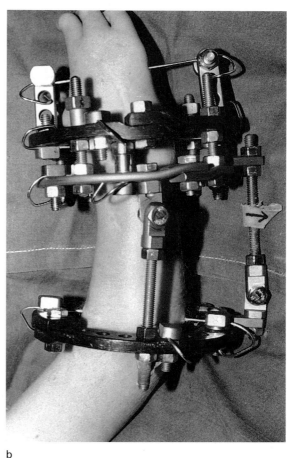

b

Figure 5

(a,b) Ilizarov lengthening of short ulna.

improved since this time.[5-7] However there is little in the literature to compare with Vilkki's long-term review of Heikel's work. Therefore it is understandable that doubts remain about the efficacy of centralization.

Radialization attempts to attend to some of the disadvantages of centralization. The carpus is mobilized and placed at the ulnar side of the ulna by release of the tight radial structures. A portion of carpus is not excised. The wrist is rebalanced by transfer of radial musculotendinous units to extensor carpi ulnaris. Of course, this rebalancing should also accompany centralization. It

remains unclear as to whether radialization will in the long term protect the physis from premature closure, overcome the problem of recurrent deformity and therefore lead to a longer forearm with a stable, mobile wrist joint. In the short term motion is improved—from neutral extension to between 40 and 90° of flexion (Figure 4).[8] This is of benefit, particularly when the elbow has a limited range of motion. However the deformity of radial longitudinal deficiency has a component of flexion, which becomes more apparent at the time of correction of radial deviation. Increasing flexion deformity is a possible consequence of

Table 1 Patients treated by realignment without preoperative distraction.

Patient	Age at operation (months)	Age at follow up (months)	Operation	Angulation preop/postop (improvement)	Translation (mm) preop/postop (improvement)
1	5	27	Centralization Wedge	−12°/5°` (−17°)	9/−4 (13)
2	8	36	Centralization Wedge	42°/33° (9°)	15/2 (13)
3	15	53	Centralization Wedge	87°/10° (77°)	16/−4 (20)
4	17	36	Radialization	−30°/−35° (5°)	14/−9 (23)
5	24	96	Centralization Wedge	30°/25° (5)	15/3 (12)
6	28	30	Centralization Wedge	47°/11° (36°)	15/0 (15)

Note: Negative figures indicate degree of ulnar deviation and ulnar translation.

Table 2 Patients who underwent preoperative distraction before realignment.

Patient	Age at operation (months)	Age at follow up (months)	Operation	Angulation preop/postop (improvement)	Translation (mm) preop/postop (improvement)
7(L)	12	30	Centralization Wedge	90°/32° (58°)	16/−4 (20)
(R)	10	30	Failed radialization Centralization Wedge	90°/37° (53°)	15/2 (13)
8(L)	10	23	Radialization	40°/−10° (50°)	15/−9 (24)
(R)	7	23	Radialization	43°/0° (43°)	14/0 (14)
9	5	20	Radialization	70°/17° (53°)	14/0 (14)
10	5	7	Radialization	15°/12° (−27°)	12/−4 (16)

Note: Negative figures indicate degree of ulnar deviation and ulnar translation.

stabilization in the radio-ulnar plane. The tendency for this to occur is increased when the ulnocarpal joint is mobile following radialization.

Failure to attend to the deforming forces of the soft tissues is the prime reason for recurrence of deformity. Indeed, even with both aggressive mobilization of the carpus and release of the extrinsic muscles proximally, it may not be possible to achieve correction without shortening the skeleton. Tension within the median nerve, in particular, may demand skeletal shortening. More recently distraction methods have been used to stretch the soft tissues across the concavity of the deformity prior to surgical realignment of the carpus.[12,16,17] This offers a means of decreasing soft-tissue tension in neural, musculotendinous and fibrous structures, and the skin. Stretching of neural tissues may result in intraneural damage and therefore distraction methods should not be undertaken lightly. Neither the rate of neural lengthening nor the absolute increase in length allowable have been determined. The ability to stretch fibrotic soft tissue with minimal elasticity is also limited.

A surgical release at the time of placement of the distractor may be necessary to achieve adequate distraction prior to realignment.

Nevertheless, even without surgical release, distraction would appear to allow easier correction without resection of the carpus. Tables 1 and 2 compare two small groups of patients reported by Nanchahal and Tonkin, in whom preoperative distraction proved beneficial.[17]

Concomitant bone lengthening, with or without correction of radial bowing of the ulna, is also possible, but may better be performed secondarily. Ilizarov techniques are now being used to correct failed early surgical management or neglected cases (Figure 5).[16,18–21] The advantages of a longer, straighter forearm must be balanced against the high complication rate, which includes nerve injury and finger contractures.

Conclusion

The deformity of radial longitudinal deficiency and the loss of function resulting remain a challenge to the clinician. A combination of previously described techniques is optimal in achieving a satisfactory result. Preoperative distraction, with or without radial release, followed by radialization or centralization depending on availability of tendons for transfer, offers a rational approach for surgical management.

References

1   Bayne LG, Klug MS, Long-term review of the surgical treatment of radial deficiencies, *J Hand Surg* (1987) **12A**:169–79.

2   Bora FW Jr, Nicholson JT, Cheema HM, Radial meromelia. The deformity and its treatment, *J Bone Joint Surg* (1970) **52A**:966–79.

3   Lamb DW, The treatment of radial club hand, *Hand* (1972) **4**:22–30.

4   Lamb DW, Radial club hand, *J Bone Joint Surg* (1977) **59A**:1–13.

5   Bora FW Jr, Osterman AL, Kaneda RR, Esterhai J, Radial club-hand deformity. Long-term follow-up, *J Bone Joint Surg* (1981) **63A**:741–5.

6   Manske PR, McCarroll HR Jr, Swanson K, Centralization of the radial club hand: an ulnar surgical approach, *J Hand Surg* (1981) **6**:423–33.

7   Watson HK, Beebe RD, Cruz NI, A centralization procedure for radial club hand, *J Hand Surg* (1984) **9A**:541–7.

8   Buck-Gramcko D, Radialization as a new treatment for radial club hand, *J Hand Surg* (1985) **10A**:964–8.

9   Riordan DC, Congenital absence of the radius, *J Bone Joint Surg* (1955) **37A**:1129.

10 Sawaizumi M, Maruyama Y, Okajima K, Moteei M, Free vascularized epiphyseal transfer designed on the reverse anterior tibial artery, *Br J Plast Surg* (1991) **44**:57–9.

11 Netscher DT, Scheker LR, Timing and decision-making in the treatment of congenital upper extremity deformities, *Clin Plast Surg* (1990) **17**:113–31.

12 Kessler I, Centralization of the radial club hand by gradual distraction, *J Hand Surg* (1989) **14B**:37–42.

13 Evans DM, Gateley DR, Lewis JS, The use of a bilobed flap in the correction of radial club hand, *J Hand Surg* (1995) **20B**:333–7.

14 Heikel HVA, Aplasia and hypoplasia of the radius, *Acta Orthop Scand (Suppl)* (1959) **39**:1–55.

15 Vilkki S, Distraction lengthening and microvascular epiphyseal transfer in radial club hand. In: *Proceedings of 6th Congress of IFSSH*. Helsinki, July 1995.

16 Ilizarov GA, Clinical application of the tension-stress effect for limb lengthening, *Clin Orthop* (1990) **250**:8–26.

17 Nanchahal J, Tonkin MA, Pre-operative distraction lengthening for radial longitudinal deficiency, *J Hand Surg* (1996) **21B**:103–7.

18 Dick HM, Petzoldt RL, Bowers WR, Rennie WRJ, Lengthening of the ulna in radial agenesis. A preliminary report, *J Hand Surg* (1977) **2**:175–8.

19 Villa A, Catagni MA, Bell D, Cattaneo R, Lengthening of the forearm by the Ilizarov technique, *Clin Orthop* (1990) **250**:125–7.

20 Catagni MA, Szabo RM, Cattaneo R, Preliminary experience with Ilizarov method in late reconstruction of radial hemimelia, *J Hand Surg* (1993) **18A**:316–21.

21 Tonkin MA, Nanchahal J, An approach to the management of radial longitudinal deficiency, *Ann Acad Med Singapore* (1995) **24**(Suppl):101S–7S.

53
Delta phalanx

David W Vickers

Introduction

'Delta phalanx' is the general term applied to a heterogenous group of anomalies of the small bones of the hands or feet where asymmetric development and reduced growth of tubular bones are the principal features, usually producing a clinodactyly. A tether linking the proximal and distal epiphyses on one side prohibits normal growth so parallelism of the proximal and distal joint surfaces is lost. Asymmetric progression in the secondary centres of ossification produces a delta phalanx. The bone of the diaphysis appears triangular on a radiograph (Figure 1). The proximal and distal epiphyses are inclined towards each other on one side, being linked by a soft tissue, cartilaginous or sometimes bony isthmus, which prohibits symmetrical longitudinal growth. The distal epiphysis often has fused incompletely with the metaphysis. The use of the term delta phalanx is attributed to Jones.[1] Wood has suggested 'delta bone' would be more appropriate as the anomaly is also seen in metacarpals and metatarsals.[2] Blevens and Light have classified this anomaly into five types.[3] The overall shape of most delta phalanges on a radiograph is more typically trapezoidal rather than triangular

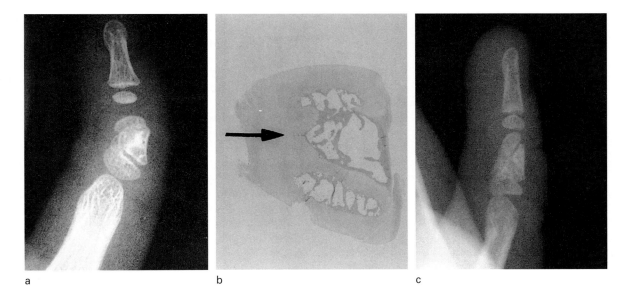

a   b   c

Figure 1

(a,b) Delta phalanx in a finger demonstrating a triangular diaphysis/metaphysis, a continuous physis, not yet fully ossified, and partial fusion of the distal epiphysis and metaphysis. (c) Lateral radiograph demonstrating the narrowed isthmus of the continuous epiphysis.

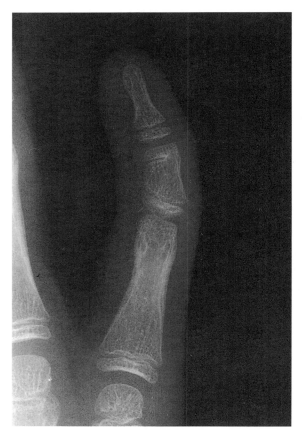

Figure 2

A 'typical' delta phalanx in the author's series had a trapezoidal shape, a nonossified isthmus with a clinarthrosis at the proximal end.

(Figure 2). The appearance of the whole specimen is like a cylinder with one or both ends truncated obliquely. In some extreme examples the shape of the bone on X-ray examination is semicircular.

Clinodactyly of the little finger is the most frequent presentation, with a delta anomaly in the middle phalanx. Less frequently, clinodactyly of the thumb occurs with a delta anomaly in the proximal phalanx, or in the case of a triphalangeal thumb, in the middle phalanx of the digit. Curiously, the anomaly occurs in the second most distal phalanx in these cases, but there are exceptions elsewhere in other digits and in rare cases the metacarpals or metatarsals are involved. The anomaly in the little finger is frequently familial (dominant with variable penetrance) with some sporadic cases. Clinodactyly of the thumb in the proximal phalanx is often part of a syndrome (especially Rubenstein–Taybi), or in the case of triphalangeal thumb is usually familial. A delta phalanx may be associated with many other syndromes but these are less common. The more bizarre shapes or multiple delta phalanges are often related to polydactyly which may be overt or pernicious. For example, in some cases of delta anomaly of the proximal phalanx of the thumb, the distal phalanx will be broad, with evidence of a duplex tuft—subtle evidence of polydactyly. Watson and Boyes reported that the majority of cases of delta phalanx in their survey were associated with polydactyly, but this is not the case in other gene pools.[4]

The unilateral continuity or isthmus joining the epiphyses has been termed 'continuous epiphysis' by Jones,[1] 'longitudinal bracketed diaphysis' by Carstam and Theander,[5] and 'longitudinal epiphyseal bracket, LEB' by Light and Ogden.[6] In the case of the 'classical' delta phalanx as described by Jones, epiphyses are linked on one side by a bone bridge, but in a 'typical' delta phalanx (which is more common) the isthmus is usually nonossified, especially in the young in whom the tissue forming the tether is periosteum, articular cartilage and physis, or if bone is present it is often a barely visible thin layer. The author believes that even soft tissue tethers of this kind maintain the deformity or cause slow progression. Ossification of the isthmus clearly will prohibit longitudinal growth on one side, either causing increasing clinodactyly if limited, or prohibiting proper growth if more substantial. However some growth is observed in even the most extreme examples of delta phalanx with an ossified isthmus, but this must be epiphyseal and appositional.

Clinical management

Bony tethers can form in long bones following trauma, causing progressive angular deformity if peripheral, or no growth if substantial or central.

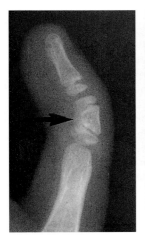
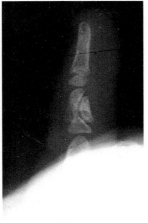

a

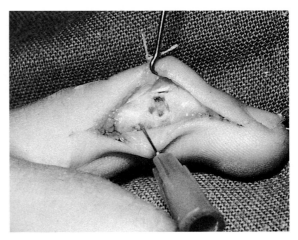

b

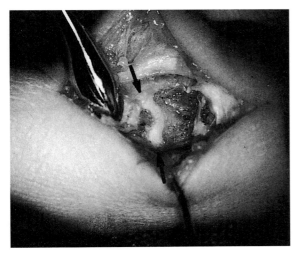

c

Figure 3

(a) A 'classic' delta phalanx with an ossified isthmus joining the proximal and distal epiphyses. (b) After the bone of the isthmus of the continuous epiphysis is excised the grey/blue longitudinal continuous physis is seen with the bony nuclei of the epiphysis at each end and diaphyseal bone above and below. (c) At the completion of removal of the anomalous longitudinal isthmus and some additional metaphysis, the normally orientated physis is clearly seen from the dorsal to the palmar perichondrial ring (arrow). (Reproduced with permission from reference 8.)

It is now well established that excision of these bone bridges, and prevention of their recurrence with interposition material fat, can allow natural restoration of alignment, length and articular surfaces.[7] Langenskiold[7] was the first to advocate fat for interposition, and further experience has shown that this is the most suitable material. It has been observed that congenital deformity can reverse in the same way if the tether is removed.[8,9] The author uses the term 'physiolysis' for this surgical procedure.

The accepted approach in management has been to ignore minor clinodactyly, or correct more obvious deformity with some form of osteotomy. Jones summarized his experience of osteotomy during growth by saying that 'the deformity needs radical treatment by repeated surgery because there is no tendency to spontaneous correction, and growth of the phalanx is prevented by the epiphyseal deformity'. Osteotomy during growth is not favoured and osteotomy after maturity is not simple surgery. There is now an intermediate choice—to restore growth in the anomalous phalanx. This approach is ideal in young children in whom deformity is apparent, and especially in whom there is a family history of significant deformity. Older children can still obtain a worthwhile benefit if more than one year of growth is possible before maturity. The ideal age is about 4 years when the phalanx is large enough for precision surgery, with plenty of growth remaining for progressive correction. Growth restoration (physiolysis) is simple, virtually painless and requires no specific aftercare. This procedure should always be considered in the immature skeleton, especially in clinodactyly of the little finger. Early physiolysis will remove the need for osteotomy later on. Clinodactyly of the thumb is less common, and more difficult to treat as the deformity is much greater, so associated osteotomy is always required. When a delta phalanx is supernumerary, especially in the triphalangeal thumb, there is no place for physiolysis—traditional procedures remain the method of choice. Likewise after maturity, physiolysis is no longer available so traditional methods prevail.

Surgical technique: physiolysis

Growth restoration surgery for clinodactyly of a digit secondary to a delta phalanx is performed under general anaesthesia using a pneumatic tourniquet inflated to 180 mm of mercury. The use of a quality loupe of 3.5× diameter magnification is recommended. A midlateral incision slightly greater than the length of the phalanx is made on the concave side of the deformity, and after the subcutaneous fat has been mobilized the longitudinal tether linking the proximal and distal epiphyses of the phalanx is excised with a No 15 scalpel blade (Figure 3). First the periosteal layer, then the white cartilage of the continuous epiphysis with underlying lamellae of bone and grey/blue physis are easily excised. In some more extreme cases the fibrous flexor sheath is also very thick and should be partially excised. Only rarely is the bony continuous epiphysis hard enough to require the use of a rongeur at this stage. As the excision proceeds to a deeper plane at the proximal end, one can see the vertical line developing of grey/blue cartilage of the physis, in contrast to the white epiphyseal cartilage. Further careful excision with the scalpel or a very fine rongeur (1 mm tip) will bring the bony epiphyseal nucleus into view. The bony margin of the physis should be further defined on the metaphyseal side with the rongeur so the physis stands a little above the bony terrain. In less extreme deformity, such as a trapezoidal phalanx with a nonossified isthmus, it is not necessary to expose the epiphyseal nucleus to any extent, if at all, as long as the surgeon is sure there is no longitudinal physeal

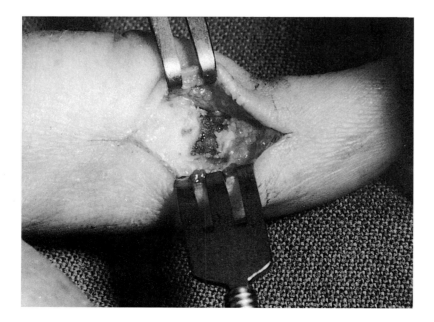

Figure 4

The more typical finding where a nonossified longitudinal physeal layer has been removed with a scalpel along with some metaphyseal bone (1 mm rongeur) so the proximal epiphyseal nucleus is just visible. With magnification the surgeon can ensure that there is no distal continuity of the physis, so further exposure of the bony epiphysis is unnecessary.

or bony tissue linking the epiphysis to the distal bony structures including the zones well dorsal and ventral to the midline (Figure 4). The periosteal margins must be cleanly incised dorsally and ventrally at the perichondral ring as flaps of this tissue could lead to a recurrence of the fusion across the physis.

A small piece of subcutaneous fat is excised from the forearm along the midulnar border— enough to fill the surgical void. It is usual to treat both hands under the one anaesthetic so a single piece of fat large enough to treat both digits is harvested. After some subcutaneous bupivacaine (0.25% plain) has been injected into the wound edges of the donor and recipient sites, the donor site wound is closed with 5/0 or 6/0 plain catgut, and the tourniquet is deflated. After haemostasis occurs the tourniquet is reinflated, and the surgical cavity in the finger is washed out and completely filled with a piece of fat. The fat graft is stabilized with the catgut skin sutures and a nonadhesive dressing, some cotton padding and 2.5 cm crepe bandage is loosely applied for 10 days or so. The bandage is more likely to survive the rigours of childhood if the skin is sprayed with an aerosol adhesive before application, and if the dressings are extensively taped down with micropore. Apart from an attempt to keep the dressings dry, no restrictions are placed upon the child, and rigid splintage is not required.

An associated osteotomy has only been necessary in the thumb. In the very young, a physiolysis has been performed first, so that after some years of longitudinal growth an osteotomy is then possible. In an older child the two procedures can be performed concurrently. A closing wedge osteotomy has been employed. It is arguable whether the surgical approach should be from the concave or convex side, or both. The physiolysis is best performed from the concave side, but the osteotomy is easiest from the convex side. The ideal procedure would be a combination of physiolysis and open wedge osteotomy performed from the concave side, but it is believed that the skin length would be inadequate even with a Z-plasty.

Clinical applications and results

Little finger clinodactyly may be visible at birth, but more commonly presents in early childhood.

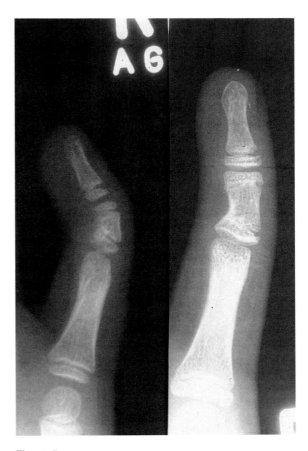

Figure 5

Spontaneous reformation over a 5-year period following physiolysis in a 'classical' delta phalanx (also illustrated in Fig. 3). The inclination of the interphalangeal joints reduced from 55° to 15°. (Reproduced with permission from reference 8.)

Families with the gene will be aware, and present earlier. There is an opinion that these cases do not warrant surgery, but the owners of the fingers and their parents often disagree with this advice. In some cases a persistent clinodactyly with asymmetric interphalangeal joints causes uneven loading and osteoarthritis in the fourth decade, requiring arthrodesis.

Since 1980 the author has performed a physiolysis on the middle phalanx of a little finger clinodactyly 52 times. All cases demonstrated growth (Figures 5, 6 and 7). In one case the fusion redeveloped later, but the finger remains

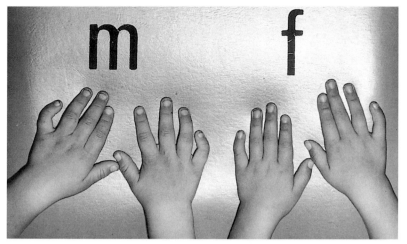

a

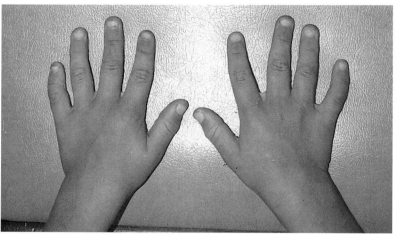

b

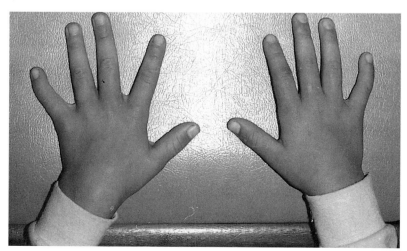

c

Figure 6

(a) The male member only of this family duo had a physiolysis of both little fingers: (b) three years later he demonstrates improvement, whereas his sister (c) remains unchanged.

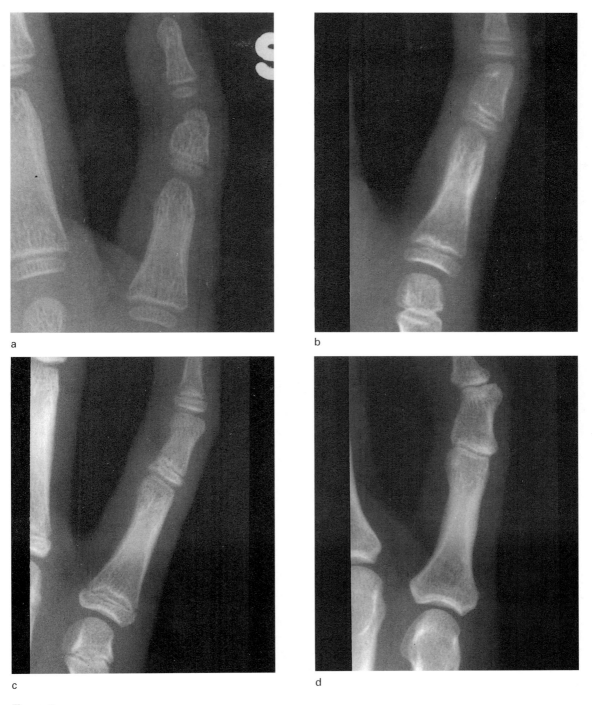

a

b

c

d

Figure 7

(a) Aged 4, routine radiograph because a sibling was treated for significant clinodactyly. (b) Aged 8.5: physiolysis requested by mother. (c) Aged 13: some improvement in length and alignment. (d) The mother of this patient (who had no surgery herself): arthritis developing.

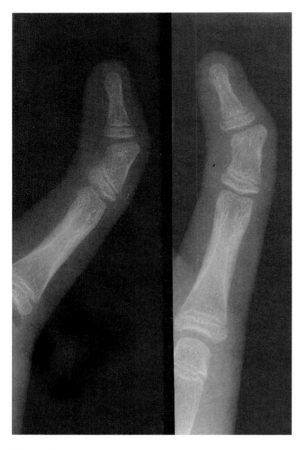

Figure 8

The clinodactyly is a result of proximal and distal clinarthrosis. Since the distal physis was fused no change is possible here, however at the proximal physis growth in length occurred and the clinarthrosis decreased by 20° over a 15-month period following physiolysis. Osteotomy was still necessary in this one case.

satisfactory so repeat surgery was not performed. In one case a granuloma developed as some bone wax was tried as an interposition material instead of fat. This technique has since been abandoned. There was no loss of range of motion in any case. In one case bilateral osteotomy at maturity was indicated. This was not a failure of the physiolysis as the clinarthrosis was at the distal interphalangeal joint (Figure 8). Since the distal physis was closed at the time of

physiolysis there was no possibility of spontaneous correction here, however the proximal clinarthrosis did improve, and the phalanx did grow in length at the proximal end.

The need for physiolysis in the thumb is less common as these cases are quite rare. The surgery is more difficult but with persistence the stubby, crooked little thumbs can be improved enough to make the effort worthwhile. Since 1980 the author has treated 11 thumbs in this way. Two thumbs in one patient were managed with physiolysis alone initially, with a view to osteotomy as a second stage (Figure 9). Another case is illustrated where a closing wedge osteotomy was performed concurrently (Figure 10). Light and Ogden have also advocated this method.[6] In one patient multiple epiphyseal dysplasia was the associated pathology, and in this case the phalanx developed normally after physiolysis and osteotomy (Figure 11).

Conclusion: comparison to classical techniques

The mild clinodactyly sometimes seen with trapezoidal phalanx could be ignored, especially in later childhood. The gross anomalies or multiple delta phalanges may be more amenable to osteotomy or reduction of the bony elements. The author favours physiolysis in all cases of delta phalanx with clinodactyly of the little finger in the immature skeleton. A relatively large series with a maximum follow-up of 16 years has indicated good outcomes with a high level (universal) of satisfaction in the children and parents. Families with the gene now watch for the lesion and present affected children early expecting surgery. The offer to remove the tether then 'let nature finish the job' is appealing. The simplicity of the surgery is also appreciated. Conversely, osteotomy is more complex, more prone to complications, and if performed on immature bones can actually cause a bony fusion with progressive deterioration. Overcorrection of the osteotomy is not uncommon which is completely unacceptable. Stiffness in the finger is more likely. Bilateral osteotomies at one sitting are not as acceptable because of the need for internal fixation and rigid casting. The

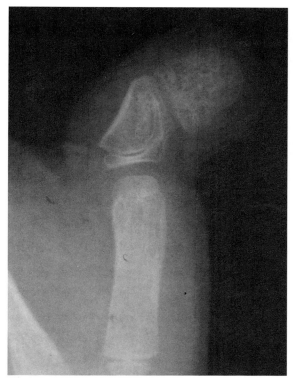

a

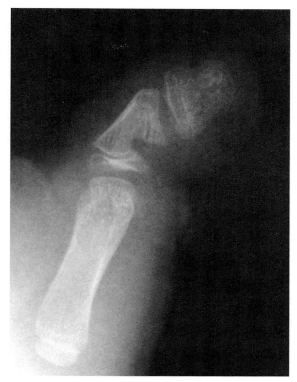

b

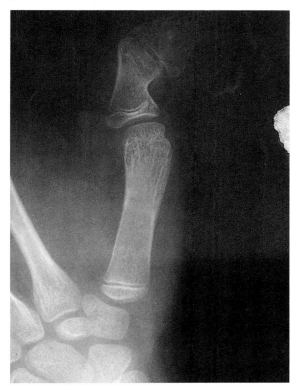

c

Figure 9

(a) Rubenstein–Taybi thumb. (b) Physiolysis. (c) Four years later: some growth, clinarthrosis reduced 20°, but may be fusing at radial condyle.

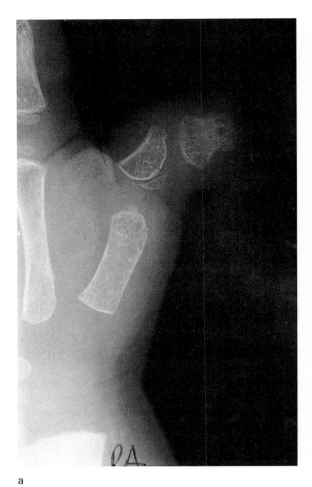

a

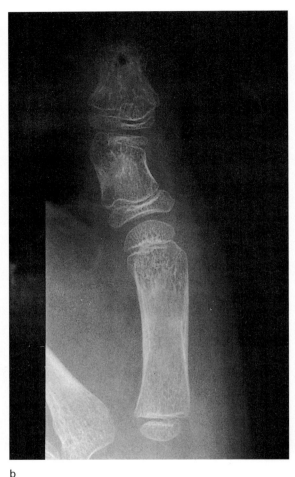

b

Figure 10

(a) Delta phalanx in thumb with subtle evidence of polydactyly in distal phalanx. (b) Nine years after physiolysis and osteotomy the thumb is longer and well aligned, and still growing.

only advantage of osteotomy is immediate correction of the deformity, but this is only guaranteed in the mature skeleton where physiolysis is not indicated in any case. The advantages of physiolysis are its surgical simplicity, natural recovery of alignment and length, and restoration of joint surfaces preventing the development of arthrosis.

References

1   Jones GB, Delta phalanx, *J Bone Joint Surg* (1964) **46B**:226–8.
2   Wood VE, Congenital hand deformities. In: Green D, ed, *Operative Hand Surgery* (Churchill Livingstone: New York, 1993) 430.
3   Blevens A, Light T, Crooked fingers—delta bones. In: Flatt AE, ed, *The Care of Congenital Hand Anomalies*, 2nd edn. (Quality Medical Publishing: St Louis, 1994) 212–13.

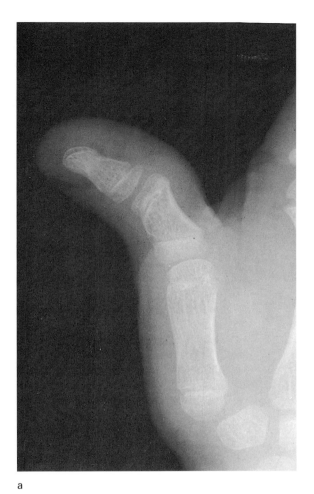
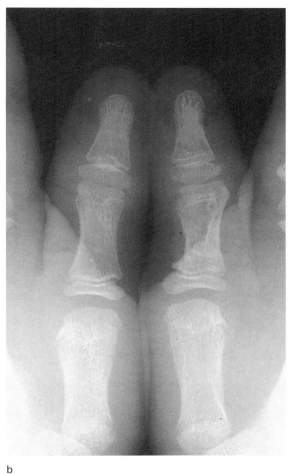

a   b

Figure 11

(a) Delta phalanx with associated epiphyseal anomalies elsewhere. (b) Two years after physiolysis and osteotomy growth is restored and both thumbs have a similar appearance clinically.

4   Watson HK, Boyes JH, Congenital angular deformity of the digits, delta phalanx, *J Bone Joint Surg* (1967) **49a**:333–8.

5   Carstam N, Theander G, Surgical treatment of clinodactyly caused by longitudinally bracketed diaphysis ('delta phalanx'), *Scand J Plast Reconstr Surg* (1975) **9**:199–202.

6   Light TR, Ogden JA, The longitudinal epiphyseal bracket: implications for surgical correction, *J Paed Orthop* (1981) **1**:299–305.

7   Langenskiold A, An operation for partial closure of an epiphyseal plate in children and its experimental basis, *J Bone Joint Surg* (1975) **57B**:325–30.

8   Vickers DW, Clinodactyly of the little finger: a simple operative technique for reversal of the growth abnormality, *J Hand Surg* (1987) **12B**:335–42.

9   Vickers DW, Epiphyseolysis, *Curr Orthop* (1989) **3**:41–7.

54

Classification and techniques in thumb hypoplasia

Paul R Manske

Introduction

There are five types of thumb hypoplasia, as noted in Table 1. The classification system[1,2] reflects the progressive stages of arrested development associated with longitudinal radial deficiency, and is useful in directing treatment principles. The features of each category are quite well defined, particularly with the sub-classification of Type III thumbs.[3,4]

Type I

The thumb is generally decreased in size, specifically the median innervated thenar muscles

Table 1 Thumb hypoplasia classification.

Type I: Minimal shortening and narrowing   • Thenar muscle hypoplasia (APB/Opp P)

Type II: Moderate underdevelopment
           • Narrow thumb–index web space
           • Thenar muscle hypoplasia (APB/Opp P)
           • MP joint instability

Type III: Extensive underdevelopment
           • Narrow thumb–index web space
           • Thenar muscle hypoplasia (APB/Opp P)
           • MP joint instability
           • Extrinsic tendon abnormalities
           • Metacarpal hypoplasia, CMC stable (IIIA)
           • Proximal metacarpal aplasia, CMC unstable (IIIB)

Type IV: *Pouce flottant*
           • Rudimentary phalanges
           • Thumb attached to hand by skin bridge containing vessels and nerves

Type V: Absent thumb

(abductor pollicis brevis, APB and opponens pollicis, Opp P).

Type II

There are three specific features:

(1) Narrowing of the thumb–index web space.
(2) Aplasia of the median innervated thenar intrinsic musculature, usually sparing the deeper ulnar innervated muscles.
(3) Instability of the ulnar collateral ligament (UCL) at the metacarpal phalangeal (MP) joint.

Type III

Type III hypoplastic thumbs represent more extensive deficiencies. The three manifestations of the Type II thumb are present, frequently in more severe form. The narrow thumb–index web space may present as a distal take-off of the thumb from the hand. The MP instability may be more global and involve the radial collateral ligament in addition to the UCL laxity.

Type III hypoplastic thumbs also include extrinsic tendon deficiencies, in addition to the intrinsic muscle deficiencies and hypoplasia or partial aplasia of the proximal thumb metacarpal.[3,4] Type IIIA hypoplastic thumbs have the extrinsic tendon abnormalities, but the thumb metacarpal (although hypoplastic) is present, and the carpal metacarpal (CMC) articulation is stable. Type IIIB thumbs also have extrinsic tendon abnormalities, but the proximal thumb metacarpal is absent, and the CMC joint is unstable.

The most frequently observed extrinsic tendon abnormalities include absent extensor pollicis longus (EPL), absent or aberrant flexor pollicis longus (FPL) and/or a tendon interconnection between the FPL and the extensor hood; several deficiencies may be present in the same thumb. The 'pollex abductus' thumb described initially by Tupper[5] is a form of IIIA hypoplasia; there is an aberrant FPL on the radial side of the thumb, which in conjunction with laxity of the UCL causes marked abduction at the MP joint.

Type IV

Type IV hypoplasia is the classic *pouce flottant*. The thumb is attached to the hand only by soft tissue, primarily skin and neurovascular elements. There are no significant musculotendinous structures, and no stable osseous unit between the thumb and the hand.

Type V

Type V represents complete absence of the thumb. There may be rudimentary thumb muscles, tendons, or neurovascular structures along the radial border of the index metacarpal.

Indications

Thumb hypoplasia constitutes a significant functional deficiency for the child. The intrinsic muscle deficiency interferes with the child's ability to rotate the thumb in front of the fingers, and contributes to an inefficient pinch mechanism. The narrowed thumb–index web space and unstable ulnar collateral ligament interfere significantly with the child's ability to pinch or grasp objects.

Type I

Often, no treatment is necessary for Type I, because the thumb hypoplasia and muscle atrophy are minimal and constitute no significant functional deficit. However, the surgeon should specifically evaluate the opponens function.

In the case of deficient opponens function, the abductor digiti quinti (ADQ) opponensplasty[6] is preferred to other opponensplasties in the treatment of the hypoplastic thumb. The muscle is on the ulnar side of the hand. It is reliably and predictably present in radial deficiencies. It is an expendable muscle, and there is no appreciable functional deficit after transfer. The muscle is the same length and is of equal strength to the abductor pollicis brevis (APB) and opponens pollicis (Opp P) muscles that it replaces. Pulley reconstruction is not required to alter the direction of pull. After transfer, the appearance of the thumb is improved by the added muscle mass in the deficient thenar area.

Type II

The three features of Type II hypoplasia must all be addressed. The narrow thumb–index web space requires deepening and widening, usually by a standard three- or four-flap Z-plasty. On occasion it is necessary to use a rotation or transposition flap from the dorsum of the hand or thumb. We have not found it necessary to use a distant vascularized pedicle flap, but this may be indicated in severe narrowing.

The MP joint must be stabilized. In the case of Type II hypoplasia, this is usually accomplished by imbrication or reefing the ulnar capsule.[6] The ulnar capsule can be further reinforced using the distal end of the opposition transfer tendon.

An opponensplasty is necessary to restore opposition function, as described for Type I hypoplasia. The abductor digiti quinti is preferred,[6,7] but some authors recommend the ring finger sublimis tendon.[8]

Type III

It is important to differentiate between Type IIIA and Type IIIB hypoplastic thumbs because IIIA thumbs are reconstructible, while IIIB thumbs require ablation and pollicization of the index finger. Functionally, there are significant advantages to a reconstructed thumb compared to a pollicized index finger. A reconstructed thumb is usually stronger than a pollicized digit. Additionally, the CMC joint of the reconstructed Type IIIA thumb will have two axes of motion in the flexion/extension and abduction/adduction planes which allows full circumduction of that joint. In contrast, the basal joint of the pollicized index finger (i.e. the MP joint) has only one primary axis of motion in the flexion/extension plane, which limits the ability to circumduct the pollicized digit.

Type IIIA thumbs must meet four requirements for adequate thumb function; these conditions must be inherently present in the thumb preoperatively or accomplishable by various reconstructive operative procedures:

(1) Development of an adequate thumb–index web space (as described for Type II thumbs).
(2) Thumb length must be sufficient to accomplish grasp and pinch activities. The normal thumb tip reaches the proximal interphalangeal joint of the adjacent digit; although the reconstructed thumb may be somewhat shorter, it should at least reach the mid-proximal phalanx of the adjacent digit.
(3) The thumb ray needs to be stable. If there is instability at the MP joint, stabilization can be accomplished by ulnar capsular imbrication, as described for Type II thumbs. If there is global instability, radial and ulnar capsulodesis or epiphyseal arthrodesis[9] (which can be performed after an ossification center is radiographically apparent in the epiphysis of the proximal phalanx—usually by 2–4 years of age) can be performed. If CMC joint stability is not inherently present (as in Type IIIB hypoplasia), surgical reconstruction is usually not possible.
(4) Muscles to extend, flex, abduct, and adduct the thumb must be inherently present or provided by tendon transfer.

The specific reconstruction procedures for Type IIIA thumbs include those described previously for the Type II thumb (i.e. deepening of the thumb–index web, stabilizing the MP joint, and opponens transfer). In addition, the extrinsic tendon abnormalities must also be addressed. This is accomplished in part by release of the tendons which cause deformities or limit motion, in particular the aberrant FPL which results in the severe ulnar deviation of the MP joint, and the tendon interconnection between the flexor and extensor mechanisms.

Additionally, IIIA thumbs require tendon transfers to address deficient extrinsic tendon function. Extension deficiency is treated by extensor indicis proprius transfer. Flexion deficiency can be addressed by rerouting the aberrant FPL to a more volar position on the thumb, by transferring the ring finger sublimis tendon and reconstructing fibro-osseous pulleys, or by accepting the functional deficiency of absent interphalangeal (IP) joint flexion and allowing the flexion force of the flexor pollicis brevis at the MP joint to be sufficient. Abduction deficiency is accomplished by opposition transfer as described. Adduction deficiency is rarely a problem since the adductor pollicis is usually present, except in the most severe hypoplastic thumbs; in these instances, the thumb usually has enough other deficiencies to make it not reconstructible.

Type IIIB hypoplastic thumbs usually do not meet these requirements for adequate thumb function, particularly the instability at the CMC joint. Unless there are social or cultural reasons for preserving a five digit hand, the Type IIIB thumb is best treated by ablating the hypoplastic thumb and index ray pollicization.

Types IV and V

These hypoplastic thumbs are treated by pollicization, which is the transposing and repositioning of the index finger, as the radial post, to the position of the thumb.

Variations on classical techniques

There are a few minor variations in the recommended technical aspects of these procedures.

Opponensplasty

Although in the original description of the procedure of the ADQ opponensplasty Huber[10] and Nicholaysen maintain the ADQ origin attached to the pisiform, Littler and Cooley[7] detached the origin of the ADQ from the pisiform and based the transfer on the extended attachment to the flexor carpi ulnaris (FCU). We prefer to keep the muscle origin attached to the pisiform to serve as a stable base, and prevent undue tension on the neurovascular pedicle. Experimentally, the vascular perfusion of the ADQ muscle is maintained more effectively if the muscle is not detached from the pisiform origin.[11] Littler and Cooley reported muscle fibrosis in one of four patients.[7] We noted fibrosis in one of 21 children,[6] and in one more of approximately 100 additional unreported patients. Oberlin and Gilbert reported no fibrosis in the series of 14 children when the muscle was not detached.[12]

Littler and Cooley also recommended dissection and identification of the neurovascular bundle on the radial side of the origin of the ADQ.[7] We prefer to assume that these structures are dependably present and do not require identification at surgery. Therefore, we do not applicate their identification on a routine basis.

Several authors use a ring finger sublimis opponensplasty because it is more substantial and potentially supplements the capsular imbrication more effectively.[9] The shorter length of the ADQ tendon requires that the surgeon include a portion of the extensor hood as an extension to the tendon, but this does not impair extension of the small finger.

MP stabilization

An alternative to epiphyseal arthrodesis is chondrodesis, which is the apposition of adjacent cartilaginous surfaces.[13] This technique is more likely to result in pseudarthrosis with a potential for long-term instability, and carries with it the same potential risk to the growth plate. We prefer chondrodesis only when there is gross joint instability in conjunction with an epiphysis that is not yet ossified.

Conclusion

The thumb is the most significant digit of the hand. Consequently, the surgical treatment of the hypoplastic thumb is extremely important. The classification system describes the various stages of developmental deficiency and serves as a guide to the surgical concepts and procedures which are necessary for thumb reconstruction.

References

1   Blauth W, Schneider-Sickert F, Numerical variations. In: Blauth W, Schneider-Sickert F, eds, *Congenital Deformities of the Hand. An Atlas on Their Surgical Treatment* (Springer-Verlag: Berlin, 1981) 120.

2   Buck-Gramcko D, Hypoplasia and aplasia of the thumb. In: Nigst H, Buck-Gramcko D, Millesi H et al, eds, *Hand Surgery*, Vol 2 (Thieme: Stuttgart, 1981) 12.93.

3   Manske PR, McCarroll HR, Reconstruction of the congenitally deficient thumb, *Hand Clin North Am* (1992) **8**:177–96.

4   Manske PR, McCarroll HR Jr, James M, Type IIIA hypoplastic thumb, *Am J Hand Surg* (1995) **20A**:246–53.

5   Tupper JW, Pollex abductus due to congenital malposition of the flexor pollicis longus, *J Bone Joint Surg* (1969) **51A**:1285–90.

6   Manske PR, McCarroll HR Jr, Abductor digiti minimi opponensplasty in congenital radial dysplasia, *J Hand Surg* (1978) **3**:552–9.

7   Littler JW, Cooley SGE, Opposition of the thumb and its restoration by abductor digiti quinti transfer, *J Bone Joint Surg* (1963) **45A**:1389–96.

8   Lister GD, Reconstruction of the hypoplastic thumb, *Clin Orthop Rel Res* (1985) **195**:52–65.

9   Kowalski MF, Manske PR, Arthrodesis of digital joints in children, *J Hand Surg* (1988) **13A**:874–9.

10 Huber E, Hilfsoperation bei medianuslhung, *Dtsch Z Chir* (1921) **162**:271–5.

11 Dunlap J, Manske PR, McCarthy JA, Perfusion of the abductor digiti quinti after transfer a neurovascular pedicle, *J Hand Surg* (1989) **14A**:992–5.

12 Oberlin C, Gilbert A, Transfer of the abductor digiti minimi (quinti) in radial deformities of the hand in children, *Ann Chir Main* (1984) **3**:215–20.

13 Neviaser RJ, Congenital hypoplasia of the thumb with absence of the extrinsic extensors, abductor pollicis longus, and thenar muscles, *J Hand Surg* (1979) **4**:301–3.

55
Ulnar deficiency

Dieter Buck-Gramcko

Congenital deformities of the ulnar border of the hand and forearm, extending up to the shoulder, are described under several different terms: congenital absence of the ulna; congenital defect of the ulna; aplasia/hypoplasia of the ulna; ulna hemimelia; ulnar club hand; longitudinal arrest of development of the ulna. In this chapter, the general term 'ulnar deficiency' is used.

Incidence

Ulnar deficiencies are much less frequent than the other longitudinal deficiency of the arm, the radial club hand. Flatt (1994) reported only 28 patients with this deformity and 127 with radial club hands of his 2758 patients with congenital malformations. In my own clinical material of about the same number of patients as Flatt, there are 104 patients with ulnar and 240 with radial deficiencies. Birch-Jensen (1949) reported an incidence at birth of 1:100 000; he described 19 ulnar and 73 radial defects from his investigations in Denmark.

Bilateral involvement is reported at a frequency of 25% (Bayne 1993; Flatt 1994; Masson et al 1995), but seems to be quite different in the reviews, depending on the hospitals from which the patients' data were collected. While in my own patients bilateral involvement is only 22%, it is reported elsewhere as high as 40% (Blauth and Hippe 1990) or even 60% (Ohnesorge 1987). The ratio between male and females is about 2:1 in my patients, but has been reported elsewhere as 3:2.

Almost all cases of ulnar deficiencies are sporadic. Genetic and environmental factors are

discussed, but remain obscure. In the cases in which the ulnar defect is part of a syndrome (for example some cases of the Cornelia de Lange or the FFU (Femur Fibula Ulna) syndrome, which was described by Kühne et al (1967) and is the European synonym for the American PFFD (Proximal Femoral Focal Deficiency), described by Aitken in 1969), the inheritance shows autosomal dominant patterns (Temtamy and McKusick 1978). In my own patients, the family history was negative in all cases, with the exception of two twin brothers with bilateral identical deformities.

Classification

With regard to the great variability of the pathological findings in ulnar deficiencies, it is almost impossible to collect all their different combinations in a classification system. Therefore, all previously published trials are inaccurate, incomplete and of little clinical value. Some are based only on the length of the ulna, others more on the elbow deformity. Hand and shoulder involvement are often ignored. The most popular classification is that of Bayne (1993, first published in 1982).

Clinical picture

Because this deformity involves the hand, wrist, forearm and elbow as well as the shoulder in different extents and combinations, the description follows this order of the parts of the arm.

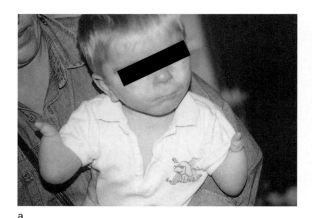

a

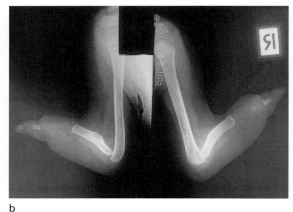

b

Figure 1

(a,b) Typical facial expression and deformity of both arms with complete aplasia of the ulna and a monodactylous hand in a boy with Cornelia de Lange syndrome.

Hand

The hand involvement is characterized by aplasia of one or more digital rays. A full complement of digits is present in about 11%. The digital rays, including their carpal bones, are missing mostly at the ulnar border of the hand. The thumb may also be absent or hypoplastic, but not as frequently as reported by Broudy and Smith (1979). In many hands, some of the remaining fingers are hypoplastic, have unstable joints or flexion contractures of the proximal interphalangeal joint, and show anomalies of their tendons, especially their extensors. An adactylous

hand is very rare; its incidence is reported mainly in papers which include cases with congenital amputation at the wrist such as Swanson et al (1984). The monodactylous hand is in most cases combined with severe flexion contracture of the elbow, pterygium cubitale and complete absence of the ulna as in the Cornelia de Lange syndrome (Figure 1). In about half of the involved hands, three digits are present (Table 1).

As already demonstrated in a single case by Jones and Roberts (1926), in my own series bones of additional, mostly rudimentary digits were seen in 24 hands (19%). All were located in the phalangeal level (Figure 2; see also Figure

Table 1 Number and percentage of digits present in three series of patients with ulnar deficiences.

Number of digits present	Johnson and Omer (1985)		Masson et al (1995)		Buck-Gramcko	
	Hands	%	Hands	%	Hands	%
None	6	3	2	1.4	—	—
1	26	14	13	9.1	8	6
2	58	31	35	24.5	20	16
3	53	29	63	44.0	65	51
4	22	12	11	7.7	23	18
5	20	11	19	13.3	11	9
Total	185	100	143	100	127	100

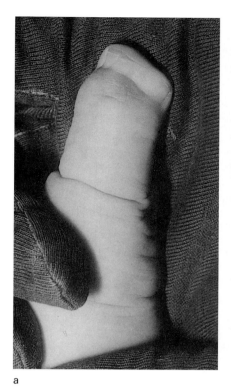

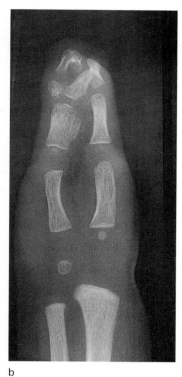

a

b

Figure 2

(a,b) Ulnar hypoplasia with oligo-syndactyly as a two-finger hand with additional bones of a rudi-mentary finger and brachymeso-phalangia of the ulnar digit.

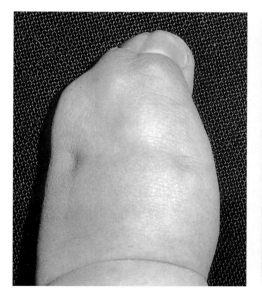

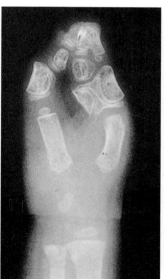

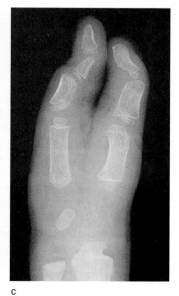

a

b

c

Figure 3

(a,b) Ulnar hypoplasia with oligosyndactyly: two digital rays with additional bones of a rudimentary finger and multiple bones with longitudinal bracketed epiphyses. (c) Radiological appearance after syndactyly separation and removal of the supernumerary bones.

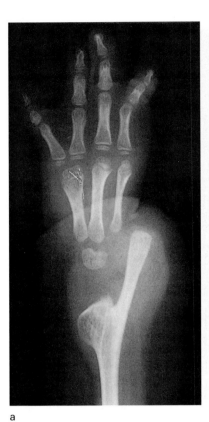
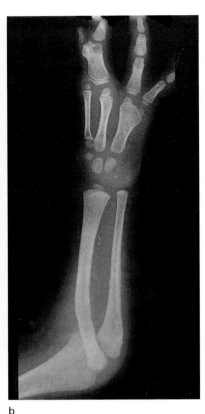

a   b

Figure 4

Bilateral ulnar deficiency with
ulnar aplasia and radiohumeral
synostosis in the left arm (a) and
ulnar hypoplasia with dislocation
of the radial head in the right
arm (b). There are synostoses of
phalanges in the right hand, of
metacarpals in both, and of carpal
bones in the left hand.

13). Sometimes they seemed to be similar to
duplications, as in polydactyly; in other cases
there was a combination with bones with longitudinal bracketed epiphyses or with synostosis
(Figure 3). Two-phalangeal fingers were found in
my patients in 20 hands (16%) and absent
metacarpals in the presence of three phalanges
in eight hands (6%) (see Figures 6, 15 and 16).
Phalanges were deformed as (delta) bones with
longitudinal bracketed epiphyses only in four
hands, but as short triangular or trapezoidal
middle phalanges (brachymesophalangia) in 30
hands (24%). The clinodactyly, caused by these
bones, had to be corrected in only a few cases,
because the angle of inclination was mostly not
more than 15–20°.

Further bone deformities in the hand are
synostoses (Figures 4 and 5), seen in the phalangeal level in 13 hands (10%) and between
metacarpals in 18 hands (14%). While a
phalangeal synostosis was separated—besides
the excision of additional bones—only twice, this
procedure was performed in 11 metacarpal
synostoses (see Figure 7b), mostly combined
with bone grafting, as recommended by Buck-
Gramcko and Wood (1993).

Syndactyly is the most frequent soft-tissue
deformity and was found in my patients in 67
hands (53%). In some cases it is only a partial
syndactyly, but in the majority of hands complete syndactylies are seen. Bony bridges of the
terminal phalanges were found in several hands,
especially in hands with only two digital rays
(see Figures 2 and 13). The thumb is—with or
without syndactyly—often fixed in an adducted
position to the index finger and lies in the level
of the other metacarpals without any rotation,
although thenar muscles are present, mostly in

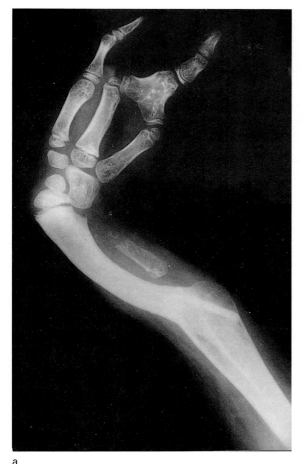

a

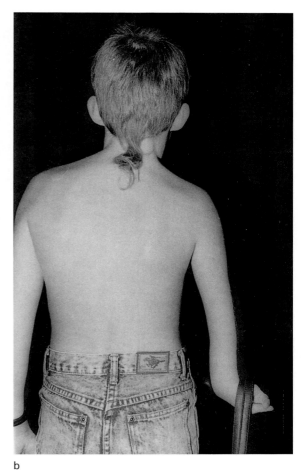

b

Figure 5

(a) Severe ulnar deviation at the wrist in a case of partial ulnar aplasia and radiohumeral synostosis without resection of the anlage. Note the slant of the radial epiphysis, the deformed synostotic carpal bones, and the rare type of osseous syndactyly. The boy has refused any surgical correction of the ulnar deviation, because he uses this deformity for carrying objects (b).

a hypoplastic state. Therefore, rotational osteotomies with widening of the first web space are often necessary to improve the function of the hand.

Wrist

The carpal bones are absent in correlation to the missing digital rays. Only in cases of hypoplasia of the ulna with a full complement of digits is their number normal; however a delay in the appearance of their ossification centers is almost always seen.

Synostoses of the carpal bones are very frequent (about 30–40%). The correct frequency is not known, because many patients were treated in their first years of life and not followed to an age with full carpal ossification. If seen at this age, the X-ray films often show the carpal

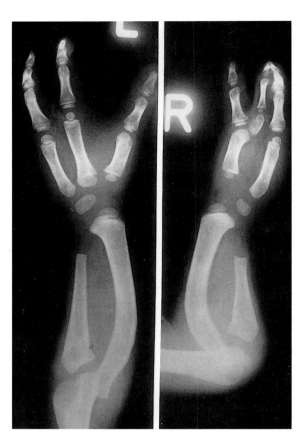

Figure 6

Bilateral involvement with ulnar deficiencies of the same type: partial aplasia of the ulna, dislocation of the radial head, bowing of the radius with slant of its epiphysis, carpal synostosis, reduced number of digits, and absent metacarpal in the right hand.

bones to have a shape which differs considerably from normal anatomy (see in Figures 5, 9, 13, and 17). In one hand we have seen a synostosis between the trapezoid bone and the radial base of the second metacarpal bone.

Ulnar deviation at the wrist is a finding in almost all cases of partial or complete aplasia of the ulna. It is caused both by bowing of the radius and by a slant of the distal articular surface of the radius. Riordan (1978) believes that the slowly growing fibrocartilaginous anlage of the distal ulna tethers the distal radius by its

insertion and contributes to bowing of the radius, dislocation of the radial head, ulnar slant of the distal radius (Figures 5 and 6), and to an increase of the ulnar deviation. He recommended, therefore, excision of the anlage at the age of 6 months (Riordan et al 1961). Others (Broudy and Smith 1979; Marcus and Omer 1984; Johnson and Omer 1985) have shown that excision of the anlage will influence the ulnar deviation only very slightly and that it is warrantable only in the rare cases of progressive deviation, to perform an early excision. This seems to be an acceptable policy, all the more as in most cases the deviation will not exceed 30°. In exceptional cases, the severely deviated wrist may be used to carry some objects (Figure 5).

Forearm

The deformities of the forearm are responsible for the collection of all associated malformations of the upper extremity in one group. In the forearm, it is easy to classify and differentiate three types: hypoplasia, partial, and complete aplasia of the ulna. But there are so many different combinations with deformities of the hand, wrist, and elbow that it is not possible to find a relatively simple and clinically applicable classification system. Interestingly, the extent of the ulnar deformity does not correlate to the deformities of the hand.

Hypoplasia of the ulna was present in my patients in 77 arms (61%), partial aplasia in 26 (20%), and complete aplasia in 24 (19%). While in ulnar hypoplasia (Figure 7a) the elbow was normal in all cases, partial aplasia was combined in 20 out of 26 arms with dislocation of the radial head (Figures 6 and 8). A radiohumeral synostosis was seen in 11 (46%) of the 24 arms with complete aplasia of the ulna (Figures 4 and 8). The length of the forearm is in all cases shorter than normal: in ulnar hypoplasia, only 2–4 cm, but considerably more in cases with partial and complete aplasia of the ulna (see Figure 12). The role of the cartilaginous anlage of the distal ulna and the bowing of the radius has already been mentioned in the section on the wrist. In bilateral cases, the distribution between arms with the same type (Figure 6) and different types of ulnar deficiencies (Figures 4 and 8) is equal.

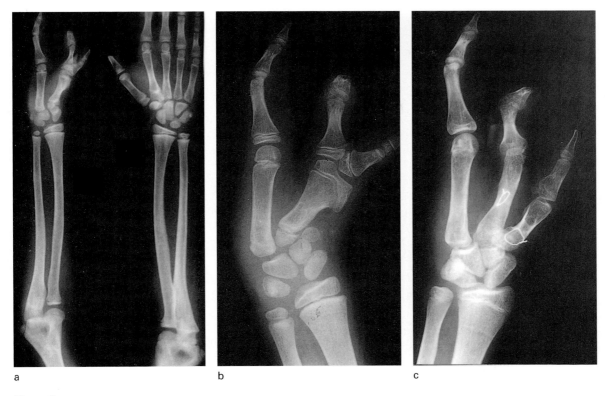

a   b   c

Figure 7

Hypoplasia of the left ulna with a normal elbow, slight forearm shortening, and reduction in the number of digits (a). The metacarpal synostosis of the two radial digits was separated in combination with rotational osteotomy of both halves: X-ray films (b) preoperatively and (c) 4.5 years postoperatively.

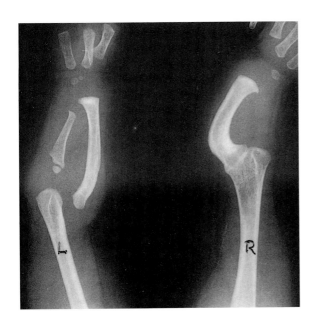

Figure 8

Bilateral ulnar deficiency with partial ulnar aplasia and dislocation of the radial head on the left side and complete aplasia of the ulna with radiohumeral synostosis on the right side.

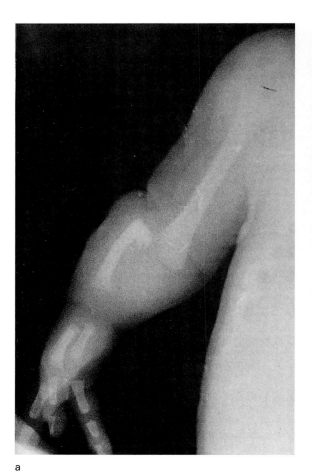

a

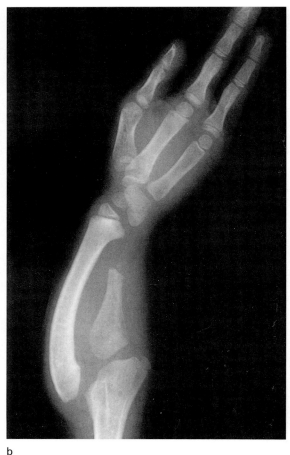

b

Figure 9

(a) The X-ray film 1 week after birth shows no ossification of the ulna, while (b) 7 seven years later the proximal half of the ulna was well developed in an osseous state.

Only in a few publications are the muscles, tendons, nerves, and arteries mentioned. The reason is probably the limited number of operations which were performed at the forearm level, at least in former years. There are only a few reports of dissections: Wierzejewski (1910) mentioned in his review the paper of Priestley of 1856, in which some anatomical defects were described. Other dissection reports are from Strecker (1892), Stoffel and Stempel (1909), and Watt (1917). In the few cases in which I have performed surgery on the wrist and forearm, both ulnar wrist extensor and flexor muscles, a small ulnar artery, and an ulnar nerve were present.

An interesting detail may lead to a wrong classification in the groups of partial and complete ulna aplasia: the delayed ossification of the cartilaginous ulna anlage in its proximal parts. In about the first year of life, the diagnosis seems to be 'complete aplasia of the ulna', while some years later the proximal third of the ulna is well developed in an osseous state as 'partial aplasia of the ulna' (Figure 9).

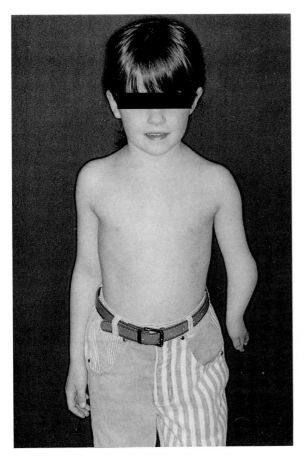

Figure 10

Typical for the more severe cases of ulnar deficiencies is the short and hypoplastic arm with nner rotation, elbow deformity, and pronation of the hand.

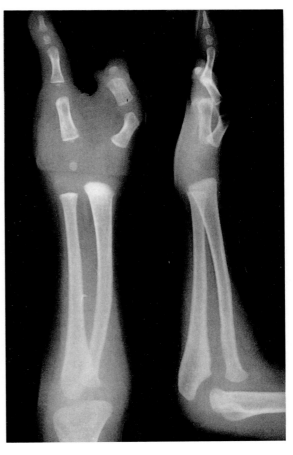

Figure 11

Combination of hypoplastic ulna with congenital dislocation of the head of the radius and with a reduced number of digits. Note the brachymesophalangia of the ulnar finger.

Elbow

Only in combination with ulnar hypoplasia do the articular surfaces of the elbow joint have a normal configuration. The other extreme is the absence of any joint, as in radiohumeral synostosis (see Figures 4 and 8). In my 104 patients radiohumeral synostosis was seen in 20 of 127 involved arms (16%). In 11 arms (8.6%) synostosis was combined with complete aplasia of the ulna and in 9 arms (7%) with partial aplasia. No patient with bilateral radiohumeral synostosis was seen.

The radiohumeral synostosis is almost always associated with a hypoplastic humerus and especially a rotational deformity. The position of the synostosis is in extension or even hyper-extension and often in marked pronation (Figure 10). This malrotation is esthetically and function-ally disturbing and requires surgical correction.

Congenital dislocation of the radial head is mostly combined with ulnar deficiencies. It was found in my material in 41 elbows (32% of all arms). Although the association with partial ulnar aplasia seems to be 'typical' (49% of all

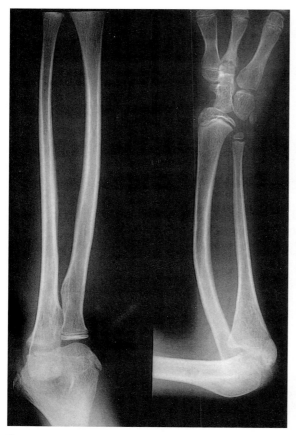
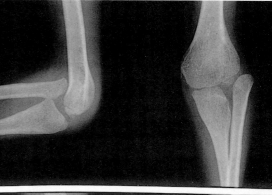
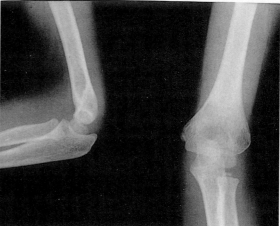

a   b

Figure 12

Comparison of the length of the normal left forearm with the right forearm with ulna hypoplasia, dislocation of the radial head, and bowing of the radius (a). Note also the synostotic carpal bones with abnormal shape. The articulating parts of the elbow show severe deformation (b, upper part), in comparison with the normal left elbow (b, below).

dislocations, but in 20 of 26 arms (77%) with partial aplasia (see Figures 6, 8, and 9)), it is also combined with ulnar hypoplasia (Figures 11 and 12) in 19 arms (46% of the dislocations and 25% of the arms with hypoplastic ulna).

In only two arms with complete aplasia of the ulna did we find radial head dislocation (5% of the dislocations and 8% of the arms with complete aplasia). The function is relatively little impaired, although pro- and supination are limited and extension is not complete. Experience has shown that operative reduction

will not improve the range of motion, because the articular surfaces are dysplastic (Figure 12). It is not possible to construct a normal joint under these conditions.

Upper arm and shoulder

The proximal part of the arm was often ignored in the description of ulnar deficiencies. The shoulder was also not mentioned in the records of several of my patients, or its mobility was described as normal or barely reduced. Only in a few cases were the hypoplasia of humerus, scapula, and clavicle, the hypoplasia or aplasia of muscle, and the resulting limitation of the mobility recorded. In their review, Masson et al (1995) found 19 patients (16%) with afflictions of the shoulder girdle; in most cases the functional problems were insignificant.

Associated anomalies

Several authors have reported a high incidence of associated anomalies outside of the involved limbs. The majority were restricted to the musculoskeletal system. Swanson et al (1984) have mentioned in 41.5% associated anomalies of the lower extremities and 47.6% of the contralateral arm (in unilateral involvement). Masson et al (1995) reported in their collective review an incidence of 55%. In my own patients, there were 24 patients (23%) with associated anomalies in the extremities not involved by ulnar deficiencies. Exactly half belonged to the FFU syndrome. Two other patients had a Cornelia de Lange syndrome, three club feet, two severe scoliosis, and one patient each an anal atresia, an aplasia of the whole arm, and an aplasia of forearm and hand.* One patient showed on the opposite arm an aplasia of the thumb and a proximal radioulnar synostosis, another a duplication of the big toe and a Fanconi anemia.

Surgical treatment and results

Three decades of my own experience have shown that there is no place for conservative treatment of ulnar deficiencies. Although splintage was often recommended, especially for the prevention of progressive ulnar deviation at the wrist, it is useless and bothers both mother and child.

Interestingly, 91% of all operations in my patients with ulnar deficiencies were performed on the hand. This is in accordance with most

*Cases of phokomelia and of aplasia of both forearm bones are not included in the personal series of the author.

reports in the literature. The most frequent operations were syndactyly separations (in 46 hands), widening of the first web space (34 hands), often combined with a rotational osteotomy of the first metacarpal bone (21 hands), or of both metacarpal bones in the case of a hand with two fingers (14 hands), and the removal of additional bones of rudimentary digits (26 hands). By these procedures, the function of the hands was always improved considerably.

This was particularly important in hands with two syndactylized digits (Figure 13). It is possible to convert a primitive 'paddle' into a pinching hand by syndactyly separation with removal of the additional bones, rotational osteotomy of the radial metacarpal, and widening of the web space. These procedures should be performed in two or three steps, as was demonstrated in another patient. His right hand consisted of three digits: index and middle fingers were bound together by syndactyly with a distal bone bridge, the thumb was lying in an adducted position and at the level of the other two metacarpals without any rotation (Figure 14a,b). The separation was performed in the first stage, including pulp plasties (Buck-Gramcko 1988) for skin cover of the exposed bone and construction of a good nail wall (Figure 14c,d). The second stage was the rotational osteotomy of the first metacarpal and widening of the first web space with a rotation advancement flap (Figure 14e,f). Only by this second procedure was the most important improvement in the function obtained.

A pollicization of the index finger is indicated in the rare cases of aplasia of the thumb. It was performed in five of my patients.

In hands with a two- or three-phalangeal finger without a metacarpal there is always the question of whether to retain or ablate this digit. Arguments for an amputation are the lack of flexor and extensor tendons, the instability of the joints, and the resulting minimal function of such a finger, which may sometimes disturb the function of the whole hand. In some bilateral cases, the solution is the combination of both procedures: to amputate the less functional finger and to use some of its bone for supporting such a digit in the contralateral hand by the construction of a metacarpal (Figure 15). In unilateral cases, the new metacarpal is formed by an iliac bone graft. The result may be impaired by partial resorption of the bone graft (Figure 16).

382   CONGENITAL

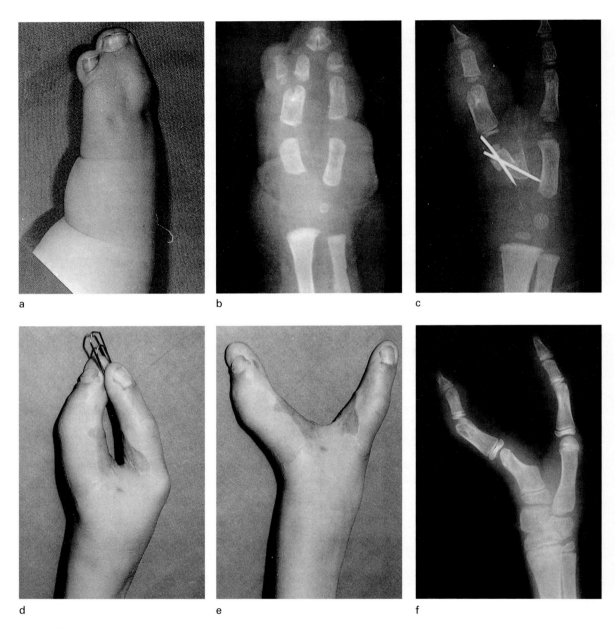

a

b

c

d

e

f

Figure 13

Ulnar deficiency with a small hand of two syndactylized digits with a distal bone bridge and an additional rudimentary radial digit with phalangeal synostosis (a and b). (c) Radiograph following syndactyly separation, removal of the additional bones, and rotational angulatory osteotomy of the radial metacarpal. The result 13 years postoperatively shows a firm pinch (d) and a wide abduction of the two digits (e). (f) Note in the radiograph the configuration of the carpal bones.

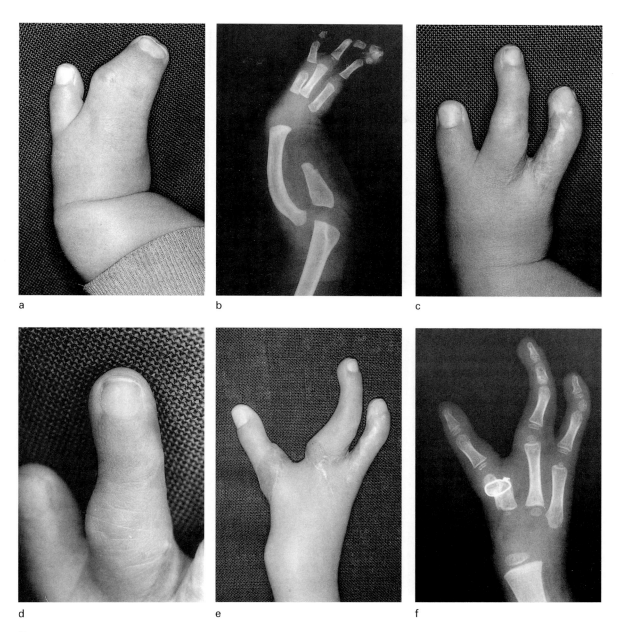

Figure 14

(a,b) Ulnar deficiency with partial aplasia of the ulna, marked bowing and dislocation of the head of the radius, aplasia of the two ulnar digits, syndactyly with a distal bone bridge of the second and third fingers, and adducted position of the thumb without rotation. (c,d) The condition following syndactyly separation: note the normal nail wall, created by the pulp plasty after separation of the bone bridge with a common nail. (e,f) Result of the second operation with rotational angulatory osteotomy of the first metacarpal; the widened and deepened first web space was covered with a rotation advancement flap and additional full thickness skin grafts.

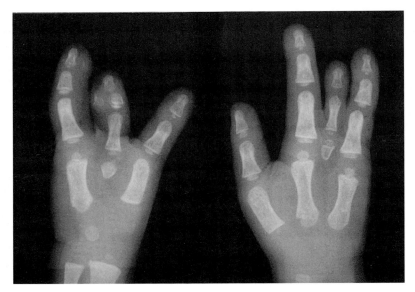

a

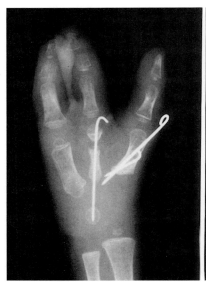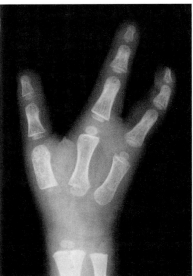

b

Figure 15

(a) Ulnar deficiency with missing metacarpals in both hands and an additional middle phalanx in the left index finger. (b) Early result after amputation of the right incomplete digit and stabilization of the left index finger with bones from the ablated digit.

The resection of the cartilaginous anlage remains controversial. We have performed this procedure in only four cases with ulnar deviation of more than 25°. Care was taken not to damage the ulnar nerve, which runs immediately anterior to the anlage. The resection was combined in our cases with some change of the muscle balance: the transposition of the tendons of the extensor carpi ulnaris and flexor carpi ulnaris to a more radial position. This weakens the strength for ulnar deviation.

In two of my cases with resection of the cartilaginous anlage, there is some evidence that in the period of postoperative growth the slant of the distal articular surface of the radius is

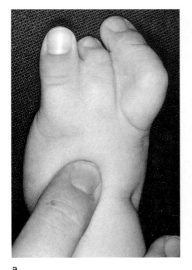

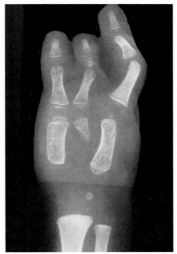

a

b

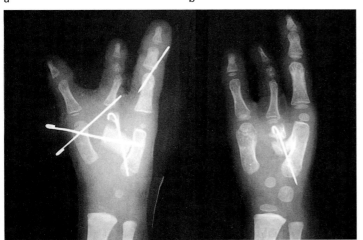

c

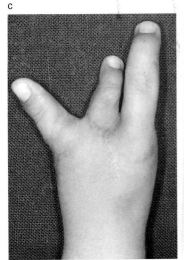

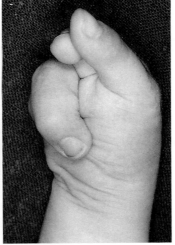

d

e

Figure 16

(a,b) Ulnar deficiency with partial absence of the metacarpal and brachymesophalangia of the index finger, flexion contracture of the proximal interphalangeal joint of the middle finger, adducted position of the non-rotated thumb, and syndactyly. (c,d,e) Result of syndactyly separation, widening of the first web space by a rotation advancement flap, arthrolysis of the proximal interphalangeal joint, and stabilization of the index finger by an iliac bone graft with some subsequent resorption. The index finger has very limited mobility, but can be used in pinching.

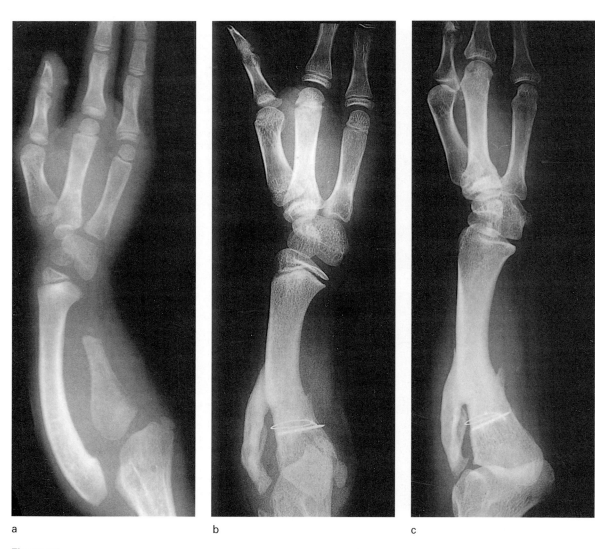

a   b   c

Figure 17

Construction of a one-bone forearm in a patient with partial ulnar aplasia, dislocation of the radial head, and elbow–forearm instability. The anlage was resected. (a) The postoperative development of the radial epiphysis is interesting, as it showed preoperatively a marked obliquity. (b) Three years later, the slant was considerably reduced, and (c) 13 years later at the age of 20, no obliquity was present.

reduced (Figures 17 and 18). In both arms a 'one-bone forearm' procedure was performed, by which the longitudinal axis of the forearm and the radial bowing were changed. The radiological controls showed that the epiphysis of the radius has grown in a straight direction, without the obliquity which was previously present.

The construction of a one-bone forearm was originally used for the stabilization of a forearm with segmental bone defects in trauma cases. In a congenital case with partial aplasia of the ulna, a forearm stabilization by lengthening of the proximal ulna by the proximal half of the dislocated radius and fascia lata arthroplasty between

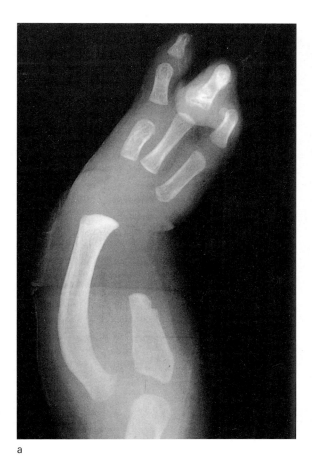

a

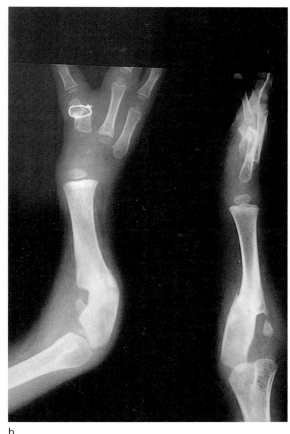

b

Figure 18

Two years after construction of a one-bone forearm with resection of the cartilaginous anlage (a), only a minimal slant of the radial epiphysis has developed (b).

the humerus and the proximal end of the distal radius was described by Goddu (1930).

More successful was the fusion of the distal radius to the proximal ulna after resection of the proximal half of the radius with its dislocated head (Figures 17 and 18). This was described at first by Vitale (1952) and later recommended by Riordan et al (1961), Lowe (1963), Straub (1965), Lloyd-Roberts (1973), Buck-Gramcko (1981), Kitano and Tada (1985), Peterson et al (1995), and others. The reason for the relatively low incidence of this procedure is its indication only in cases of unstable elbows and forearms, which are rare.

In the future, the one-bone forearm procedure will be performed more often, but in combination with a preceding distraction lengthening of the radius until its proximal shortened end can be transposed on top of the partially absent ulna (Smith and Green 1995). This method will lead to much greater lengthening of the forearm and is, therefore, also to be recommended for esthetic improvement.

At the elbow level too, the number of surgical corrections is limited. Open reduction of the dislocation of the radial head is not recommended, even early in life. Our own experience has

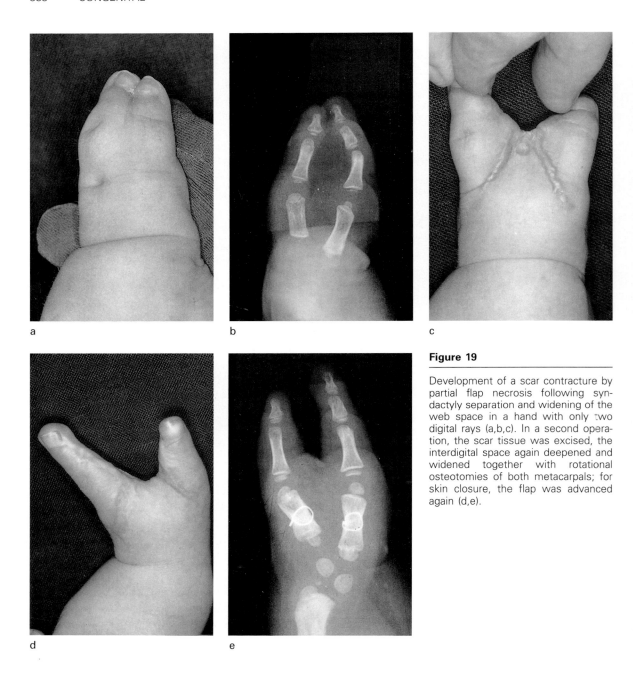

a

b

c

d

e

Figure 19

Development of a scar contracture by partial flap necrosis following syndactyly separation and widening of the web space in a hand with only two digital rays (a,b,c). In a second operation, the scar tissue was excised, the interdigital space again deepened and widened together with rotational osteotomies of both metacarpals; for skin closure, the flap was advanced again (d,e).

shown that the radiological and functional results are generally not improved by operative reduction. This is due to disfiguration of the distal end of the humerus (see Figure 12).

Better results can be expected from rotational angulatory osteotomy for correction of the rotational deformity (see Figure 10). The forearm has to be fixed by a plate or screws in more supination and elbow flexion, so that the hand is in a more functional position.

Complications

The number of complications is limited and consists mainly in the usual problems of wound healing. Marginal skin necroses were seen in several patients with syndactyly separation. The construction of a wide interdigital space is more difficult in the presence of only two digits, because the small dorsum does not have enough skin for a large advancement flap. If it is sutured under too much tension, the tip of the flap may become necrotic, so that the new web space is again narrowed by scar tissue (Figure 19). Fortunately, the flap can be mobilized a second time after scar excision, so that it can cover the widened and deepened web.

Other complications which occurred in our patients were iliac bone graft resorption (see Figure 16), ulnar nerve damage during excision of the anlage, and damage of the brachial artery in its abnormal course at the elbow during a rotational osteotomy.

References

Aitken GT (1969) *Proximal Femoral Focal Deficiency. A Congenital Anomaly* (National Academy of Science: Washington).

Bayne LG (1993) Ulnar club hand (ulnar deficiencies). In: Green DP, ed, *Operative Hand Surgery*, 3rd edn (Churchill Livingstone: New York) 289–304.

Birch-Jensen A (1949) *Congenital Deformities of the Upper Extremities* (Andelsbogtrykkeriet i Odense and Det Danske Forlag: Odense).

Blauth W, Hippe P (1990) Klassifikationsversuch von Fehlbildungen am ulnaren Strahl. In: Flügel M, Landsleitner B, eds, *Zum 60sten. Ein Lesebuch für Jürgen Geldmacher* (Druckhaus Mayer: Erlangen) 29–40.

Broudy AS, Smith RJ (1979) Deformities of the hand and wrist with ulnar deficiency, *J Hand Surg* **4**:304–15.

Buck-Gramcko D (1988) Angeborene Fehlbildungen. In: Nigst H, Buck-Gramcko D, Millesi H, eds, *Hand-chirurgie*, Vol I, (Thieme: Stuttgart; English edition Thieme Medical Publications: New York, 1988).

Buck-Gramcko D, Wood VE (1993) The treatment of metacarpal synostosis, *J Hand Surg* **18A**:565–81.

Flatt AE (1994) *The Care of Congenital Hand Anomalies*, 2nd edn (Quality Medical Publications: St Louis).

Goddu LAO (1930) Reconstruction of elbow and bone graft of rudimentary ulna, *New Engl J Med* **202**:1142–4.

Johnson J, Omer GE (1985) Congenital ulnar deficiency. Natural history and therapeutic implications, *Hand Clin* **1**:499–510.

Jones HW, Roberts RE (1926) A rare type of congenital club hand, *J Anat, Lond* **60**:146–7.

Kitano K, Tada K (1985) One-bone forearm procedure for partial defect of the ulna, *J Pediatr Orthop* **5**:290–93.

Kühne D, Lenz W, Petersen D, et al (1967) Defekt von Femur und Fibula mit Amelie, Peromelie oder ulnaren Strahldefekten der Arme. Ein Syndrom, *Humangenetik* **3**:244–63.

Lloyd-Roberts GC (1973) Treatment of defects of the ulna in children by establishing cross-union with the radius, *J Bone Joint Surg* **55-B**:327–30.

Lowe HG (1963) Radio-ulnar fusion for defects in the forearm bones, *J Bone Joint Surg* **45-B**:351–9.

Marcus NA, Omer GE (1984) Carpal deviation in congenital ulnar deficiency, *J Bone Joint Surg* **66-A**:1003–1007.

Masson MV, Bennett JB, Cain TE (1995) Congenital absence of the ulna. Paper read at the 50th Meeting of the American Society for Surgery of the Hand, San Francisco, California, 15 September 1995. *J Hand Surg* (in press).

Ohnesorge W (1987) *Ulnare Reduktionsfehlbildungen*, Inaugural Dissertation, University of Göttingen.

Peterson CA, Maki S, Wood MB (1995) Clinical results of the one-bone forearm, *J Hand Surg* **20A**:609–18.

Riordan DC (1978) Congenital absence of the ulna. In: Lovell WW, Winter RB, eds, *Pediatric Orthopaedics* (JB Lippincott: Philadelphia) 714–19.

Riordan DC, Mills EH, Alldredge RH (1961) Congenital absence of the ulna, *J Bone Joint Surg* **43-A**:614.

Smith AA, Greene TL (1995) Preliminary soft tissue distraction in congenital forearm deficiency, *J Hand Surg* **20A**:420–24.

Stoffel A, Stempel E (1909) *Anatomische Studien über die Klumphand* (Enke: Stuttgart).

Straub LR (1965) Congenital absence of the ulna, *Am J Surg* **109**:300–305.

Strecker C (1892) Eine angeboren vierfingerige rechte Hand, *Archiv pathol Anat Physiol klin Med* **127**:181–7.

Swanson AB, Tada K, Yonenobu K (1984) Ulnar ray deficiency: its various manifestations, *J Hand Surg* **9A**:658–64.

Temtamy S, McKusick V (1978) *The Genetics of Hand Malformations. Birth Defects,* Original Article Series, Vol XIV, No 3 (AR Liss: New York).

Vitale CC (1952) Reconstructive surgery for defects in the shaft of the ulna in children, *J Bone Joint Surg* **34-A**:804–10.

Watt JC (1917) Anatomy of a seven months' foetus exhibiting bilateral absence of the ulna accompanied by monodactyly (and also diaphragmatic hernia), *Am J Anat* **22**:385–437.

Wierzejewski I (1910) Ueber den kongenitalen Ulnadefekt, *Zschr Orthop Chir* **27**:101–31.

56
Triphalangeal thumb

Clayton A Peimer

Introduction

The thumb develops from the preaxial (radial) border of the limb bud hand plate in the fifth through eighth weeks of gestation. The apical ectodermal ridge and zone of polarizing activity focuses and modulates the specific (three-dimensionally oriented) morphogenesis of the upper limb.[1] It now appears that genetic information critical to normal (thumb) morphologic development is located throughout the genetic code.[2] Although congenital deformities of the thumb are relatively common, thumb triphalangism is not the most frequent.[3–12]

The first reported case of triphalangeal thumb was by DuBois in 1826.[13] Of the approximately 800 additional cases described since, almost 90% were bilateral, and many were associated with hereditary and syndromic abnormalities.[14–28] Associated anomalies of the cardiac, ophthalmic, otic, facial, gastrointestinal, genitourinary, muscular/skeletal (including spinal) and the hematopoietic systems have been recorded.

The triphalangeal thumb is long and awkward (Figure 1). The terminal portion is most frequently angulated (usually ulnarward), and sometimes widened. This congenital abnormality significantly diminishes both hand function and thumb appearance. Triphalangeal thumb may occur alone or associated with polydactyly;[16,27,29–32] the exact etiology of the abnormality remains speculative.[12,15,33–35]

Classification

Thumb triphalangealism has been described in different ways, generally based on the ability to functionally oppose, or based on the shape of the extra phalanx.

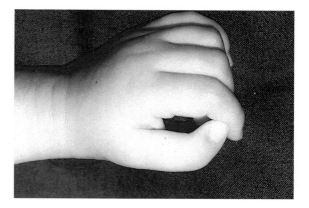

Figure 1

This 2-year-old boy with bilateral thumb triphalangism has a slightly lengthened, ulnarly angulated deformed thumb. Attempts at pinch and small object manipulation are difficult and awkward (see Figure 2 for radiographs).

The 'opposable triphalangeal thumb' has adequate thenar muscles and a satisfactory first web space (tissues) and can therefore actively abduct, pronate, and oppose to the fingers. The 'unopposable triphalangeal thumb' occurs as a part of the pentadactylous (five-fingered) hand. This is a hand in which each of the five digits consists of three phalanges plus a metacarpal with a distal physis. The most radial of the digits lies in the plane of the other four fingers, and it is nonopposable, lacking both thenar muscles and a usefully generous first web.[9,29,36] Other than by their clinical appearance, these two different functional types of thumb triphalangealism are also best distinguished by the location of the (first) metacarpal physis. In the five-fingered hand, the most radial metacarpal physis is distal,

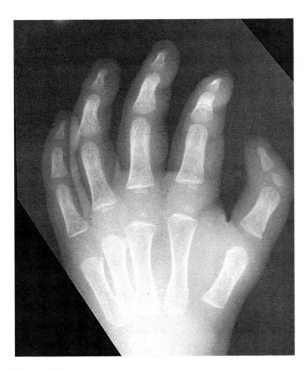

Figure 2

Radiographs of a 2-year-old boy (Figure 1) show thumb triphalangism with ulnar deviation. The extra phalanx is eccentric (radial) to the axis of the first ray; arguably, the shape of the extra bone makes this a 'small Type II' in the Wood classification.

birthday. However, the diagnosis should be suspected by X-rays that show widening of the space between the ossified proximal and distal phalanges (often as an 'empty space', and especially if the thumb is angulated at or near the interphalangeal region). At times, the primary ossification center of the extra phalanx is located eccentric to the axis of the first ray (Figure 2). Buck-Gramcko classifies thumb triphalangism into seven types, based on the combination of size and shape of the extra bone, thenar muscle and first web adequacy, and presence/absence of polydactyly in the first ray.[37]

Treatment

Unopposable

For the true pentadactylous/five-fingered hand, the triphalangeal thumb must be transposed to a position more radial, palmar, and pronated with respect to the digits. In such hands, the method of pollicization described by Buck-Gramcko,[38] with modifications by Flatt,[39] is the most efficacious single-stage approach.

In my experience, however, considering all cases of pollicization, I find that nearly half need later augmentation of intrinsic abduction and opposition; and I most typically use the abductor digiti minimi (quinti) muscle transfer (of Huber) elucidated by Littler and Cooley,[40] if poor grasp patterns become dependably evident after pollicization through occupational therapy evaluations. In most such patients, the need for muscle transfer is definable within 18–24 months following pollicization.

In truth, some children have 'relatively unopposable' thumbs: the first web is inadequate but not as narrow as the other four, and the plane of the first ray is not as palmar and pronated as it should ideally be. The majority will also have capsular laxity at the metacarpal phalangeal (MP) joint of the thumb; usually the ulnar collateral is worst, but often the MP joint is globally unstable. This constellation may be remedied by the combination of first metacarpal shortening, with rotation (into pronation) and slight palmar angulation. The first web is simultaneously widened with a four-flap Z-plasty. The

whereas the opposable triphalangeal thumb has a metacarpal physis at its proximal end (like a thumb).

Classification based on the shape of the extra phalanx was proposed by Wood.[6,7] Type I has a smaller delta (triangular) middle phalanx; Type II has a rectangular extra phalanx (actually, a trapezoidal shape); and Type III includes a full extra phalanx whose proximal and distal ends are parallel to each other and both perpendicular to the long axis of the ray. The presence of an additional phalanx adds excessive length and an unneeded joint. It is the shape of this extra bone that determines the angular deformity.

A small delta (Type I/triangular) middle phalanx will not ossify until after the child's first

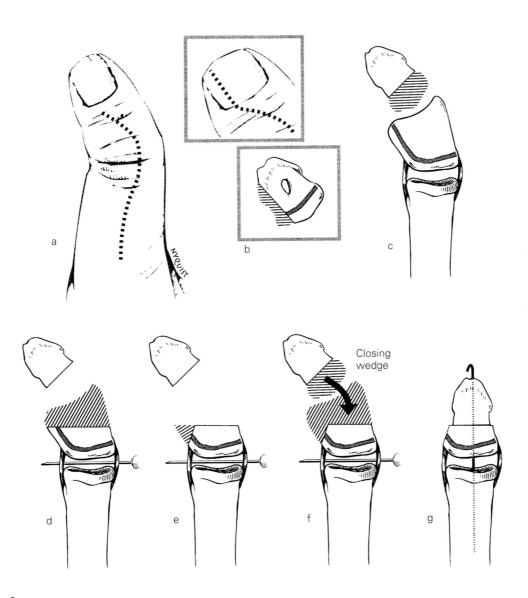

Figure 3

Reduction osteotomy surgical technique.

(a) Curvilinear longitudinal dorsal incision as marked; skin flaps are elevated and the extensor tendon transected barely proximal to its dorsal lip insertion in the true distal phalanx. Reflecting the extensor proximally exposes the distal phalanx and supernumerary bone. (b) (insets) If the nail and distal phalanx are duplicated or abnormally widened, narrowing will improve the final esthetics. (c) The distal phalangeal physis is excised with a scalpel blade. (d) A fine Kirschner wire or hypodermic needle is passed across the true (i.e. proximal) interphalangeal joint to orient the transverse osteotomy parallel to the proximal phalangeal condyles. (e) The final bone cut in the true proximal phalanx is used to excise the abnormal, longitudinal portion of the (C-shaped) physis; the collateral ligament is kept intact. (f,g) A combination of the several osteotomies creates a closing wedge which shortens and realigns the thumb, eliminating the extra, abnormal joint and abnormal, longitudinal physis. The bone ends are fixed with Kirschner wires and the extensor tendon shortened and repaired to the distal stump. (Modified and redrawn from reference 48.)

MP joint capsule is imbricated, and the joint is pinned for 8 weeks.

Having said all this, one must remember that such a thumb is still one segment and one joint too long! The best way to address this last problem (in what is now an 'opposable' thumb) is described in the section that follows, under reduction osteotomy.

No matter which of the primary surgical methods is chosen, these children should be followed until adolescence, and carefully evaluated by a physician and hand therapist skilled in functional analysis. Where problems of inadequate pinch or of active opposition positioning in any operated thumb become evident, additional remedies will need to be offered. The parents will have been told at the initial evaluation, of course, that in a growing child, the 'major reconstructive procedure' may well not be the only one necessary.

Opposable

Where first ray position is satisfactory, the goal of surgery is to reduce excessive length and abnormal angulation. In theory, several methods are available including supranumerary bone excision,[33,35] amputation of the tip,[41] and other modifications.[4,6,8,29] None of these techniques has provided a uniformly esthetic or predictably functional outcome, and of bone excision[6,8,29,42–45] combined with attempts at collateral ligament reconstruction have resulted—where documentable numbers are available in the literature—in horrendously unacceptable postoperative ligament instability and malposition; notably 71% of operated patients in Wood's retrospective series.[6] Indeed, incomplete correction, secondary angulation, and chronic ligament laxity are—most regrettably—typical outcomes in these reports. By 1944, Bunnell recommended that no surgical treatment be provided, fearing the results of attempted correction worse than the original congenital malformation.[46]

The technique I prefer is one that requires surgical diligence, but has resulted in successful correction of the problem in our patients over now more than 15 years.[47,48] The technique of reduction osteotomy is based on traditional and widely accepted treatment for correcting congenital angular deformities in fingers.[29,31] The problem in the triphalangeal thumb is, after all, really excessive length plus angulation where the extra (middle) segment contains a delta or C-shaped physis; plus the one additional problem of an extra joint.

Carstam and Theander considered the delta or trapezoidal physis to be a 'longitudinally bracketed diaphysis'.[49] Watson and Boyes believed that a delta phalanx represents a syndactylous supernumerary digit.[32] They and others routinely excised the abnormal, longitudinal portion of the epiphysis in the C-shaped finger phalanx, with deangulation by (opening or closing) wedge osteotomy. The reduction osteotomy technique merely adapts this method to the problem of triphalangeal thumb by removing excess length via bone and (extra) joint excision.

The surgical technique (Figure 3) includes marking the preoperative X-rays and making a sketch of the phalangeal and growth plate deformities to approximate the location of the proposed bone cuts and resections. The curvilinear dorsal incision may include removal of a portion of the nail matrix if the terminal segment is excessively wide. Two or three longitudinal or crossed Kirschner wires are used to fix the final bone positions.

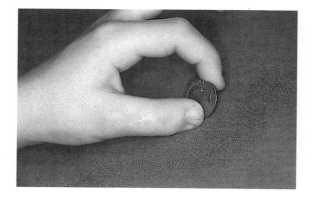

Figure 4

Five years after reduction osteotomy, thumb length, alignment, stability, and proportionate growth has been maintained; fine motor skills—including pinch—have been enhanced. (Same case as Figures 1 and 2.)

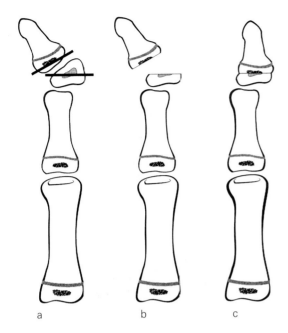

a   b   c

Figure 5

Skeletally immature triphalangeal thumb with radiographically evident secondary ossification centers in the three phalanges and metacarpal.
(a) Bone and cartilage excision is planned through the ossific nuclei of the distal and 'middle' phalanx; each cut is perpendicular to the long axis of that phalanx, as drawn.
(b) Osteocartilaginous excision perpendicular to the long axis creates a closing wedge to allow skeletal realignment.
(c) Realignment is maintained with Kirschner wires, preserving and coapting the secondary ossification centers; much of the longitudinal portion of the middle phalangeal physis (when C-shaped) is also removed simultaneously. (Modified, adapted, and redrawn from reference 50.)

Wires are removed in the office after about 5–6 weeks, when there is X-ray evidence of union at the osteotomy. Once the bone has healed, splint protection is not necessary since ligament reconstruction was not performed (because the congruous and stable, normal, proximal joint is retained) (Figure 4).

I find this method even simpler in patients with already closed physes or Wood Type III triphalangeal thumbs.

Light has noted in older children, in whom the extra phalanx has already ossified, that it is possible to fuse the secondary ossification center

of the distal phalanx to the ossified portion of the middle phalangeal epiphysis, still preserving the distal phalangeal physis (Figure 5).[50] His approach shortens the digit, eliminates one phalanx, and attempts to preserve longitudinal distal phalangeal growth in the realigned thumb. However, he clearly notes that his procedure 'still leaves the thumb longer than normal', but feels that this problem is better addressed by later (i.e. secondary) distal phalangeal epiphysiodesis. I disagree.

In any event, if a joint resection/osteotomy procedure is planned, the surgery needs to be delayed until epiphyseal ossification patterns are radiographically clear, and this will be after the child is 24–36 months old;[51] Buck-Gramcko waits until age 6–8 years.[37] After one has used reduction osteotomy technique with some frequency, the age at operation may be lowered if care is taken.

Conclusion

Thumb triphalangealism is an uncommon but significantly dysfunctional disorder and a cosmetic failure. The anomaly may arise as an isolated finding or with syndromic variants. Children should be carefully screened for serious associated hematopoietic and other abnormalities of the cardiac, renal, GI, and GU systems before surgery is done. With care and skill, the method of reduction osteotomy can achieve the desired diminution of length and deangulation, restoring functional prehension in the opposable triphalangeal thumb; and pollicization can be reproducibly utilized for the unopposable variant.

References

1 Upton J, Congenital anomalies of the hand and forearm. In: McCarthy JG, ed, *Plastic Surgery*, Vol 8 (WB Saunders: Philadelphia, 1990) 5213.
2 Zaleske DJ, Tsukurov O, Boehmer A et al, A complex bilateral polysyndactyly disease locus maps to chromosome 7_q36, *Nature Gen* (1994) **6**:282–6.
3 Wassel HD, The result of surgery for polydactyly of the thumb: a review, *Clin Orthop* (1969) **64**:175–93.

4   Tada K, Yonenobu K, Tsuyuguchi Y, Kawai H, Egawa T, Duplication of the thumb, *J Bone Joint Surg* (1983) **65A**:584–98.

5   Marks TW, Bayne LG, Polydactyly of the thumb: abnormal anatomy and treatment, *J Hand Surg* (1978) **3**:107–16.

6   Wood VE, Treatment of the triphalangeal thumb, *Clin Orthop* (1976) **120**:188–99.

7   Wood VE, Polydactyly and the triphalangeal thumb, *J Hand Surg* (1978) **3**:436-44.

8   Wood VE, Congenital anomalies. In: Green DP, ed, *Operative Hand Surgery*, 3rd edn (Churchill Livingstone: New York, 1993) 461–5.

9   Miura T, Triphalangeal thumb, *Plast Reconstr Surg* (1976) **58**:587–94.

10 Palmieri TJ, Polydactyly of the thumb: incidence, etiology, classification, and treatment, *Bull Hosp Jt Dis Orthop Inst* (1973) **34**:200–21.

11 Swanson AB, Brown KS, Hereditary triphalangeal thumb, *J Hered* (1962) **53**:259–65.

12 Lapidus PW, Guidotti FP, Coletti CJ, Triphalangeal thumb—report of six cases, *Surg Gynecol Obstet* (1943) **77**:178–86.

13 Dubois P, *Arch Gen Med* (1826) **11**:148.

14 Aase JM, Smith DW, Congenital anemia and triphalangeal thumbs: a new syndrome, *J Pediatr* (1969) **74**:471–4.

15 Abramowitz I, Triphalangeal thumb—a case report and evaluation of its importance in the morphology and function of the thumb, *S Afr Med J* (1967) **41**:104–6.

16 Castilla E, Paz J, Mutchinick O, Munoz E, Giorgiutti E, Gelman Z, Polydactyly: a genetic study in South America, *Am J Hum Genet* (1973) **25**:405–12.

17 Diamond LR, Allen DB, Magill FB, Congenital (erythroid) hypoplastic anemia: a 25-year study, *Am J Dis Child* (1961) **102**:403–15.

18 Holmes LB, Congenital heart disease and upper extremity deformities: a report of two families, *N Engl J Med* (1965) **272**:437–44.

19 Holt M, Oram S, Familial heart disease with skeletal malformations, *Br Heart J* (1960) **22**:236–42.

20 Juberg RC, Hayward JR, A new familial syndrome of oral, cranial, and digital anomalies, *J Pediatr* (1969) **74**:755–62.

21 Minagi H, Steinbach HL, Roentgen appearance of anomalies associated with hypoplastic anemias of childhood, *Am J Roentgenol* (1966) **97**:100–9.

22 Murphy S, Lubin G, Triphalangeal thumbs and congenital erythroid hypoplasia: report of a case with unusual features, *J Pediatr* (1972) **81**:987–9.

23 Pozanski AK, Garn SM, Holt JF, The thumb in the congenital malformation syndromes, *Radiology* (1971) **100**:115–29.

24 Rath F, Triphalangia of the thumb as a manifestation of thalidomide embryopathy, *Wein Klin Wochenschr* (1966) **78**:181–3.

25 Temtamy SA, McKusick VA, The genetics of hand malformations, *Birth Defects* (1978) **14**:393–439.

26 Woolf CM, Myrianthopoulos NC, Polydactyly in American Negroes and whites, *Am J Hum Genet* (1973) **25**:397–404.

27 Woolf CM, Woolf RM, A genetic study of polydactyly in Utah, *Am J Hum Genet* (1970) **22**:75–87.

28 Ogino T, Ishii S, Kato H, Opposable triphalangeal thumb: Clinical features and results of treatment, *J Hand Surg* (1994) **19A**:39.

29 Flatt AE, *The Care of Congenital Hand Anomalies* (Quality Medical Publishing: St Louis, 1994) 136–45, 207–17.

30 Jones GB, Delta phalanx, *J Bone Joint Surg* (1964) **46B**:226–8.

31 Smith RJ, Osteotomy for 'delta-phalanx' deformity, *Clin Orthop* (1977) **123**:91–4.

32 Watson HK, Boyes JH, Congenital angular deformity of the digits: delta phalanx, *J Bone Joint Surg* (1967) **49A**:333–8.

33 Haas SL, Three-phalangeal thumbs, *Am J Roentgenol* (1939) **42**:677–82.

34 Milch H, Triphalangeal thumb, *J Bone Joint Surg* (1951) **33A**:692–7.

35 Shiono H, Ogino T, Triphalangeal thumb and dermatoglyphics, *J Hand Surg* (1984) **9B**:151–2.

36 Chan KM, Lamb DW, Triphalangeal thumb and five-fingered hand, *Hand* (1983) **15**:329.

37 Buck-Gramcko D, Triphalangeal thumb. In: Buck-Gramcko D, ed, *Congenital Malformations of the Hand and Forearm* (Churchill Livingstone: London) in press.

38 Buck-Gramcko D, Thumb reconstruction by digital transposition, *Orthop Clin North Am* (1977) **8**:329–42.

39 Flatt AE, *The Care of Congenital Hand Anomalies*. (Quality Medical Publishing: St Louis, 1994) 96–112.

40 Littler JW, Cooley SGE, Opposition of the thumb and its restoration by abductor digiti quinti transfer, *J Bone Joint Surg* (1963) **45A**:1389–96.

41 Kristjansen A, Supernumerary phalanx in the thumbs, 'hyperphalangeal pollis', *Hosp-Tid* (1926) **69**:109–19.

42 Schrader E, Three-joint thumbs, *Fortschr Geb Roentgenstr Nuklearmed Erganzungsband* (1929) **40**:693.

43 Grobelnik S, Triphalangeal thumb (supernumerary distal phalanx of the thumb), *Z Orthop* (1951) **80**:294–8.

44 Jaeger M, Refior HJ, Congenital triangular deformity of tubular bones in hand and foot, *Clin Orthop* (1971) **81**:139–50.

45 Burke F, Flatt AE, Clinodactyly: a review of a series of cases, *Hand* (1979) **2**:269–80.

46 Bunnell S, *Surgery of the Hand*, 1st edn (JB Lippincott: Philadelphia, 1944) 641.

47 Peimer C, Combined reduction osteotomy for triphalangeal thumb, *J Hand Surg* (1985) **10A**:376–81.

48 Jennings JF, Peimer CA, Sherwin FS, Reduction osteotomy for triphalangeal thumb: an 11-year review, *J Hand Surg* (1992) **17**:8–14.

49 Carstam N, Theander G, Surgical treatment of clinodactyly caused by longitudinally bracketed diaphysis, *Scand J Plast Reconstr Surg* (1975) **9**:199–202.

50 Light TR, Congenital anomalies: syndactyly, polydactyly and cleft hand. In: Peimer CA, ed, *Surgery of the Hand and Upper Extremity* (McGraw-Hill: New York, 1996).

51 Poznanski AK, ed, *The Hand in Radiologic Diagnosis* (WB Saunders: Philadelphia, 1984) 77–8.

57

Arthrogryposis multiplex congenita: Techniques and indications for early corrective surgery of the wrist and elbow

Ulrich Mennen

Introduction

Arthrogryposis multiplex congenita (AMC) is a specific, well-defined congenital syndrome which affects muscles of the limbs resulting in 'deformed joints'. The muscles are fibrotic, fewer in number and shortened, causing the characteristic bilateral symmetrical deformities. In the classical form the elbows are in hyperextension, wrists in flexion, thumbs adducted and flexed in the palm and the fingers stiff and slightly flexed. Secondary deformities due to the primary muscular pathology result in ligamentous and capsular shortening with intra-articular adhesions and displastic joints of the affected limbs.

Arthrogryposis multiplex congenita does not refer to all the conditions which produce deformed joints.[1] It is important that the AMC referred to in this chapter fits the original description in its classical form described by Otto (quoted by James[2]), using the term coined by Rocher.[3] Much confusion exists because of the indiscriminate grouping of congenitally stiff limbs and deformed joints which are caused by a variety of etiological factors into one group. Although the etiology of AMC is still unknown, the characteristic features of the deformed limbs and even the face make this an entity by itself. A number of causative agents have been implicated as the cause of the primary muscle pathology, such as viral infections. Inherited chromosome involvement has been excluded by the findings of Mennen et al.[4]

Previous treatment included physiotherapy and splinting. Symptomatic corrective surgery was often delayed until preschool age or even puberty. Fortunately this indecisive attitude has been replaced by the realization that definitive and early surgical intervention may improve the lot of these congenital deformities.[5–8]

The purpose of this chapter is to encourage early active and specific surgery for the deformities of the elbow and wrist.

Technical aspects

At the age of about 3 to 6 months, surgery is recommended as a one-stage procedure to the elbow and wrist. A lazy S-incision is made over the dorsum of the wrist to expose the extensor retinaculum which is incised lengthwise. The extensor tendons are retracted sideways to expose the dorsal capsule of the carpal joint. The capsule is incised transversely, leaving a proximal and distal flap of equal width. The mostly cartilaginous scaphoid, lunate and triquetrum are very carefully removed, by a scalpel blade or a bone nibbler. Great care should be taken to avoid any damage to the articular cartilage of the radius and the TFCC ligament. If 40° of wrist extension is not achieved by this proximal carpectomy, the proximal parts of the trapezium, trapezoid, capitate and hamate are removed in thin slices until the desired degree of extension is achieved. These slices should be thicker

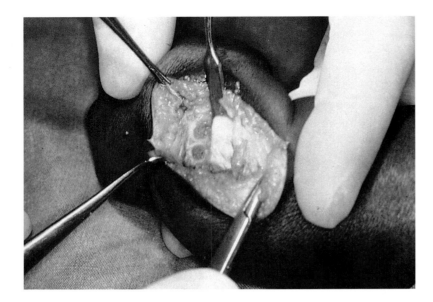

Figure 1

Intra-operative view of the removed proximal carpal ray and half of the distal ray, exposing the ossification centres of the distal carpal bones.

dorsally, creating a trapezoid shape gap. It is important that less carpal material is removed from the ulnar side to avoid ulnar deviation (Figure 1).

The resultant removal of the carpal bones will leave a trapezoid shaped gap, i.e. a gap which is wider dorsally than volarly. This will not only allow slight proximal migration of the whole hand and wrist, releasing the tension on the volar side, but will also allow the wrist and hand to be placed in a more normal dorsiflexed position.

Once the desired position of 40° of wrist extension is achieved, a 1.4 mm diameter Kirschner wire is passed retrograde through the remaining carpus towards the third metacarpal bone. Ideally the wire should exit distally between the heads of the third and fourth metacarpals. The wrist is now held in the corrected position, i.e. 40° dorsiflexion and 10° to 15° radial deviation (third metacarpal/radius 0° angle). The Kirschner wire is carefully pushed proximally into the radius. In order to protect the single wire, the capsule is now sutured tightly with absorbable sutures in an overlapping fashion.

Two longitudinal volar incisions are made over the shortened wrist flexors. The tendons are carefully identified as either very short, tight, thin and even absent. Care should be taken not to confuse these tendons with the median and/or ulnar nerves. The flexor carpi ulnaris (FCU), palmaris longus and flexor carpi radialis (FCR) should be severed as far distally as possible. The palmaris longus tendon is excised. The FCU and the FCR are carefully transferred subcutaneously to the dorsal aspect and sutured to the basis of the appropriate metacarpals via the preserved capsule, or to the extensor carpi radialis longus and extensor carpi ulnaris when the tendons are too short. Often only one flexor tendon is available which should then be sutured to the base of the third metacarpal using some form of tissue augmentation as described above.

The elbow is approached through a lateral incision. The triceps insertion is released from the olecranon with a periosteal tongue for extra length and is transferred subcutaneously anterior to the axis of the elbow joint to reach the anterior aspect of the elbow. Care should be taken to release the triceps muscle from the humerus to allow adequate elasticity or 'give' in the muscle. The triceps is usually too short to be inserted into the bicepital insertion on the radius. If this could be achieved the classical triceps flexor plasty is done. However, in most cases the triceps is too short. We have inserted the triceps with equally good results into the common extensor tendon about 2 cm distal to its lateral epicondyle insertion. A posterior capsulotomy of the elbow joint is done carefully to achieve full flexion of the elbow. Once the triceps is sutured into position, the 90° flexed position of the elbow is held with one Kirschner wire across the elbow joint from the olecranon to the humerus.

After meticulous haemostasis and skin closure an above elbow volar plaster-of-Paris splint is applied for 1 week. This splint is replaced with an above-elbow circular cast for another 5 weeks. The Kirschner wires are then removed and the wrist is protected by a removable volar night splint for another 3–6 months.

The resultant removal of the carpal bones will leave a trapezoid trough, i.e. a gap which is wider dorsally than volarly. This will not only allow slight proximal migration of the whole hand and wrist, releasing the tension on the volar side, but will also allow the wrist and hand to be placed in a more normal dorsiflexed position.

Results

We use a clinical classification of AMC which is purely based on observation pre- and postoperatively. Patients are grouped into the 'loose' type with an optimistic prognosis for a good range of motion and near normal function. The second group is classified as the 'stiff' type, with a better cosmetic appearance but a predictably reduced range of motion and function. In pathological terms there is a direct relationship with the number of muscles, amount of fibrous tissue present and the function of the remaining muscle fibres. The overall appearance of the upper limbs of these children approaches near normal and differs radically from the pre-operative position. Table 1 summarises the number of patients operated on, age, sex and side.

The motion and function of these upper limbs will have a wide range of measurements. The following active ranges of motion were recorded for the whole group:

Elbow   30–100° flexion (average 49° active flexion)

Table 1 Number of patients operated on, age, sex and side.

Age	
0–3 months	5
3–6 months	7
6–9 months	5
9–12 months	5
1–5 years	5
5–10 years	2
Total	29 patients
Sex	
boys	15
girls	14
Total	29 patients
Side	
Right	28
Left	27
Total	55 operated limbs

Wrist   10° flexion to 30° extension (average 27° active motion)

Fingers   MP joint 20–85° flexion (average 65° active flexion)
PIP joints 20–80° flexion (average 45° active flexion)
DIP joints 15–35° flexion (average 20° active flexion)

Neglected patients who did not have the operation were brought to the clinic at a late age, showed no movement in the elbow and wrist joints and minimal movement in the finger joints (Figure 2).

In one patient, aged 7 years, a distal osteotomy of the radius and ulnar was performed to correct the flexion deformity of the wrist. However, the corrected position was lost within 2 years due to remodelling. This type of surgery, propounded in text books and many papers, was definitely not indicated. The loss of correction made the operation unnecessary and eventually the little improvement that was gained in appearance and function was also lost.

Discussion

The ideal age for this operation is between 3 and 6 months. The operative technique at this age is

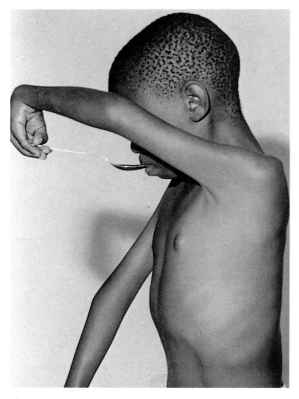

Figure 2

Neglected boy with no elbow and wrist function and minimal active movement of his fingers. The appearance and function are not acceptable.

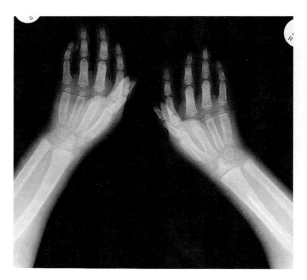

Figure 3

The radiographic appearance of a bilateral proximal row carpectomy done between the age of 3 and 6 months. This led to a functioning carpus with a development of carpal bones from the carpal remnants after the carpectomy.

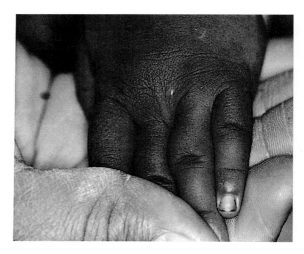

Figure 4

Skin creases develop over the finger joints of the hand, allowing good extension and flexion of the fingers.

much easier than at a later stage as a sharp knife is usually sufficient to excise the soft cartilaginous carpal bones. Since magnification with an operating loop is used, the small size of the structures which are operated on should pose no problem.

The advantage of early surgery is the development of a near normal bilateral body image which is usually fully developed by the age of 18 months to 2 years. At this early age recovery is rapid and the young patient's natural activities are sufficient to make intensive physiotherapy or occupational therapy unnecessary. Another advantage of early surgery is more active motion in the postoperative period. This could be due to greater remodelling ability of the joint surfaces with less adhesion formation. The earlier congenital deformities are operated on, the less

bony correction and removal is usually needed. In the very young patients remnants of the carpal bones that are left behind after the carpectomy

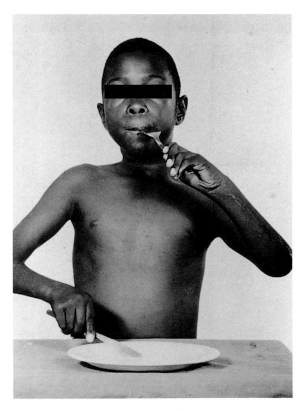

Figure 5

Wrist stability and function have been restored. The cosmetic appearance is near normal. Elbow flexion allows full use of the upper limbs for activities of daily living.

will develop ossification centres which then develop into functional carpal bones (Figure 3).

Loss of correction was seen in our first few cases, until the introduction of the one-step carpectomy plus tendon transfer at the elbow. The deforming wrist flexors are transferred to the dorsum to act as either dynamic wrist extensors when functional or as a static tenodesis when nonfunctional. This procedure is imperative because deforming forces are removed and utilized as correcting or 'holding' forces. Not only is a balance across the wrist achieved, but adaptation to the new position occurs in one stage.

A typical finding of AMC is the lack of skin creases on the dorsum of the fingers. These skin creases develop over the finger joints, probably due to the more functional position of the fingers and thus more movement (Figure 4).

It is important that the wrist flexors are only removed after the carpectomy and fixation with the Kirschner wire has been done. The intact wrist flexors prevent unnecessary tension on the neurovascular bundles on the volar side.

We do not advocate the Steindler flexor plasty of the elbow on these children because the flexors of the fingers and wrists are not only shortened and abnormal, but have too little power and excursion for elbow flexion. The triceps flexor plasty advocated by Bunnell[9] and Carroll[10] has been very rewarding in our cases.

Because of their normal or above-normal IQ, these patients can become useful members of society. In spite of having fewer muscle units, muscle fibres replaced by fibrous tissue, less muscle bulk, reduced muscle excursion and bilateral and general involvement of the entire upper limbs which makes them severely handicapped, they have an improved appearance, improved function and improved body image which makes it all so much more socially acceptable (Figure 5).

References

1   Gericke GS, Hall JG, Nelson MM, Beighton PH, Diagnostic considerations in arthrogryposis syndromes in South Africa, *Clin Gen* (1984) **25**:155–62.

2   James T, Multiple congenital articular rigidities, *Edin Med J* (1951) **58**:565–97.

3   Rocher HL, Les raideurs articulaires congénitales multiples, *J Méd Bord* (1913) **43**:772–815.

4   Mennen U, Williams E, Arthrogryposis multiplex congenita in only one of a monozygotic twin, *J Hand Surg (B&E)* (1996) **21**:647–8.

5   Thompson GH, Bilenker RM, Comprehensive management of arthrogryposis multiplex congenita, *Clin Orthop Rel Res* (1985) **194**:6–14.

6   Wenner SM, Barry S, Proximal row carpectomy in arthrogrypotic wrist deformity, *J Hand Surg* (1987) **12A**:523–5.

7   Williams PF, Management of upper limb problems in arthrogryposis, *Clin Orthop Rel Res* (1985) **194**:60–7.

8   Bayne LG, Hand assessment and management of arthrogryposis multiplex congenita, *Clin Orthop Rel Res* (1985) **194**:68–73.

9   Bunnell S, Restoring flexion to the paralysed elbow, *J Bone Joint Surg* (1951) **33A**:566–71.

10 Carroll RE, Restoration of flexor power to the flail elbow by transplantation of the triceps tendon, *Surg Gynecol Obstet* (1952) **95**:685–8.

58
Pollex abductus

Richard K Green, William H Holmes and Graham D Lister

Introduction

Pollex abductus is a congenital anomaly in which the flexor pollicis longus (FPL) attaches to the extensor pollicis longus (EPL) by means of an aberrant tendon passing around the radial aspect of the thumb. Tupper (1969) first coined the phrase 'pollex abductus' for this condition in his description of four patients with Blauth Type II thumb hypoplasia. He encountered a malposition of the FPL in which the tendon passed radial to the metacarpophalangeal (MP) joint bifurcating at the midphalangeal level. The major limb passed obliquely into the palmar base of the distal phalanx, while the lesser limb passed dorsally into a conjoint insertion with an otherwise normal EPL tendon.

This 'lesser limb' is the primary feature of pollex abductus because it effectively eliminates normal flexor pull on the interphalangeal (IP) joint (Fitch et al 1984). Either by contraction of the FPL or by a tenodesis effect of the proximal tendon, only abduction forces on the MP and IP joint are produced. This may cause marked deviation, especially at the MP level because of the ulnar collateral ligament laxity associated with the hypoplastic thumb. The abnormal intertendinous connection in pollex abductus prevents active flexion of the IP joint, although passive motion remains intact. In addition to the association of this anatomic anomaly with the hypoplastic thumb (Tupper 1969, Blair and Omer 1981, Fitch et al 1984) it has also been noted in patients with radial polydactyly (Lister 1991a) and, rarely, as an isolated finding (Salama and Weissman, 1975).

Those patients in whom pollex abductus is associated with Blauth Type II hypoplastic thumb present with some constant findings. These include the characteristic Type II features (Figure 1): narrowing of the first web space, laxity of the ulnar collateral ligament, and deficiency of the thenar muscles. In addition, they all have an intertendinous connection at the level of the metacarpal, MP or proximal phalanx that defines the condition of pollex abductus. The hypoplastic thumbs may also have other anatomic anomalies such as abnormal origin, route, and insertion of the FPL tendon. Reported anomalous insertions of the FPL tendon include into the thenar muscles, transverse carpal ligament, and into the index finger (Miura 1981, Linburg and Comstock 1979, Murakami and Edashige 1980, Blair and Buckwalter 1983). Additional anomalies include absence of a flexor pulley system, as well as anomalous local muscles. A previous report has described an anomalous lumbrical muscle, the

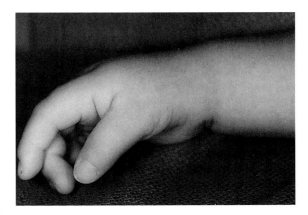

Figure 1

Blauth Type II hypoplasia. This demonstrates the narrowing of the first web space and the deficiency of the thenar muscles. In addition, it should be noted that there are no creases on the extensor surface of the interphalangeal joint of the thumb, suggesting a pollex abductus.

musculus lumbricalis pollicis, which passes from the FPL tendon in the region of the MP joint and passes across the first web space to join the lumbrical belly of the index (Lister 1991b).

As is common in duplicate thumbs, the flexor and extensor tendons to the two digits may arise from a common, single, proximal tendon on each surface. Pollex abductus associated with radial polydactyly typically demonstrates an aberrant tendinous band that passes from the common flexor, through the cleft between the duplicates to insert into the extensors, usually of both thumbs, as an aponeurotic sheet. In contrast to the hypoplastic thumb, the flexor pollicis longus of the polydactylous thumb typically appears normal in all other respects.

Diagnosis

The diagnosis of pollex abductus is made by observation, examination, and finally by exploration of the hand. Although the term 'pollex abductus' suggests that the thumb is in the abducted position, the majority of patients do not demonstrate frank radial deviation of the MP joint at rest. The universal finding among these patients is poor definition or absence of the interphalangeal creases of both the flexor (Figure 2) and extensor surfaces. No motion of the IP joint is noted either with active attempts or by compressing the musculotendinous junction at the level of the wrist. In contrast, near normal passive IP motion is noted in the vast majority of these patients (Figure 3). Clear delineation of any intertendinous connection between the FPL and EPL, as well as any associated anatomic abnormalities, must await surgical exploration.

Treatment

The key to treatment of pollex abductus lies in making a diligent search for evidence of its presence during the preoperative examination, and for the abnormal tendon at the time of surgical exploration. In patients who present with Blauth Type II hypoplasia, correction of the anomalous intertendinous connection should be performed at the time of thumb reconstruction.

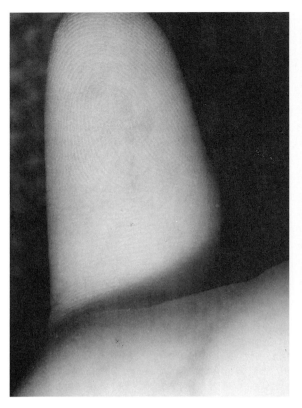

Figure 2

The complete lack of a flexion crease corresponding with the interphalangeal joint of the thumb is the most obvious evidence of pollex abductus.

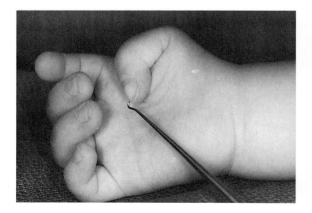

Figure 3

In the same thumb as in Figs 1 and 2 full passive flexion can be demonstrated, illustrating that the problem must lie with the tendon and not with the joint structure.

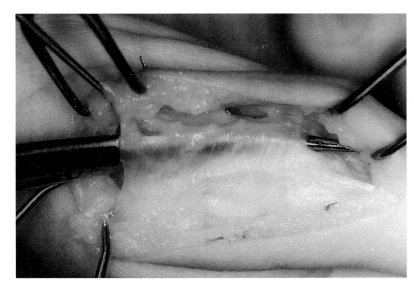

a

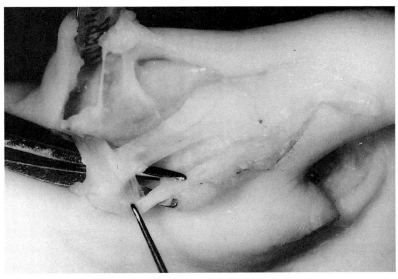

b

Figure 4

Two of the many varieties of inter-tendinous connection between flexor and extensor to be found in pollex abductus. (a) A fairly lengthy band of fascia-like material joining flexor to extensor. (b) A more narrow junction in which the extensor shown to the top of the picture (the tip of the thumb is to the right) receives a very significant contribution from a flexor which continues as a vestigial tendon, the lower tendon in the photograph.

Hypoplastic thumb reconstruction includes widening of the first web space using local flaps of differing designs, reinforcing the deficient ulnar collateral ligament (UCL), and doing an opponensplasty as needed. The flexor digitorum superficialis (FDS) of the ring finger is usually chosen over the abductor digiti minimi for opposition both because it is believed to be stronger and because it can be passed through the neck of the metacarpal, using its distal end to reconstruct the deficient UCL. The MP joint should be pinned in the correct position before ligament reconstruction. One must then explore the radial border of the thumb for a tendinous interconnection between the FPL and the EPL (Figure 4). Those identified as having this

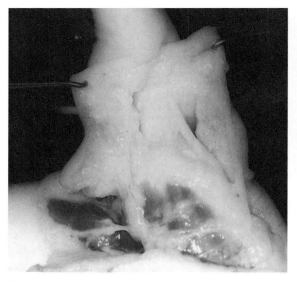 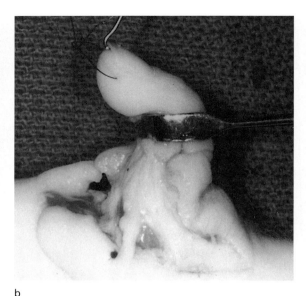

a   b

Figure 5

(a) The flexor tendon in this thumb is the structure running from upper left to lower right across the center of this photograph. Clearly it is anomalous and arises from the extensor surface of the thumb. (b) After this was traced onto the dorsum of the thumb and found to arise from no significant muscle, the tendon was divided proximally. Traction shows good flexion at the interphalangeal joint. An appropriate reconstruction was performed.

anomaly require excision of that connection, centralization of the distal insertion of the FPL and/or EPL as needed, and confirmation that there is an adequate motor to power the extrinsic tendon. The existing flexor may suffice, but often requires construction of a competent pulley at the level of the proximal phalanx using the extensor retinaculum from either the wrist or ankle. An alternative for pulley reconstruction in those patients who have already undergone opponensplasty using the FDS tendon is to utilize the distal end of this tendon for both UCL reconstruction and for pulley reconstruction (Lister 1985).

In some cases, the FPL may not originate from a suitable muscle belly as judged by the absence of normal elastic excursion of the tendon (Figure 5). In such instances, the FDS of the middle finger may be transferred, although occasionally it may be prudent to insert a silastic rod beneath the pulley reconstruction, returning later to complete the reconstruction of the long flexor of the thumb.

In contrast to the subtleties of recognizing thumb hypoplasia in infancy, radial polydactyly is immediately apparent to even the most casual observer. Detection of the presence of the intertendinous connection between flexor and extensor, so that it may be divided at the time of surgery to remove the duplicate, is more difficult. However, the absence of normal skin creases over the IP joint will be evident when sought.

In infants presenting with radial polydactyly, each thumb must be assessed preoperatively for size, deviation, function, and passive mobility. At the time of surgery, the lesser developed of the duplicate thumbs is removed, taking from it whatever tissue is required to create the best remaining thumb. This may include extensor tendon, collateral ligament, periosteum, and intrinsic muscle attachments as needed. Exploration of the extensor and flexor tendons is

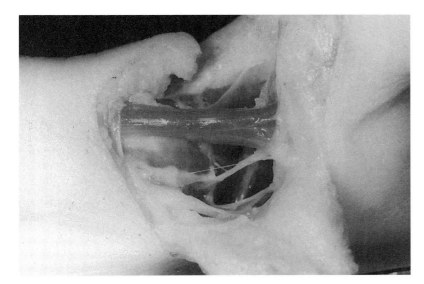

a

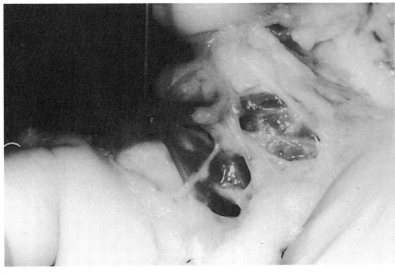

b

Figure 6

(a) and (b) The musculus lumbricalis pollicis. In (b) the two origins of this muscle are seen, one from the flexor digitorum profundus to the index finger and the other, anomalous, muscle belly from the flexor pollicis longus.

mandatory. In a similar manner as that described for the hypoplastic thumb, any intertendinous connection between the FPL and EPL must be excised with realignment of the insertion of these tendons as necessary.

Previously described surgical therapy for this condition has universally recommended release of the FPL–EPL intertendinous connection. In Tupper's description of four cases of patients presenting with hypoplastic thumb, he recommended four means of therapy depending on the individual case. This included detachment of the bifurcated tendon insertion and reattachment to the metacarpal neck in a patient felt to be deficient in the abductor pollicis brevis. In two other patients, the FPL was detached at its insertion, withdrawn to the level of the wrist, and rerouted to the normal course of the FPL where it was reattached to the distal phalanx. The insertional slip of the EPL was detached and shifted ulnarward at the MP joint in a patient with minimal deformity. In all cases, the radial collateral ligament was released at the MP joint level, and reefing of the UCL was performed.

Blair and Omer (1981) recommended releasing the FPL from its abnormal tendinous insertion, and centralizing it by moving it ulnarward. This was achieved by dividing the abductor pollicis brevis musculotendinous junction, transferring the FPL under that intrinsic muscle, and then reattaching the abductor pollicis brevis (APB) so that it acted as a pulley. This procedure allows the FPL to be moved to a mechanically advantageous position, while avoiding tenorrhaphy of the extrinsic flexor.

All described surgical therapies for pollex abductus include excision of the aberrant intertendinous band. Our emphasis is on defining and correcting the routing of the tendon, identifying and excising other aberrant bands or intrinsic muscles, and evaluating the status of the proximal muscle belly. We perform tendon transfer as needed. In those patients without an adequate pulley system, we recommend construction of the pulley, rather than passing the FPL tendon under the divided APB, as described by Blair and Omer (1981), because it does not require dividing an already compromised thenar muscle.

Personal series

Over the 20 years from 1976 to 1995, the senior author treated 55 cases of radial polydactyly and 43 cases of Blauth Type II or Type III thumb hypoplasia. An abnormal connection between the FPL and the EPL was observed in 27 of these thumbs in 23 patients. Thirteen of the hypoplastic thumbs were Blauth Type II and two were Type III with marked hypoplasia of the first metacarpal. The ages of the patients ranged from 2 months to 40 years, with an average of 4.25 years. The average age at operation was 13 months excepting the two oldest patients who were not treated primarily. The anomalous intertendinous connection was found incidentally in the 40-year-old patient while a partially lacerated FPL tendon was being repaired. The 12-year-old was seen for radial deviation and lack of IP

flexion following removal of a duplicated thumb in infancy.

In eight of the hypoplastic thumbs and one of the thumb duplications, an anomalous lumbrical muscle passed from the bifid FPL tendon to the index finger across the first web space. This musculus lumbricalis pollicis (Figure 6) arose in the region of the MP joint of the thumb and inserted at the musculotendinous junction of the index lumbrical on the radial aspect of the index MCP joint. Stimulation of this muscle produces adduction of the thumb when the index finger is restrained, thereby narrowing an already deficient first web space. It should be routinely excised when encountered.

Other anomalies were noted in many of the patients, including congenital dislocation of the hip, ipsilateral dislocation of the radial head, bilateral inguinal hernia, esophageal fistula, and atrial septal defect. Six patients (not including those with bilateral duplication or hypoplasia) had radial anomalies on the opposite upper extremity such as radial club hand, triphalangia, floating thumb, and complete thumb aplasia.

As part of the preoperative examination in these patients, an attempt was made to produce IP flexion by applying pressure over the musculotendinous junction at the wrist. No motion of the thumb distal phalanx was observed with this maneuver in any of the thumbs later shown to have pollex abductus. Also noted in all of these patients was the absence or poor definition of normal IP joint skin creases on either the palmar or dorsal surfaces. Passive motion of the IP joint remained nearly normal in the infant thumbs, exceeding 60° in all cases.

Conclusion

The anomalous intertendinous connection between the FPL and EPL, most commonly associated with hypoplastic thumb and radial polydactyly, typically presents in a patient with an active or passive abduction deformity at the MP joint of the thumb and lack of active motion at the IP joint. Other causes of congenital inability to flex the IP joint of the thumb include symphalangia, congenital tendovaginitis of the flexor sheath, congenital absence of the FPL, and anomalous insertion of the FPL (Fitch et al 1984). The cornerstone of treatment for pollex abductus lies in suspecting the condition preoperatively, and recognizing any associated anatomic anomalies at the time of surgical exploration. The procedures undertaken for correction specifically of the FPL anomaly include:

(1) Division of the anomalous connection to the extensor.
(2) Rerouting of the FPL if it is radially or dorsally deviated.
(3) Construction of pulleys.
(4) Tendon transfer where indicated.

Most studies demonstrate good resolution of the abductor tendencies following treatment, but active IP joint motion remains disappointing. It may be that unrecognized anomalies located more proximally, i.e. at the muscle/motor unit, or unrecognized additional tendon insertions (e.g. to index lumbrical) may have a negative bearing on the surgical outcome of this condition. Alternatively, the less than full range of IP motion may simply be a reflection of the multiplicity and complexity of the variations, and the steps necessary to correct them.

References

Blair WF, Buckwalter JA (1983) Congenital malposition of flexor pollicis longus—an anatomy note, *J Hand Surg* **8**:93–4.

Blair WF, Omer GE (1981) Anomalous insertion of the flexor pollicis longus, *J Hand Surg* **6**:241–4.

Fitch RD, Urbaniak JR, Ruderman RJ (1984) Conjoined flexor and extensor pollicis longus tendons in the hypoplastic thumb, *J Hand Surg* **9A**:417–19.

Linburg RM, Comstock BE (1979) Anomalous tendon slips from the flexor pollicis longus to the flexor digitorum profundus, *J Hand Surg* **4**:79–83.

Lister GD (1985) Reconstruction of the hypoplastic thumb, *Clin Orthop* **185**:52–65.

Lister GD (1991a) Musculus lumbricalis pollicis, *J Hand Surg* **16**:622–5.

Lister GD (1991b) Pollex abductus in hypoplasia and duplication of the thumb, *J Hand Surg* **16**:626–33.

Miura T (1981) Congenital anomaly of the thumb—unusual bifurcation of the flexor pollicis longus and its unusual insertion, *J Hand Surg* **6**:613–15.

Murakami Y, Edashige K (1980) Anomalous flexor pollicis longus muscle, *The Hand* **12**:82–4.

Salama R, Weissman SL (1975) Congenital bilateral anomalous band between flexor and extensor pollicis longus tendons, *The Hand* **7**:25–6.

Tupper JW (1969) Pollex abductus due to congenital malposition of the flexor pollicis longus, *J Bone Joint Surg* **51A**:1285–90.

59
Camptodactyly

Guy Magalon, Frédéric Tomei, Dominique Casanova, Jacques Bardot

Introduction

Camptodactyly is a deformity that is classified as a frontal malposition (group III in Swanson's classification). It applies to a nontraumatic flexion deformity of the proximal interphalangeal (PIP) joint of one or several of the long fingers. The ulnar fingers are more frequently affected, particularly the small finger, and the deformity is usually bilateral, but not necessarily symmetrical. Unilateral forms are more commonly found in the dominant hand. Camptodactyly may be an isolated or primary deformity, or it may form part of a more complex syndrome. Many associated deformities have been described, such as syndactyly, radial clubhand, oro-digito-facial dystosis or arthrogryposis. Moreover camptodactyly is considered by some authors as a minor form of arthrogryposis.[1]

Most authors draw a distinction between two forms:

- An early onset (or congenital) form which is mostly present at birth or appears before the age of one. Both sexes are equally affected.
- A later onset (or acquired) form which is usually found in girls before puberty.

Engber and Flatt[2] reported that in a series of 66 patients, 84% developed the deformity during their first year, whereas only 13% of the forms occurred after the age of 10. Familial forms are frequent, and occur as an autosomal dominant trait. There are also sporadic cases which are not hereditary.

The clinical examination reveals a flexion contracture of the PIP joint, often associated with hyperextension of the metacarpopha-

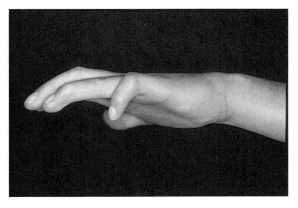

Figure 1

Severe camptodactyly of the fifth digit, 90° deficit in active extension of the PIP joint and hyperextension of the MP joint.

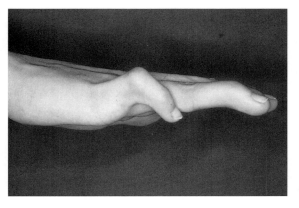

Figure 2

Severe camptodactyly of the fifth digit. Note the extreme shortage of palmar skin.

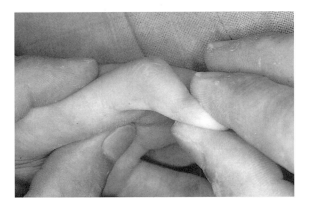

Figure 3

Severe fixed camptodactyly of the fifth digit. The shortage of palmar skin does not allow passive extension of the PIP joint.

langeal (MP) joint (Figure 1). MacFarlane even defines MP extension as being part of the clinical features of camptodactyly.[3,4] In contrast to a posttraumatic, 'buttonhole' type deformity, there is no fixed hyperextension of the distal interphalangeal (DIP) joint. The authors recorded a shortage of skin on the palmar side of the long fingers (Figures 2 and 3). There is usually no modification in the size of the affected joint and it is generally painless. It is important to note that active flexion of the finger remains possible with a full range of movement, allowing the joint to lock normally when a strong grip is required. Passive extension is not always possible. In two-thirds of the cases the contracture was set in MacFarlane's series.[4] The extent of the flexion deformity varies from case to case and can sometimes lead to functional disability; however it is not usually a major handicap, rather a slight functional hindrance, with a deficit in extension of less than 30°. Patients with this type of camptodactyly usually consult for cosmetic reasons. However, it does become a handicap above 60°.[5] For the same extension deficit the degree of disability is more noticeable when it affects the middle fingers. However, even with severe deformity the functional deficit remains only moderate.[6]

Radiological data should include a strictly lateral X-ray film of the affected fingers which will show any abnormalities such as narrowing of the neck and the flattened aspect of the head of the first phalanx. Palmar subluxation of the base of the second phalanx is found in forms that have evolved and erosion of the joint surfaces of the first and second phalanxes can sometimes be detected, although it does not usually develop into osteoarthritis.

Pathophysiology

The exact pathophysiology of camptodactyly is unknown. Since it was first described in 1906 by Landouzy,[7] who considered it as a stigma or 'neuroarthritism', many hypotheses have been put forward. Thus, MacCash[8] attributed the deformity to a shortage of the skin on the palmar side of the long fingers, associated with bands of congenital fibrous tissue on the palmar side of the finger; Miura[9] mentioned fibrosis of the subcutaneous tissue and the theory according to Siegert et al[10] is that the soft tissue of the palm of the hand has not developed and lengthened in proportion to the underlying bone structure. Petit et al[11] described a weakness of the midbands of the extensor muscles. For Smith and Kaplan,[12] almost all the structures of the fingers are involved in the deformity.

The hypothesis which is generally accepted by most contemporary authors is that camptodactyly is due to a disorder in the balance between the flexion and extension forces in the PIP joint.[2,3] Modifications in the joint capsule, ligaments and underlying bone structures seem to be a secondary pathology.

Retraction of the flexor digitorum superficialis was also reported by Smith and Kaplan,[12] who demonstrated that in some cases extension of the fingers became possible when the wrist was flexed. However, in practice this rarely proves to be the case.[4] Courtemanche[14] and Maeda and Matsui[15] reported abnormal findings in the lumbrical muscles. MacFarlane et al[4] found evidence of abnormal distal insertion of the fourth lumbrical muscle in 74 consecutive operations for camptodactyly of the fifth finger. The most frequent pathology was an abnormal capsular insertion of the fourth lumbrical muscle on the MP joint, with no connection to the extensor muscles of the finger. An associated abnormality of the fourth interosseous palmar muscle was also sometimes found.

The main cause of camptodactyly would thus seem to be the loss of normal function of the fourth lumbrical muscle which the author deems to be an intrinsic minus deformity. However, anatomical studies of the intrinsic muscles have demonstrated the wide range of possible variations in the system without any signs of camptodactyly. Siegert et al,[10] who researched into this type of anomaly, only found it in 2 out of the 17 cases of camptodactyly operated on. Goffin et al[5] found it only in 26% of all the early forms and 33% of the later forms. For Miura et al[16] and Hori et al,[17] the imbalance between extension and flexion forces may result from palmar translocation of the lateral bands of the extensor tendon due to the second phalanx being set in a flexed position. The initial flexion of the second phalanx could be caused by a fibrous subcutaneous substratum, abnormal shortness of the flexor digitorum superficialis or an anomaly in the insertion of the lumbrical muscles.

However, the number of hypotheses put forward and the wide variety of surgical findings would seem to suggest that camptodactyly is not the consequence of a single aetiological factor.[6,10,13,18]

Course

The natural course of the deformity is difficult to predict. Wood considers that if the deformity is left untreated it does not improve and is likely to become worse in 80% of cases.[19] The flexion is usually reducible at the onset, allows passive extension and subsequently stiffens and becomes set.

A wide range of different forms are found; some are severe at birth and others remain benign for life. It is not always easy to determine the exact onset of the deformity as it sometimes progresses insidiously.[4,6] The risk of aggravation increases during the phases of fast growth during infancy and the teenage period. The condition ceases to develop in young adults.

Treatment

Previous suggestions

Many pathophysiological explanations have been suggested and the surgical procedures are as varied as the indications and can sometimes be contradictory according to the authors. Treatment may be conservative or surgical.

Conservative management is based on the use of long-term splinting. The splints can either be static, designed to maintain the finger in a position of maximal extension,[4,6] or dynamic with a device to bring the finger back into extension.[16,17] Most authors recommended splinting both pre- and postoperatively.

Miura et al[16] and Hori et al[17] strongly recommend conservative management, and base their position on the assumption that the imbalance between flexion and extension on PIP level is the result of a 'long standing malposition' of the lateral bands of the extensor tendon. A splint decreases flexion and may thus readjust the function of the lateral bands and bring it back to normal. According to the authors, the treatment should be implemented as early as possible, before a contracture of the periarticular tissues and the deep transverse ligaments make readjustment difficult. A dynamic splint should be worn 24 hours a day until complete extension is obtained, then 8 hours a day until the end of the teenage period to prevent recurrence. After comparative analysis of the results of operated and nonoperated camptodactyly, Siegert et al[10] also considered conservative management to be preferable in slight and moderate cases with a deficit of less than 60° in extension. They reserved surgery for the severe or evolutive forms, only if conservative treatment had failed. The authors argued that surgical operations inevitably generate a loss of flexion, which is not observed after splinting alone or associated with stretching, which yields equivalent or even better results.

Surgery may be indicated according to the aetiology, or the presumed pathophysiology or simply based on the symptoms, when all the structures involved in the deformity are taken into account. The large number of surgical procedures proposed, either single or multiple according to the case, demonstrate that camptodactyly can be a challenge for the surgeon's imagination. Various authors have successively performed procedures to release the skin using Z-plasty or total skin grafts, release of the palmar plate and the collateral ligaments of the PIP joint.

Smith and Kaplan[12] advocated transection of the flexor digitorum superficialis muscle when the deformity can be reduced by flexion of the wrist. Millesi[13] advocated lengthening the flexor digitorum superficialis and O'Brien and Hopgson[20] suggested lengthening the flexor digitorum profundus. Miura et al[16] and Hori et al[17] recommended simple transection of the fibrous subcutaneous tissue as a complementary treatment after splinting. In compliance with his surgical findings, MacFarlane and colleagues[3,4] advocated transfer of the flexor digitorum superficialis of the fifth digit, or even better of the fourth digit, to the extensor muscles, completed by release of the periarticular tissues when a residual contracture of more than 30° persists. Z-plasties can be used to correct the shortage of palmar skin. However, it is interesting to note that although the mean deficit fell from 69° to 25°, only one-third of all their patients recovered complete flexion postoperatively. Flatt[6] used a release procedure on the soft tissues, associated with Z-plasty and tendon transfer in surgical management of camptodactyly and he also recorded a loss of active flexion in the joint.

Tendon transfers are probably more effective in transferring the range of movement of the joint towards extension rather than actually improving the active mobility of the PIP joint. Siegert et al[10] stressed the importance of early postoperative mobilization and recommended avoiding any surgical procedure that requires long postoperative immobilization, likely to lead to a loss of flexion mobility.

Gupta and Burke[21] reported promising early results after transfer of the extensor indicis proprius to the radial side of the extensor muscles of the fifth digit. Glicenstein and colleagues[22,23] advocated total anterior teno-arthrolysis of the finger (TATA), using the procedure described by Saffar, which involved lengthening the skin by use of a rotation flap harvested on the lateral side of the finger. Flatt[6] performs an osteotomy to correct the angle of the neck of the first phalanx in forms with severe

contracture and abnormal radiographic findings. Iselin and Pradet[1] proposed a Swanson arthroplasty in severe cases.

Our procedure

Our team chose to use the procedure described by Petit et al[11] in 1968. Their procedure deals with all the structures involves in camptodactyly. Without refuting the basic principle stating that the primary reason for the deformity is an imbalance between the flexion and extension forces in the PIP joint, we would like to point out that once the deformity becomes set, the skin of the palm often shortens considerably together with retraction of the median fibres of the palmar aponeurosis, retraction of the palmar plate and contracture of the collateral ligaments. Complete extension of the finger can only be achieved when these structures are completely released. Our treatment is based on these findings.

We perform a quadrangular flap, harvested on a proximal pedicle from the palmar side of the second phalanx, extending up to the flexion fold of the distal interphalangeal (DIP) joint (Figure 4). The tendon of the flexor digitorum superficialis is then transected and PIP palmar capsulotomy is performed if necessary. The capsulotomy is

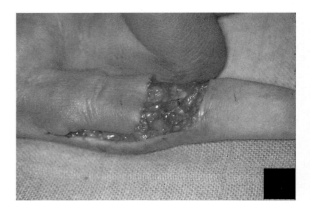

Figure 4

Quadrangular skin flap harvested from the palmar side of P2.

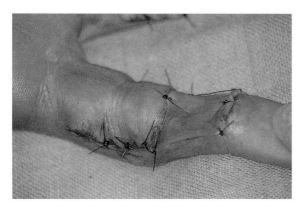

Figure 5

A skin graft is required to repair the skin defect resulting from the extension of the PIP joint when the flap is mobilized.

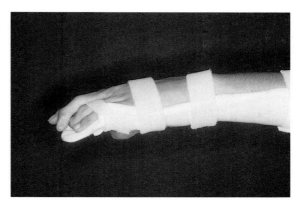

Figure 6

Static splint in maximal extension of the PIP joint.

achieved by resection of the palmar plate and the collateral ligaments until complete extension of the PIP is obtained. Very drastic release of the joint is inadvisable as it may lead to ankylosis.

We also draw attention to the extremely short vasculo-nervous pedicles; few authors have stressed this aspect. This seems to us to be the main limiting factor for any possible surgical treatment. The extension obtained during surgery may create vascular disorders because of tension applied to the collateral pedicles. Postoperative immobilization should be designed to leave the PIP joint in slight flexion and allow the extremity of P3 to be monitored for any signs of ischaemia or venous stasis. A full thickness skin graft is then used to cover the skin defect left on the second phalanx at the donor site when the flap is mobilized (Figure 5).

This operation will only yield satisfactory results if it is combined with static and dynamic splinting before and after surgery and we devote particular attention to this point (Figures 6 and 7). The features of the dynamic splint are designed:

- To avoid hyperextension of the metacarpophalageal joint and block the MP at an angle of 45° of flexion.
- To exert traction on P2, not on P3, to act efficiently on the PIP joint.

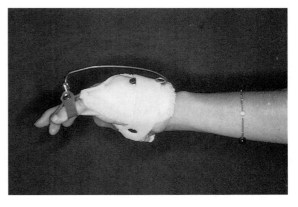

Figure 7

Dynamic splint with spring device for camptodactyly of the fifth digit.

The splint must be worn as often as possible in the daytime and replaced at night by a static splint in order to maintain the angle gained. A splint should be worn preoperatively for 2 months to assess the patient's degree of cooperation.[5] If the patient is unable to comply with the postoperative treatment, we feel that it is preferable not to attempt the operation.

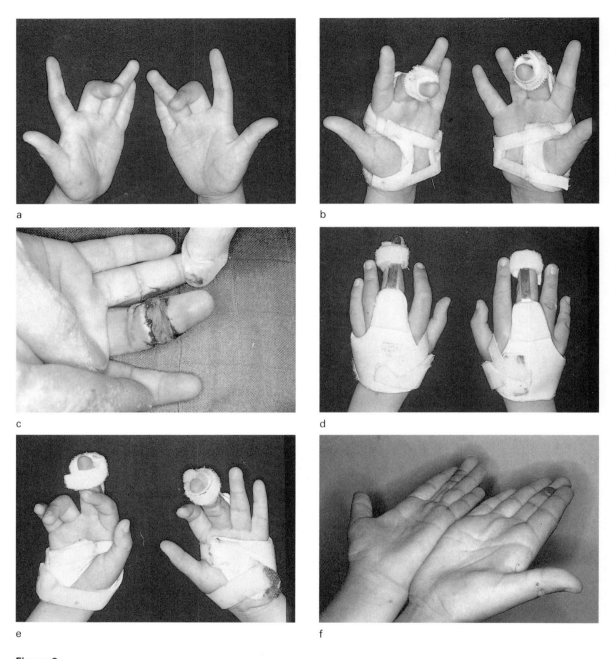

Figure 8

Patient who presented with severe camptodactyly of both middle fingers. (a) Extension deficit of about 90°. (b) Pre-operative dynamic splinting. (c) Peroperative coverage of the skin defect left behind after mobilization of the flap on P2. (d,e) Postoperative dynamic splinting. (f) Result 6 months later.

Postoperatively, the same postural treatment should be continued for 6 months. This will allow progressive recovery of the extension obtained during surgery without any risk of damage to the vascular and nerve structures.

Indications

Although some authors operate from angles of 30° or 40° upwards,[4,6] we feel that surgery is only indicated in severe cases with about 90° of extension deficit. Camptodactyly of the middle fingers is more of a functional disability and is always worth operating on, whereas cases involving the ulnar fingers are more readily tolerated (Figure 8).

References

1 Iselin F, Pradet G, Indications du traitement chirurgical des camptodactylies sévères, *Ann Chir Plast* (1979) **24**:165–72.

2 Engber W, Flatt AE, Camptodactyly: an analysis of 66 patients and 24 operations, *J Hand Surg* (1977) **2**:216–24.

3 MacFarlane RM, Curry GI, Evans HB, Anomalies of the intrinsic muscles in camptodactyly, *J Hand Surg* (1983) **8**:531–44.

4 MacFarlane RM, Porte AM, Botz JS, The anatomy and treatment of camptodactyly of the small finger, *J Hand Surg* (1992) **17A**:35–44.

5 Goffin D, Lenoble E, Marin-Braun F, et al, Camptodactylies: classification et résultats thérapeutiques, *Arch Chir Main* (1994) **13**:20–5.

6 Flatt AE, Crooked fingers. In: *The Care of Congenital Anomalies*, 2nd edn (Quality Medical Publishing: St Louis, 1993).

7 Landouzy L, Camptodactylie: stigmate organique précoce du neuroarthritisme, *Press Méd* (1906) **14**:251–3.

8 MacCash CR, Congenital contractures of the hand. In: Stack HG, Bolton H, eds, *The Proceedings of the Second Hand Club* (British Society of Surgery of the Hand: London, 1970) 399–401.

9 Miura T, Non traumatic flexion deformity of the proximal interphalangeal joint: its pathogenesis and treatment, *The Hand* (1983) **15**:25–34.

10 Siegert JJ, Cooney WP, Dobyns JH, Management of simple camptodactyly, *J Hand Surg* (1990) **15B**:181–9.

11 Petit P, Malek R, Docquier JC, A propos des camptodactylies congénitales chez l'enfant, *Lyon Chir* (1968) **64**:923–9.

12 Smith RJ, Kaplan EB, Camptodactyly and similar atraumatic flexion deformities of the proximal interphalangeal joints of the fingers, *J Bone Joint Surg* (1968) **50A**:1187–1203.

13 Millesi H, Camptodactyly. In: Littler JW, Cramer LM, Smith JW, eds, *Symposium of Reconstructive Hand Surgery*, Vol 9 (CV Mosby; St Louis, 1974) 175–7.

14 Courtemanche AB, Camptodactyly: etiology and management, *Plast Reconstr Surg* (1969) **44**:451–4.

15 Maeda M, Matsui T, Camptodactyly caused by a abnormal lumbrical muscle, *J Hand Surg* (1968) **10B**:95–6.

16 Miura T, Nakamura R, Tamura Y, Long standng extended dynamic splintage and release of a abnormal restraining structure in camptodactyly. *J Hand Surg* (1992) **17B**:665–72.

17 Hori M, Nakamura R, Inoue G, et al, Nonoperative treatment of camptodactyly, *J Hand Surg* (1987) **12A**:1061–5.

18 Magalon G, Camptodactylies. In: Magalon G, Chancholle AR, eds, *Chirurgie Plastique de L'Enfant: Pathologie Congénitale* (Maloine: Paris, 1987) 282–6.

19 Wood VE, Camptodactyly. In: Green DP, ed, *Operative Hand Surgery*, 2nd edn, Vol 1 (Churchill Livingstone: New York, 1988) 409–16.

20 O'Brien JP, Hopgson AR, Congenital abnormality of the flexum digitorum profondus: a cause of flexion deformity of the long and ring fingers. *Clin Orthop* (1974) **99**:154–67.

21 Gupta A, Burke D, Correction of camptodactyly: preliminary results of extensor indicis transfer, *J Hand Surg* (1990) **15B**:168–70.

22 Glicenstein J, Haddad R, Guero S, Traitement congénital ds camptodactylies, *Arch Chir Main* (1995) **14**:264–71.

23 Leclercq C, Glicenstein J, Traitement chirurgical de la camptodactylie. In: Gilbert A, Buck-Gramcko D, Lister G, eds, *Les Malformations Congénitales du Membre Supérieur* (Expansion Scientifique Française: Paris, 1991) 91–9.

60

The surgical approach to the cleft hand

Joseph Upton

Introduction

One of the most difficult problems treated by those interested in congenital malformations of the upper limb is the median defect or cleft hand.[1-16] True cleft hand deformities with a characteristic V-shaped central cleft are unusual and have been separated from symbrachy-dactylies, which are characterized by a U-shaped central deficiency and the presence of rudimentary digital nubbins. Other distinguishing characteristics of the 'typical' cleft hand include: bilateral limb involvement, syndactyly, campto-dactyly, foot involvement, and in many children a positive family history.

The major anatomic problem presented in these hands is created by the index ray which may be absent, joined to the thumb in an incomplete or complete simple syndactyly, or positioned inappropriately somewhere between the thumb and the next ulnar digit of the hand. Many excellent classifications have been proposed, each was based upon skeletal morphology and each presented a different method of management. We have concentrated separately upon the skeletal and soft tissue deficiencies in an effort to establish several basic principles for treatment. This short chapter concentrates upon

(1) skin incisions,
(2) adductor pollicis muscle preservation,
(3) index ray transposition,
(4) closure and creation of the first web space and
(5) skin grafts.

We have concentrated in this chapter on the child with a median cleft and an index ray which is worth saving but must be repositioned.

Before describing in some detail a complicated reconstruction for a very complicated congenital malformation, one should consider the words of Adrian Flatt: '... the untreated cleft hand is a functional triumph and an aesthetic disaster'. Often the best treatment is to do nothing. Each hand in each child is different and treatment must be carefully individualized.

Technical aspects

Skin incisions (Figure 1)

Keep it simple! Do not sacrifice dorsal or palmar skin and do not potentially compromise tissue with narrow transposition or rotation flaps. First, a small commissure flap based on the radial side of the digit across the cleft is outlined. This flap is located at the midproximal phalangeal level and is oriented on a 45° volar-to-dorsal angle to the longitudinal axis of the ray. The incision is then extended down into the depth of the cleft in the midlateral longitudinal axis of the rays. Next, the incision is continued circumferentially around the index ray at the level of the new commissure. A straight incision is then made between the index finger and thumb. When a syndactyly is present incisions are designed with equal distribution to both partners on both dorsal and palmar surfaces. With very tight simple syndactylies preference is given to the ulnar pulp surface of the thumb. Skin grafts may be needed and will be addressed later.

Dorsal and palmar flaps are then carefully elevated with complete preservation of both

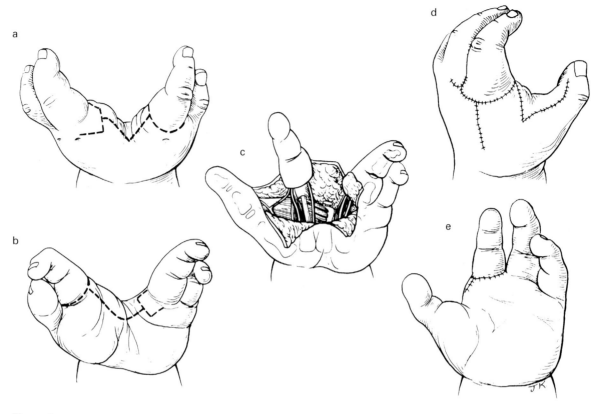

Figure 1

Incisions. (a,b) Outline of incisions on dorsal and palmar surfaces shows a radially based commissure flap on the ring digit and equal division of tissue within the depth of the central cleft. (c) After flap mobilization there is wide exposure of all neurovascular structures and the adductor pollicis muscle (if present). (d,e) Following transfer as a vascular island, the index ray is positioned adjacent to the ring ray. No additional Z-plasties have been performed to improve the contour of the thumb–index web space.

dorsal and palmar neurovascular structures to the index finger and thumb. Dorsal sensory nerves and veins are preserved and elevated off the extensor tendons and interosseous muscles. With relatively shallow central clefts a large princeps pollicis artery is present with its bifurcation to the radial side of the index ray. These vessels can be mobilized and usually will easily span the new web space without division of either branch (see Figure 1b). Careful mobilization of these flaps provides excellent access to the entire dorsal and palmar metacarpal region of the hand. The palmar structure will be located palmar to the broad adductor pollicis muscle (if

present) (see Figure 1c). Tight fascial bands between the thumb and index rays at the metacarpal level are first isolated, then excised. These may extend down to the thumb carpometacarpal (CMC) level.

Adductor pollicis muscle preservation (Figure 2)

All adductor intrinsic muscles are preserved. Preoperatively the location and size of a third metacarpal correlates well with the presence and

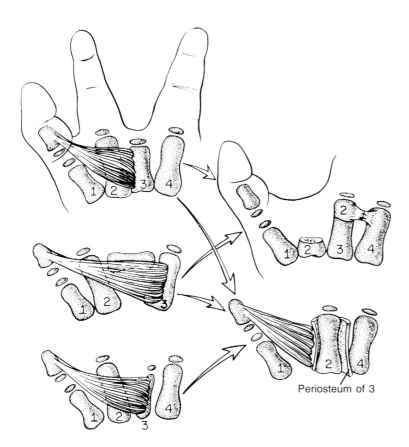

Periosteum of 3

Figure 2

Adductor pollicis muscle. A strong adductor muscle should be saved as a weak pinch is one of the most prominent functional deficits in these children. Two alternatives are possible: (1) transposition of the index metacarpal at the distal diaphysis of a well formed long metacarpal as shown in the top left and center left, or (2) subperiosteal removal of a hypoplastic long metacarpal and transposition of the index metacarpal into its periosteal sleeve. Transverse phalanges at the distal metacarpal level as seen in the center left are excised.

size of this important pinch muscle. The mid-palmar exposure allows accurate visualization of both the origin and insertion of the adductor pollicis and identification of all neurovascular structures. A decision is next made about a third metacarpal. If a normal metacarpal is present, the muscle attachment is left intact and the index ray transposed onto its distal diaphysis. If the metacarpal is hypoplastic, the muscle is left attached to its periosteum and the index metacarpal is transposed within this sleeve following removal of the deficient third metacarpal. In very deep clefts extending to the carpal level, the entire third ray with the adductor pollicis muscle is absent and the index is transposed at the CMC level.

In some cleft hands with transversely oriented abnormal phalanges the adductor pollicis muscle may originate from the fourth (ring) metacarpal.

We have never seen an origin from the fifth (small) metacarpal.

The first dorsal interosseous muscle will usually present with a bipennate origin from both the first and second metacarpals. Release from the thumb metacarpal must be completed before the index ray can be transposed across the cleft.

Index ray transposition (Figure 3)

In the majority of hands the index ray may or may not be deficient but is usually situated in a 'no man's land' between a good thumb and the next ulnar ray of the hand. The markedly hypoplastic ray is often best ablated, but this recommendation may not be popular with

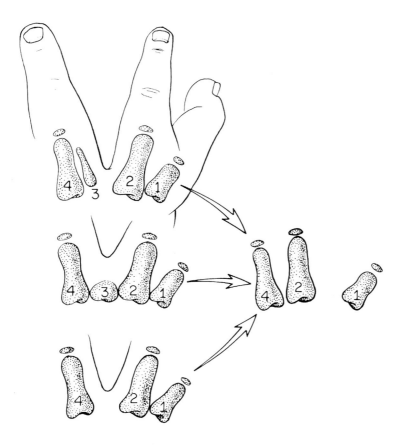

Figure 3

Metacarpal transposition. Hypoplastic long metacarpals near the depth of the cleft (top, left) and very short metacarpals at the base of the cleft (center, left) with no or very hypoplastic adductor muscles should be excised. Metacarpal transposition is best accomplished at the CMC joint level with trimming of the joint surfaces to ensure a precision fit.

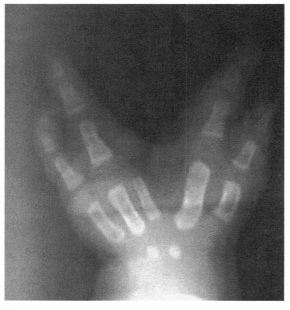

a

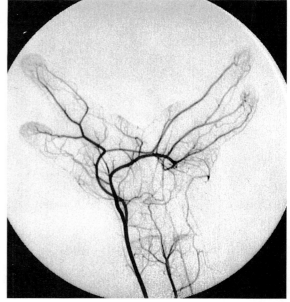

b

parents. This ray should be transposed at the metacarpal level adjacent to the ray across the cleft. The metacarpophalangeal joints of both digits should be at the same level.

The transposition is best accomplished at the CMC joint level as the second metacarpal is disarticulated from the trapezoid and capitate and advanced ulnarwards into the slot previously occupied by the deficient third metacarpal (if present). Minimal shaving of the articular surfaces will provide an excellent fit. An inter-metacarpal ligament (transverse metacarpal head ligament) is reconstructed either with a large nonabsorbable suture passed through periosteum or a more secure interwoven tendon; a small wire (C wire) fixation at the base of the metacarpal is sufficient.

The side-to-side placement and fixation of the index and next adjacent metacarpal is important because there is a tendency for the index to abduct and pronate excessively. Tight fixation of the new intermetacarpal ligament is mandatory and rotation is controlled with C wire fixation. Careful trimming of the hyaline cartilage at the CMC level will ensure a precision fit with correction of rotation.

Skin closure and creation of a first web space (see Figure 1d, e)

Once the skeletal rays have been properly positioned, wound closure can then be performed. The commissure flap is sutured to the ulnar side of the index finger (now in the long position). The clefts in the dorsal and palmar flaps are next closed. Incisions around the index finger are next approximated under no tension. A skin deficiency on the palmar surface may exist with deep clefts and should be replaced with a glabrous full thickness skin graft. After a C wire is placed between the thumb and index metacarpals the straight incision across the new thumb–index web space is closed. In many hands more than enough skin is present for an excellent web space (Figure 4). At this point appropriate Z-plasties or other preferred variations of transposition or advancement flaps can be incorporated in order to interrupt the straightline incision and to properly contour the depth of the web space.

The most appropriate time to make these modifications is after the syndactyly has been released and the index ray properly positioned. Only after this flap mobilization and skeletal repositioning has been completed can the surgeon then design smaller contouring flaps with full utilization of both skin excesses of the more distensible dorsal skin and deficiencies of the immobile palmar skin. When these flaps are closed without any tension the existing straight incision is not altered. Z-plasties can be performed at an older age if contracture is a problem with growth.

Skin grafts

Skin deficiencies may exist on the palmar surface of the index finger and along both the thumb and index phalanges with tight complete syndactylies. Complex syndactyly with osseous union has not been seen. The contact pulp prehension surfaces on the ulnar side of the thumb distal phalanx and the radial pulp surface of the index finger should be preferably surfaced with local skin so incisions here should be designed appropriately. The hypothenar donor site is ideal for harvesting dorsal, palmar (glabrous), or combined full thickness skin grafts. If more skin is needed the groin donor site is used.

Advantages and disadvantages

The design of these incisions and metacarpal repositioning is similar to Littler's modification of the pollicization procedure, in which the index ray is isolated as a vascular island, the first metacarpal shortened, and the digit (with metacarpal head) recessed and rotated into the thumb position. These simple incisions preserve all available skin which is draped after the skeletal repositioning has been completed. For the cleft hand the index ray is isolated and moved as a vascular island. The exposure provided after mobilization of the dorsal and palmar flaps is excellent as all neurovascular structures, tendons and muscles can be carefully evaluated and dissected without injury.

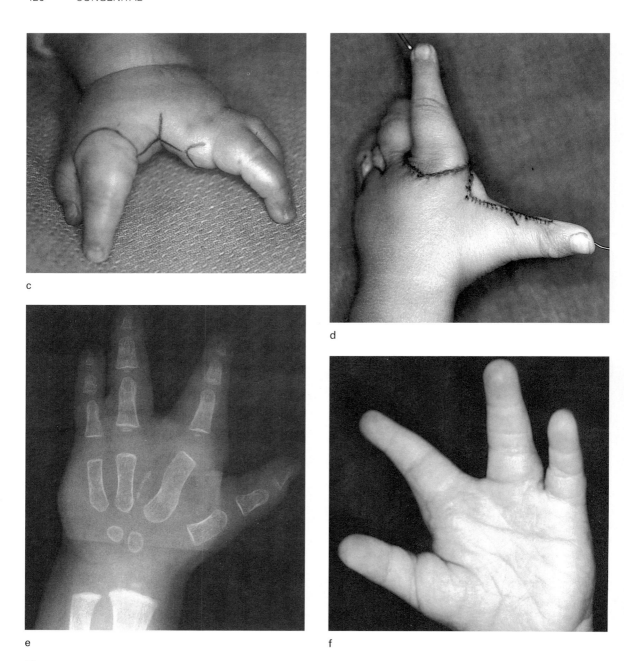

c

d

e

f

Figure 4

(a) Radiologic appearance of a central cleft with an incomplete, simple syndactyly of the thumb–index web space and a well formed third metacarpal which has a good adductor pollicis muscle. (b) An angiogram shows a prominent radial artery, a persistent interosseous artery and an absent ulnar artery. After mobilization of flaps and transposition of the index ray, neither branch of the common vessel to the first web space required ligation. (c) Outline of incisions shows an equal distribution of skin to the dorsal and palmar flaps. (d) An excellent web space has been created following transposition and primary flap closures. (e) Radiograph 1 year postoperatively shows some ossification in the periosteal sleeve into which the index metacarpal was transposed at the CMC level. The index metacarpal is much larger than the ring metacarpal in this child. (f) One year later the first web space span and contour remain excellent and the index digit has a characteristic abducted posture. The tendency for supination had been corrected at the time of transposition.

We have not seen any major disadvantages with this simple and logical approach, which avoids potential flap loss by the creation of predesigned incisions before the dorsal and palmar skin has been mobilized. After mobilization of the dorsal and palmar flaps, the index metacarpal is easily transposed in a single procedure.

Results

Sixty hands in 30 children with a diagnosis of typical cleft hand were evaluated from 1977 through 1995. Those with symbrachydactyly were not included. In 23 children (46 hands), both hands and feet were affected to some degree. Our initial surgical approach used the Snow and Littler incisions,[14] and these modifications have evolved from our experience, not with complications, but with a dissatisfaction with the limitations of the span and contour of the first web space.

In 38 hands treated with the modifications described above there were no flap losses. Visualization was excellent for dissection of the adductor pollicis muscle (if present) and index ray transposition. Secondary procedures have been performed in five children and included: excision of hypertrophic scars (N=3 hands), Z-plasties (N=3 hands), tendon transfer of the extensor carpi radialis longus plus a tendon graft to the radial base of the proximal phalanx for restoration of index digit abduction. No children lost metacarpophalangeal or interphalangeal joint motion. Excessive pronation of the transposed digit has not been a problem with key pinch, which has remained weak in all cases. No children had a normal key pinch.

Indications

This approach is applicable to those children with a central cleft with an intact index ray on the radial side of the cleft. Very hypoplastic index rays should be excised. The same approach and incisions are effective in the more complex and complicated variants of cleft hands which include thumb duplications, all variations of thumb–index syndactyly, transverse oriented phalanges at the MP joint level and Y-shaped metacarpals.

The same incision is used for correction of Types V and VI (Wassel classification) thumb duplications and other types of preaxial duplications associated with triphalangeal thumbs. In these hands the thumb–index web space is often deficient and the position of the thumb metacarpal may need to be altered with either an osteotomy or a bone graft from an excised partner. We design our skin incisions around the thumb to be retained and then move it radially into a more palmar abduction as the skin flaps are moved in the opposite direction to create a wider first web space.

We have not had difficulty performing these procedures on children between 1 and 2 years of age, primarily due to the excellent exposure afforded by these incisions. All reconstruction should be completed by the time the youngster enters kindergarten between ages 5 and 6 years. One may wish to delay this complex surgery in small children with diminutive, delicate hands. This type of reconstruction will require the operative skills and experience of a craftsman and should not be attempted by the surgical apprentice. Both the aesthetic and functional outcomes are rewarding.

References

1 Barsky AJ, Cleft hand. Classification, incidence and treatment, *J Bone Joint Surg* (1964) **46A**:1707–20.
2 Buck-Gramcko D, Cleft hands, classification and treatment, *Hand Clin* (1985) **1**:467–73.
3 David TJ, The differential diagnosis of the cleft hand and cleft foot malformations, *Hand* (1974) **6**:58–61.
4 Flatt AE, *The Care of Congenital Anomalies* (Quality Medical Publications Inc: St Louis, 1994).
5 Glicenstein J, Guero S, Haddad R, Median clefts of the hand. Classification and therapeutic indications based on a series of 29 cases (in French), *Ann Chir Main* (1995) **14**:253–363.
6 Kelikian H, *Congenital Deformities of the Hand and Forearm* (WB Saunders: Philadelphia, 1974) 467–95.
7 Lewis I, Embleton D, Split hand and split foot deformities, their types, origin and transmission, *Biometrika* (1908) **VI**:27–58.

8   Maisels DO, Lobster claw deformities of the hands and feet, *Br J Plast Reconstr Surg* (1970) **23**:269–81.

9   Miura T, Komada T, Simple method for reconstruction of the cleft hand with an adducted thumb, *Plast Reconstr Surg* (1979) **64**:65–7.

10   Nutt JN, Flatt AE, Congenital central hand deficit, *J Hand Surg* (1981) **6**:48–60.

11   Ogino T, Cleft hand, *Hand Clin* (1990) **6**:661–71.

12   Ogino T, Teratogenic relationship between polydactyly, syndactyly and cleft hand, *J Hand Surg* (1990) **15B**:201–9.

13   Sandzen SC, Classification and functional management of congenital central defect of the hand, *Hand Clin* (1985) **1**:483–98.

14   Snow JW, Littler JW, Surgical treatment for the cleft hand, *Trans Int Soc Plast Reconstr Surg* (Excerpta Medica Foundation: Rome, 1967) 888–93.

15   Wateri S, Tsuge K, A classification of cleft hands, based on clinical findings. Theory of developmental mechanism, *Plast Reconstr Surg* (1979) **64**:381–9.

16   Wood VE, Superdigit, *Hand Clin* (1990) **6**:673–84.

Commentary

Chapters 50–60

This series of chapters on congenital malformations is written by well-known international experts who have contributed to this field for many years; many of them are members of the International Study Group of Congenital Malformations.

There is no doubt that the classification adopted by the International Federation of Societies for Surgery of the Hand (IFSSH) needs to be periodically refreshed, based on advanced clinical and experimental research such as that of Toshihiko Ogino. Besides the problem of the evident relationship between syndactyly, polydactyly and cleft hand, the concept of symbrachydactyly, which has been recognized in the German literature for a long time, needs to be integrated and this has recently been accepted by the committee on congenital malformations of the IFSSH.

Many technical points are described—I already have experience of some and can recommend them: the technique of René Malek described here by Guy Magalon, the physiolysis of delta phalanx according to David Vickers, or the bi-lobed flap of David Evans to approach a radial club hand.

Michael Tonkin has stressed the relevance of the adjunction of external fixations to reduce the deformity of the radial club hand; the data are convincing but this multiplan deformity could be better corrected in the sagittal plane by a device other then the Matev distraction fixator. As in all problems of congenital malformation, only a long-term follow-up would assess the potential harm to the epiphysis after releasing the traction. This problem also applies to the recent technique described by Vilkki (personal communication) who interposes a vascularized second toe to support the radial aspect of the deformed wrist, despite an evident discrepency in potential growth.

I basically agree with Joseph Upton's concept of treating a cleft hand. However, I would add a special trick for cases with associated syndactyly of index and thumb. In such cases, I have found it useful to transfer the skin of the cleft, as an island, based on the palmar intermetacarpal artery (and vena comitantes); this pedicle has been consistently found in cases where the third metacarpal bone is present on the X-ray. The extra mobility provided by the island provides excellent positioning in the first web.

In his chapter, Paul Manske introduces an important sub-classification of the Blauth type III thumb hypoplasia. This is of relevance since the common attitude in such cases has been to propose amputation of the hypoplastic thumb with pollicization of the index, an operation sometimes strongly opposed by relatives due to the 'acceptable' aspect of the thumb. Patients and relatives have been pleased with the result of reconstruction in type IIIA cases (even if the fine pinch sometimes continues to be performed between index and middle finger) due to cosmetic improvement and the possibility to grasp large objects; this grasping was definitely improved by MP joint stabilization and first web release. I have found the four-flap technique frequently insufficient for web coverage and I have described[1] a so called 'pseudo-kite' flap which is centred on the first dorsal metacarpal artery and provides a losangic pseudo-island skin able to perfectly resurface the first web; the donor site is closed by an "LLL" plasty as described by Dufourmentel.

On the other hand, we have seen 11 cases of thumb hypoplasia type IIIB, and in five of them a classical pollicization was definitely refused by relatives despite several surgical referrals. In such circumstances, I have performed a reconstruction of the missing proximal first metacarpal and carpo-metacarpal joint through a free compound vascular joint transfer,[2] taken from the metatarso-phalangeal area of the second toe. Provisional skin is simultaneously harvested from the dorsum of the foot and fits on the thenar aspect to accommodate a Huber–Littler opponens transfer. This technique stabilizes the base of the thumb metacarpal and provides a potential for growth due to the presence of a vascularized epiphysis; in four of my cases which have been followed-up for more than five years, all the epiphyses remain opened. Despite early operations (all except one performed before two years of age), three of the children are using their index and middle finger for fine pinch but all use their thumb for grasping large objects.

Finally, a common comment on many of the malformations approached in these chapters concerns the place of free vascularized toe transfer. One of them is the monodactylous hand as seen either in symbrachydactyly or in extreme forms of cleft hand or in some ulnar deficiencies (a point which could be added to the classification proposed by Toshihiko Ogino and mentioned in the huge experience of Dieter Buck-Gramcko). In such cases I have performed a second toe transfer before body image and pinch development, at a mean 11 month of age. The results have been rewarding despite a quite disappointing range of motion (38° at IP level), due to a stable opposing ray with excellent sensibility. The worst cosmetic and functional results were observed in cleft hand and feet where the first ray is a poor substitute. An even more disappointing experiment has been our attempt to build a pincer in an adactilous symbrachydactyly with short metacarpals by distally transferring two toes from both feet. Definitely better, but limited results have been obtained in such cases

with the modification of the Furnas and Vilkki technique we have proposed,[3] transferring a second toe on the distal radial epiphysis, in front of the 'palm' to use the mobility of the wrist to come in contact with the less mobile 'thumb'. Such a more proximal transfer allows plenty of available tendons to balance the toe. Only one of our six cases (a bilateral malformation) has achieved a precise distal pinch but five are able to have a weak but useful grasp of large and medium-sized objects. Despite limited results I think that toe transfers have added possibilities, not only in congenital amputations but also in other extreme forms of malformations.

I deeply thank all the authors who have supplied the outstanding contributions to this section on congenital malformations.

GF

References

1   Foucher G, Cornil C, Braga Da Silva J, Le lambeau 'pseudo-cerf volant' de l'index avec plastie LLL dans la reconstruction de la première commissure, *Ann Chir Plast Esthet* (1992) **37**:207–9.

2   Foucher G, Vascularized joint transfer. In: Green D, ed, *Operative Hand Surgery* 2nd edn (Churchill Livingstone: New York, 1988) 1271–93.

3   Foucher G, Une modification de la technique de Furas et Vilkki dans la reconstruction des main métacarpiennes congénitales, *Ann Chir Main* (1995) **14**:103–8.

Index